Multidisciplinary Management of Sleeve Gastrectomy

Jaime Ruiz-Tovar
Editor

Multidisciplinary Management of Sleeve Gastrectomy

Springer

Editor
Jaime Ruiz-Tovar
Department of Biomedicine and Health Sciences
Alfonso X University
Madrid, Spain

ISBN 978-3-032-25643-0 ISBN 978-3-032-25644-7 (eBook)
https://doi.org/10.1007/978-3-032-25644-7

This Springer imprint is published by the registered company Springer Nature Switzerland AG
The registered company address is: Gewerbestrasse 11, 6330 Cham, Switzerland

In memory of Prof. Dr. Carlos Gamallo, MD, PhD

You were not only my Doctoral Thesis supervisor but also my mentor, and I learned everything I know about scientific research from you. More than 20 years of shared work forged not only academic collaboration, but a deep friendship that continues to guide my path.

I will never forget your wise counsel. There was only one piece of advice on which we differed: your insistence that I should always carry a backpack full of merits. "It may not serve you often," you told me, "but if the day ever comes when you need it, it will be there." What you did not say is that such a backpack can sometimes become a burden—especially when mediocre individuals in positions of power feel threatened by those who strive to move forward. These were the ones you called casposos, people who had reached their posts through family ties, political influence, religious standing, or other merits of questionable ethics.

Despite enduring these casposos for many years, your integrity and brilliance carried you to the top. Yet, for me, your greatest achievement is not your many scientific publications, but the legacy you left to us—your disciples—to pursue scientific progress and to pass knowledge on to others. You set the bar extraordinarily high, and I hope that one day we may rise to meet it.

REST IN PEACE.

Contents

Part III Postoperative Course

Part IV Mechanism of Action of Sleeve Gastrectomy and Challenges

Part I

Preoperative Evaluation

1 Preoperative Information of the Patient and Psychological Suitability

Blanca Espina-Jerez

1.1 Introduction

Morbid obesity constitutes a global health challenge, and bariatric surgery has emerged as one of the most effective treatments for achieving sustained weight loss and improving metabolic comorbidities. Among the most frequently used techniques today is the sleeve gastrectomy, characterised by its lower technical complexity and good outcome profile [4]. However, surgery alone does not guarantee success: the patient must achieve good adherence to lifestyle changes, which involves dietary, behavioural, and emotional modifications that can decisively influence long-term results. A fundamental element in this process is the preoperative information provided to the patient: being aware of the risks, benefits, lifestyle changes, postoperative management, and realistic expectations. This education not only provides technical advice but also affects the patient's psychological attitude: their emotions (anxiety, fears), beliefs (self-efficacy, expectations), motivation, and readiness for change. An adaptive psychological attitude can facilitate adherence to post-surgical instructions and improve overall outcomes [7].

In clinical practice, preoperative psychological assessment is nearly standard in most bariatric surgery centres, aiming to detect contraindications, psychological risk factors, psychiatric disorders, and emotional vulnerabilities. Nevertheless, discrepancies persist regarding its mandatory nature, its predictive utility, and its optimal design [17]. Furthermore, although reviews exist on psychological assessment in bariatric surgery in general, few specifically integrate the relationship between preoperative information and psychological attitude, especially in sleeve gastrectomy patients [11]. Therefore, the objective of this systematic

B. Espina-Jerez (✉)
Pontifical Comillas University, San Juan de Dios Foundation, Madrid, Spain
e-mail: bespina@euef.comillas.edu

J. Ruiz-Tovar (ed.), *Multidisciplinary Management of Sleeve Gastrectomy*,
https://doi.org/10.1007/978-3-032-25644-7_1

review is to analyse the existing evidence on the influence of preoperative information and the psychological attitude of patients who are candidates for sleeve gastrectomy.

1.2 Aims

1.2.1 Primary Aim

To analyse the influence of preoperative information and psychological attitude on the clinical and psychosocial outcomes of patients undergoing sleeve gastrectomy.

1.2.2 Specific Aims

- To identify the essential components of preoperative information protocols that enhance patient understanding and realistic expectations.
- To determine the relationship between the presence of pre-existing psychological pathology and the postoperative outcomes of sleeve gastrectomy (SG).
- To synthesise the validated and most frequently used psychological screening tools in the assessment of attitude for SG.
- To analyse the impact of preoperative psychological interventions on long-term adherence and quality of life.

1.3 Methods

1.3.1 Design

A systematic review was conducted following the PRISMA 2020 standard guidelines, aimed at answering the research question: *How does the preoperative information and the psychological attitude of patients who are candidates for sleeve gastrectomy influence outcomes?*

1.3.2 Sources and Search Strategy

The databases consulted were PubMed, Web of Science, PsycINFO, and the Cochrane Library. The period from January 2020 to September 2025 was considered. Articles in English or Spanish were included. The search strategy combined MeSH terms and free text words:

("Bariatric Surgery") AND ("Preoperative") AND ("Information") AND ("Psychometrics") AND ("Attitude to Health" OR "Psychological Assessment" OR "Psychosocial")

The search was complemented by reviewing the bibliographical references of the selected articles, using the "snowballing" method.

1.3.3 Inclusion and Exclusion Criteria

Inclusion:

- Studies with an adult population who are candidates for bariatric surgery (preferably sleeve gastrectomy).
- Studies evaluating the relationship between preoperative information/education and psychological variables (anxiety, expectations, self-efficacy, cognitive or emotional attitude).
- Original studies, controlled trials, qualitative, or quasi-experimental studies, published between January 2020 and September 2025.
- Language: English or Spanish.

Exclusion:

- Studies that only addressed surgical technical aspects without a psychological component.
- Studies focused exclusively on other bariatric procedures (e.g., gastric bypass).
- Narrative reviews without original empirical data.
- Studies with a paediatric population or exclusively postoperative interventions.

1.3.4 Study Selection and Data Synthesis

The PRISMA process was applied in four stages: record identification, removal of duplicates, screening by title and abstract, and full-text evaluation to determine eligibility. A PRISMA flow diagram was constructed with the final numbers.

For each study, the following were recorded: author(s), year, country, methodological design, type of informational intervention (if any), psychological instruments used, psychological variables assessed, main findings, and limitations noted by the authors.

Given the expected heterogeneity in interventions and instruments, the synthesis was thematic and narrative. Findings were organised around the following domains: (1) Impact of preoperative information on expectations and adherence. (2) Influence of psychological attitude and pre-existing psychological pathology. (3) Validated instruments for preoperative psychological assessment. (4) Efficacy of preoperative psychological interventions.

1.4 Results

1.4.1 Study Selection

Out of a total of 845 records initially identified, 312 were duplicates. After screening by title and abstract, 430 studies were discarded, leaving 103 for full-text reading. Finally, 14 studies met all inclusion criteria and were included in the review. The results extracted from the analysis of the 14 articles are summarised in Table 1.1.

1.4.2 General Characteristics

The selected studies were predominantly from Anglophone and European countries, although results from other parts of the world were also considered for their relevance. The majority used prospective observational designs.

Only a small group applied structured educational interventions before surgery or cognitive behavioural therapy (CBT). The most commonly used psychological instruments included anxiety and depression scales, such as the STAI (State-Trait Anxiety Inventory), BDI (Beck Depression Inventory), but also instruments to measure binge eating disorder, quality of life, body image, and treatment adherence ad hoc. Although some papers investigated bariatric surgery in general, few were focused exclusively on *sleeve gastrectomy.*

In general, the studies showed a high proportion of women, with a difference compared to men, and an average age ranging from approximately 35–50 years. The mean preoperative BMI was consistently high, at 45.7 kg/m^2 reflecting the typical population of SG candidates [8].

1.4.3 Emerging Themes

1.4.3.1 Impact of Preoperative Information on Expectations and Adherence

Recent research emphasises that the quality of preoperative information is a direct predictor of satisfaction and postoperative adherence [6]. The key component identified is the modification of expectations [5]. Patients who expect excessively rapid or miraculous weight loss tend to report greater dissatisfaction and depressive symptoms when faced with plateau phases or slight gains [20]. Conversely, educational programmes that employ real-life testimonials or group sessions to illustrate both successes and challenges are associated with better emotional preparation and greater resilience [18]. The evidence suggests that preoperative information should be delivered in a multimodal format (in-person, digital, support groups) to ensure

Table 1.1 Summary table of the articles used in the systematic review

Authors (year)	Study design	Country	Population (N, type of surgery)	Intervention	Main findings
Allameh et al. [1]	Study protocol (registered clinical trial)	Iran	Individuals with overweight/obesity with mild to moderate anxiety/ depression	Distance-based mindfulness-based intervention (MBI) + standard dietary treatment	The aim is to explore the effects of MBI on the intensity of food cravings and related outcomes in this population. Protocol only, no final results.
Anbara [3]	Prospective study	Iran	104 sleeve gastrectomy patients	Not applicable	Loss of control over eating and postoperative binge eating disorders are associated with poorer weight-loss outcomes and increased eating-disorder psychopathology after surgery.
Badorrek et al. [5]	Prospective longitudinal cohort	Australia	238 participants (79% women)	Not applicable	Individuals preparing for bariatric surgery reported high expectations and diverse needs for health-professional and psychosocial support. Multidisciplinary, personalised care and realistic goal-setting are required.
Chan & Vartanian [6]	Systematic review	Australia	Post-bariatric patients	Not applicable	Higher self-efficacy consistently predicts better adherence to diet and physical activity. A history of psychiatric conditions is associated with poorer adherence.
García-Redondo et al. [8]	Multicentre prospective descriptive study	Spain	70 participants (62.9% women)	Not applicable	Common comorbidities included diabetes mellitus, OSAHS, coronary ischaemic disease, and internal/ external haemorrhoids.

(continued)

Table 1.1 (continued)

Authors (year)	Study design	Country	Population (N, type of surgery)	Intervention	Main findings
Gowey et al. [9]	Original article	USA	44 women >50 with obesity	Behavioural intervention	Most individuals achieving clinically significant weight loss through behavioural intervention had average or above-average executive function (EF). Those who maintained (rather than regained) weight performed better in decision-making tasks.
Hjelmesæth et al. [10]	RCT	Norway	61 participants, BMI 43.5	Preoperative CBT (10 weeks)	Preoperative CBT was associated with a lower BMI at 4 years in patients with depressive symptoms.
Köhler et al. [12]	Cross-sectional study	Germany	110 pre/post bariatric patients	Not applicable	Highlights the importance of adequate health-specific knowledge for weight loss and prevention of adverse events, assessed pre- and post-surgery.
Law et al. [13]	Umbrella review	China	Not applicable	Not applicable	Bariatric surgery may improve mental health; however, caution is required as individuals with comorbid depression may face increased risks of suicide, self-harm, and alcohol-use disorder.
Lüscher et al. [14]	Prospective cohort	Switzerland	236 RYGB patients (81% women)	Not applicable	High preoperative anxiety (STAI-S) predicted faster long-term weight regain. Other psychiatric symptoms showed no significant impact on long-term weight loss.
Maia et al. [16]	Cross-sectional study	Brazil	124 bariatric candidates	Not applicable	Individuals with moderate or severe body dissatisfaction had high rates of food addiction.

Tolvanen et al. [18]	Qualitative study	Switzerland	16 with significant weight regain	Not applicable	Patients report "lonely struggle"—Want long-term proactive support.
Vaishnav et al. [19]	Clinical practice guidelines	India	Patients with obesity	Psychiatric pre/post intervention	Presurgical mental illness does not predict postoperative weight loss, though it worsens overall postoperative functioning. Psychological interventions (CBT, behavioural interventions, multimodal programmes) improve binge eating patterns, HRQoL, and weight loss, although effects are short- to mid-term.
Wagner et al. [20]	Qualitative (questionnaire)	Germany	164 post-bariatric patients	Not applicable	Explores patient expectations and perspectives of postoperative follow-up to identify unmet needs and ways to increase adherence to follow-up appointments.

Source: Author's own work

retention and understanding, especially in populations with lower health literacy [12].

It has also been observed that self-efficacy, the patient's belief in their ability to perform recommended behaviours, is positively related to postoperative adherence. In a recent review, preoperative self-efficacy was a consistent predictor of compliance with diet, physical activity, and attendance at follow-up appointments [6].

1.4.3.2 Influence of Psychological Attitude and Pre-existing Psychological Pathology

Preoperative psychological assessment has been redefined as a tool to identify modifiable risk factors and plan interventions, rather than as a barrier to accessing surgery.

The psychological risk factor most consistently linked to a worse weight prognosis is unresolved binge eating disorder (BED) [3].

Other relevant disorders include major depression and anxiety [14], which, if uncontrolled, can hinder adherence to diet and exercise. Caution must be exercised during the psychological assessment prior to surgery, as there may be an elevated risk of suicide and self-harm in patients with major depression symptomatology after the procedure [13].

The assessment of executive function and historical adherence to other health treatments are now considered prognostic indicators as important as the diagnosis of a mental health disorder [9].

Nonetheless, recent research on preoperative mental health [19] is clear: these conditions are not absolute contraindications, provided the patient demonstrates psychological stability and the cognitive and behavioural capacity to follow complex postoperative guidelines.

1.4.3.3 Validated Instruments for Preoperative Psychological Assessment

Preoperative psychological assessment in sleeve gastrectomy (SG) candidates is essential for identifying risk factors, planning interventions, and predicting adherence and postoperative outcomes [19]. The most commonly used instruments can be classified based on the assessment areas that have been shown to be most critical in these patients (Table 1.2).

1.4.3.4 Efficacy of Preoperative Psychological Interventions

The development of structured psychological interventions in the preoperative period is an area of increasing evidence. Cognitive behavioural therapy (CBT) adapted to obesity and the challenges of SG has proven to be the most effective strategy. However, recent studies on this are lacking. By broadening the time frame, a randomised controlled trial [10] was found that compared a group with 10 weeks of preoperative CBT (focused on coping skills and cognitive restructuring of emotional eating) with a control group without CBT. The CBT group reported having a lower weight before surgery and maintained it for 4 years after surgery.

Table 1.2 Psychological assessment instruments for patients who are candidates for sleeve gastrectomy

Pathology	Instrument	Construct evaluated	Relevance in SG
Binge eating disorder	Questionnaire on Eating and Weight Patterns: revised (QEWP-R) Binge Eating Scale (BES)	Presence and severity of binge eating disorder	Active or unresolved BED predicts lower long-term excess weight loss.
	Yale Eating Disorder Examination—Questionnaire (EDE-Q)	Frequency and severity of disordered eating behaviours (restriction, weight/shape concern, binge eating).	Provides a comprehensive overview of eating psychopathology, to adapt behavioural intervention.
Anxiety and depression	Beck Depression Inventory (BDI-II)	Severity of depressive symptoms	Preoperative depression must be treated until stabilisation before surgery to ensure coping ability and adherence.
	State-Trait Anxiety Inventory (STAI)	Severity of anxiety symptoms	High levels of anxiety may be related to emotional eating and difficulty managing postoperative stress.
	The hospital anxiety and depression scale	Detection of anxiety and depression in patients with physical diseases (useful for discriminating somatic symptoms).	Useful in the hospital setting for rapid screening and differentiation.
Quality of life and body shape	Impact of Weight on Quality of Life Questionnaire, IWQOL-Lite	Impact of weight on quality of life (physical, sexual, self-esteem, public functioning).	Is a primary outcome of SG success. Allows measurement of pre- and postoperative change.
	Body Shape Questionnaire (BSQ)	Distress and avoidance related to body image.	Is fundamental for predicting body satisfaction after weight loss, as this does not automatically improve solely with weight loss [16].
Adherence and expectations	Adherence Barriers Questionnaire (ABQ)	It assesses perceived barriers to continuing treatment, and patient motivation toward change and adherence to recommendations.	Adherence capacity is the main predictor of long-term success.
	Weight loss expectations questionnaire (ad hoc)	Realism of expectations regarding the amount of weight to be lost and postoperative life change.	Identification of unrealistic expectations is key for preoperative intervention [20].

Source: Author's own elaboration

Intervention focused on *Mindfulness* and full awareness has also emerged as a promising strategy for addressing emotional eating and stress eating [1]. These interventions strengthen the patient's self-regulation and capacity to distinguish between physiological and emotional hunger, which is crucial when the initial gastric restriction decreases. The goal is not only weight loss but the promotion of a sustainable change in the patient's relationship with food.

Furthermore, a proactive, informed, and motivated psychological attitude favours better adherence. Informational interventions that include a motivational component (psychoeducation and counselling) showed higher rates of signed commitments and appointment attendance.

1.5 Discussion

The results of this review reinforce the need for a paradigm shift: preoperative preparation must be an active and therapeutic process, not merely a collection of consent signatures. Centres that implement more robust and longer-duration informational and psychological protocols before surgery consistently report better indicators of long-term success [19]. The information should function as a therapeutic contract where responsibilities and the consequences of non-compliance are transmitted, fostering patient autonomy and personal responsibility [11].

Well-designed preoperative information positively influences the psychological attitude of the patient candidate for sleeve gastrectomy or bariatric surgery, reducing their anxiety, adjusting expectations, and increasing self-efficacy. These effects, while expected from cognitive health models, translate into a better emotional state prior to surgery, which can impact postoperative adherence and satisfaction [6].

Despite the consensus on the importance of psychological assessment, the heterogeneity of tools and cut-off points remains a methodological limitation. While the BDI-II for depression and the EDE-Q for eating pathology are routinely used, there is a lack of a standardised screening protocol [15, 16]. The future requires a minimum set of internationally validated tools and an approach that ensures all modifiable risk factors are treated until stability before surgical intervention.

The clinical implications necessitate an investment of time and resources in the preoperative phase, both in exhaustive education and psychological intervention, which translates into a greater return in the form of better long-term health outcomes. Programmes should adopt an integrated multidisciplinary approach, where the psychologist conducts an assessment accompanied by a motivational intervention, aimed at strengthening self-efficacy, exploring expectations, and detecting vulnerabilities. Subsequently, they must intervene actively with tools like CBT to equip the patient with the coping skills necessary for post-SG life.

A key direction for future research is the conduct of large-scale randomised controlled trials, with follow-up for 5 years or more, to compare the efficacy of different psychological intervention modalities (CBT vs. Mindfulness vs. Support Groups) in preventing weight regain, a challenge that becomes more evident after the second postoperative year [2].

Some limitations encountered during the review included the presence of high methodological heterogeneity. The selected studies have been conducted worldwide; however, the general findings among them are congruent. Furthermore, there is little specific evidence for the concrete procedure of sleeve gastrectomy, and the review had to broaden the search to bariatric surgery in general. Therefore, it is recommended that future research focuses specifically on patients undergoing the most common procedure, sleeve gastrectomy. It is also advised that randomised controlled trial designs be used to compare models of preoperative education and psychological intervention, tending towards their standardisation. Additionally, they should uniformly use validated and coherent psychological instruments, leading to the configuration of a general screening, conduct a longitudinal follow-up of the psychological aspects involved, and include contextual differences, previously less addressed, such as cultural factors, gender, and socioeconomic level.

1.6 Conclusions

This systematic review of recent literature confirms that the preoperative phase is crucial for the success of sleeve gastrectomy. Preoperative information must be exhaustive, address expectations realistically, and utilise multimodal approaches to maximise comprehension and adherence. Psychological suitability must be assessed with a focus on preparation and risk modification, where pre-existing conditions such as binge eating disorder, depression, or anxiety must be stabilised through structured therapeutic interventions, with CBT being the most evidence-supported. Commitment to mental health and behavioural education at this stage is a crucial prognostic factor that maximises the therapeutic potential of the surgery.

Preoperative patient information is not merely a technical informational requirement but a preventive psychological intervention that affects the emotional, cognitive, and motivational attitude of the bariatric surgery candidate. In the context of sleeve gastrectomy, although direct evidence is scarce, the reviewed findings suggest that structured education and intervention reduce anxiety, adjust expectations, and strengthen self-efficacy. These adaptive attitudes can favour long-term adherence and success. Therefore, it is recommended that bariatric teams integrate standardised protocols for preoperative psychological education and intervention. Rigorous studies focused on sleeve gastrectomy are required to consolidate this knowledge base.

References

1. Allameh SA, Mokhtari Z, Askari G. Effectiveness of a mindfulness-based intervention + standard diet treatment compared to standard diet treatment alone on food cravings in overweight/obese individuals with mild to moderate anxiety/depression: a study protocol for an open-labeled, parallel-group randomized controlled trial. Trials. 2025;26(1):283. https://doi.org/10.1186/s13063-025-08900-z.

2. Almuhtadi Y, Alageel S. Systematic review of mindfulness-based interventions for weight management among pre- and post-bariatric surgery patients. Adv Mind Body Med. 2023;37(3):15–22. https://pubmed.ncbi.nlm.nih.gov/38345771/
3. Anbara T. The impacts of eating disorders on sleeve gastrectomy outcomes. Surg Pract Sci. 2023;13:100165. https://doi.org/10.1016/j.sipas.2023.100165.
4. Anees AA, Said KA, Ayshaa Ma H, Sara Tariq AA. The impact of sleeve gastrectomy combined with lifestyle interventions on anthropometric and health outcomes in adults: a systematic review and meta-analysis. Cureus. 2025;9(17):e85587. https://pubmed.ncbi.nlm.nih.gov/40491808/?utm_source=chatgpt.com
5. Badorrek S, Franklin J, Devadas M, Williams N, Russell R, Saluja S, Batterham M, Williams K. Exploring patient perspectives: information-seeking behaviours, beliefs and support needs prior to bariatric surgery. Obes Res Clin Pract. 2025;19(5):409–16. https://doi.org/10.1016/j.orcp.2025.09.002.
6. Chan JKY, Vartanian LR. Psychological predictors of adherence to lifestyle changes after bariatric surgery: a systematic review. Obes Sci Pract. 2024;10(1):e741. https://doi.org/10.1002/osp4.741.
7. Dowgiałło-Gornowicz N, Wityk M, Lech P. Staying on track: factors influencing 10-year follow-up adherence after sleeve gastrectomy. Obes Surg. 2025;35(7):2711–8. https://doi.org/10.1007/s11695-025-07954-x.
8. García-Redondo M, Ferrer-Márquez M, Rubio-Gil F, Belda-Lozano R, RuizPardo J, Sánchez-Fuentes P, Vidaña-Márquez E, Ferrer-Ayza M, Reina-Duarte Á. Anal disease in patients who are candidates for bariatric surgery: a descriptive study. BMI J. 2023;13(1):3817–22. https://www.bmi-journal.com/articulos/download/937/en?QX4Ep29MefBoscWAuIfl6JRDWKAOy0wD
9. Gowey MA, Neumeier WH, Henry S, Wadley VG, Phillips J, Hayden KM, Espeland MA, Coday M, Lewis CE, Dutton GR. Executive function in individuals with clinically significant weight loss via behavioral intervention. Obes Sci Pract. 2021;7(1):25–34. https://doi.org/10.1002/osp4.458.
10. Hjelmesæth J, Rosenvinge JH, Gade H, Friborg O. Effects of cognitive behavioral therapy on eating behaviors, affective symptoms, and weight loss after bariatric surgery: a randomized clinical trial. Obes Surg. 2018;29(1):61–9. https://doi.org/10.1007/s11695-018-3471-x.
11. Johnston L, Jackson K, Hilton C, Graham Y. The forgotten patient: a psychological perspective on the implementation of bariatric surgery guidelines. Obes Sci Pract. 2023;9(5):538–47. https://doi.org/10.1002/osp4.670.
12. Köhler H, Dorozhkina R, Gruner-Labitzke K, de Zwaan M. Specific health knowledge and health literacy of patients before and after bariatric surgery: a cross-sectional study. Obes Facts. 2020;13(2):166–78. https://doi.org/10.1159/000505837.
13. Law S, Dong S, Zhou F, Zheng D, Wang C, Dong Z. Bariatric surgery and mental health outcomes: an umbrella review. Front Endocrinol. 2023;2(14):1283621. https://doi.org/10.3389/fendo.2023.1283621.
14. Lüscher A, Vionnet N, Amiguet M, Chartoumpekis D, Mantziari S, Frantz J, Favre L. Impact of preoperative psychiatric profile in bariatric surgery on long-term weight outcome. Obes Surg. 2023;33(7):2072–82. https://doi.org/10.1007/s11695-023-06595-2.
15. Magurano MR, Napolitano D, Bozzetti M, Lo Cascio A, Oppo L, Fernandez Tayupanta LA, Ferrazzoli S, Lopasso L, Rellini E, Raffaelli M, Chieffo DPR. Psychological assessment and psychosocial outcomes in bariatric surgery candidates: a retrospective study. Healthcare. 2025;13(11):1294. https://doi.org/10.3390/healthcare13111294.
16. Maia C, Ferreira G, Da Silveira Campos R, Dos Anjos Martins Cravo Fruet Bettini S, Panizzi LN, De Quadros Dlugosz MG, Fadanni M, Dal Molin Netto B. Association between food addiction and body image dissatisfaction in bariatric surgery candidates: a cross-sectional study. J Eat Disord. 2025;7(13 (1)):1–9. https://pubmed.ncbi.nlm.nih.gov/41204390/
17. Marek RJ, Heinberg LJ. Should presurgical psychological evaluations still be a mandated requirement for metabolic and bariatric surgery? A critique of the literature and thoughts on future directions. Surg Obes Relat Dis. 2024;20(12):1360–9. https://www.soard.org/article/S1550-7289%2824%2900720-2/abstract?utm_source=chatgpt.com

18. Tolvanen L, Svensson Å, Hemmingsson E, Christenson A, Lagerros YT. Perceived and preferred social support in patients experiencing weight regain after bariatric surgery—a qualitative study. Obes Surg. 2020;31(3):1256–64. https://doi.org/10.1007/s11695-020-05128-5.
19. Vaishnav M, Gupta S, Vaishnav P. Psychiatric intervention pre- and post-bariatric surgery. Indian J Psychiatry. 2022;64(2):473–83. https://doi.org/10.4103/indianjpsychiatry.indianjpsychiatry_1_22.
20. Wagner J, Roll M, Lautenbach A, Notz S, Plitzko G, Izbicki J, Mann O, Hackert T, Duprée A, Brodersen F, Weigel A. Patients' expectations and perspectives on follow-up care after bariatric surgery in Germany. Obes Surg. 2025;35(6):2174–84. https://doi.org/10.1007/s11695-025-07890-w.

Selection of Patients for Sleeve Gastrectomy. Indications and Contraindications

2

Manuel Medina-Pedrique, Adriana Avilés-Oliveros, Alvaro Casanova-Aparicio, Gabriela Alvarado-Carrillo, Victor Vaello-Jodra, and Jaime Ruiz-Tovar

2.1 Introduction

Vertical sleeve gastrectomy (VSG) has rapidly evolved from a staged approach in high-risk super-obesity to a dominant stand-alone operation in metabolic surgery. Over the past decade, VSG has surpassed Roux-en-Y gastric bypass (RYGB) as the most commonly performed bariatric procedure in many countries, now representing more than 50% of global case volume [1, 2]. Its expanding role reflects accumulating evidence of durable weight loss, significant metabolic improvement, and a technically streamlined surgical profile that facilitates reproducibility and widespread adoption [3, 4].

The preserved gastrointestinal continuity of VSG allows maintenance of physiological nutrient absorption and future endoscopic access to the stomach and biliary tract—features that differentiate it from RYGB and remain clinically valuable in patients at risk for peptic, pancreatic, or biliary disease [5]. At the same time, deep hormonal and metabolic shifts (notably in ghrelin, GLP-1, and insulin sensitivity) reinforce that VSG is not simply restrictive but a truly metabolic intervention [6, 7].

Nevertheless, VSG carries limitations that continue to shape operative decision-making. Increased intragastric pressure and elimination of the fundic reservoir have been associated with higher rates of de novo or worsened gastroesophageal reflux disease (GERD), erosive esophagitis, and Barrett's esophagus compared with RYGB [8–11]. Long-term randomized evidence—including the SLEEVEPASS

M. Medina-Pedrique · A. Avilés-Oliveros · A. Casanova-Aparicio · G. Alvarado-Carrillo
Department of Surgery, Henares University Hospital, Madrid, Spain
e-mail: medinamanuel1324@gmail.com; a.avilesoliveros@gmail.com

V. Vaello-Jodra · J. Ruiz-Tovar (✉)
Department of Surgery, Henares University Hospital, Madrid, Spain

Department of Biomedicine and Health Sciences, Alfonso X University, Madrid, Spain
e-mail: victorvaello@gmail.com

J. Ruiz-Tovar (ed.), *Multidisciplinary Management of Sleeve Gastrectomy*,
https://doi.org/10.1007/978-3-032-25644-7_2

trial—suggests comparable weight-loss outcomes but persistent reflux concerns after VSG [2, 10]. These anatomical and physiologic realities underscore that *procedure selection remains pivotal* to optimizing patient outcomes.

For metabolic surgeons, the clinical task is not to choose between a "better" or "worse" operation, but rather to identify which procedure best aligns with a patient's comorbidities, esophageal physiology, nutritional resilience, and long-term care needs. This chapter reviews contemporary indications and contraindications for VSG, contrasting them with scenarios where RYGB offers a superior benefit–risk profile. The ultimate objective is to support precise, individualized surgical planning that enhances durability of weight control, metabolic improvement, and quality of life.

2.2 From First-Stage Strategy to Standard of Care

VSG was initially conceived as the first stage of biliopancreatic diversion with duodenal switch in super-obese, high-risk patients. The idea was to reduce weight and operative risk before a second, more complex malabsorptive procedure. Over time, however, the favorable outcomes of VSG in terms of weight loss and comorbidity improvement led to its adoption as an independent procedure [3, 12].

Compared with RYGB, VSG offers:

- A primarily *restrictive mechanism* with significant hormonal effects, particularly through reduction of ghrelin levels [6].
- *Preserved anatomy*, which maintains easier endoscopic access to the stomach and biliary tree, an advantage in patients who may later require ERCP [5].
- *Less risk of malabsorption and micronutrient deficiency* than bypass or biliopancreatic diversion [7].
- A *simpler and shorter operation* in experienced hands, which facilitates diffusion and standardization [3, 12].

At the same time, VSG is not "neutral". The creation of a high-pressure tubular stomach is associated with an increased risk of de novo or worsened GERD, erosive esophagitis, and Barrett's esophagus [8, 9, 13–15]. Long-term randomized data, such as SLEEVEPASS, show that VSG and RYGB achieve comparable weight loss and metabolic improvements at 7–10 years, but RYGB has a more favorable reflux profile [2, 9].

The practical consequence is clear: the question is no longer simply "surgery yes or no?", but "VSG or RYGB (or another technique) for this particular patient?"

2.3 General Indications for Metabolic and Bariatric Surgery

The 2022 ASMBS/IFSO joint guidelines significantly updated the indications for metabolic and bariatric surgery, moving beyond the NIH 1991 criteria [1]. In summary, surgery is recommended:

- In patients with *BMI* ≥ *35 kg/m²*, regardless of the presence or severity of comorbidities [1].
- In patients with *BMI 30–34.9 kg/m²* and inadequately controlled type 2 diabetes or other significant metabolic disease, such as metabolic dysfunction-associated steatotic liver disease/metabolic dysfunction-associated steatohepatitis *(MASLD/MASH)*, hypertension, or dyslipidemia [1, 7].
- In *adolescents* with severe obesity under specific pediatric criteria, including BMI thresholds, comorbidities, pubertal maturity, and psychosocial readiness [16, 17].

These criteria apply to metabolic and bariatric surgery in general, not specifically to VSG. The choice of procedure depends on:

- The comorbidity profile (especially GERD, esophageal disease, diabetes, and liver disease).
- Surgical risk and previous abdominal operations.
- Age, frailty, and expected life expectancy.
- Psychiatric and psychosocial context, including family support.
- The experience and resources of the multidisciplinary team [1, 7, 16].

2.4 Specific Indications for Vertical Sleeve Gastrectomy

2.4.1 Typical Candidate Profile

In everyday practice, VSG is a good option for patients who combine:

- *Severe obesity (BMI* ≥ *35–40 kg/m²)* without significant or uncontrolled GERD.
- Need to *preserve endoscopic access* to the stomach and biliary tract (e.g., patients with a high risk of biliary disease or pancreatitis who might require ERCP) [3, 5, 12, 14].
- A clinical context in which *malabsorption is undesirable*, such as elderly patients, those at risk of protein-calorie malnutrition or with borderline nutritional reserves [7, 18].

A typical scenario might be a 45-year-old woman with BMI 42 kg/m², hypertension, and obstructive sleep apnea, with normal upper endoscopy (no esophagitis, no large hiatal hernia) and simple steatosis on liver assessment. In her case, VSG offers a reasonable balance between efficacy, safety, and technical simplicity.

2.4.2 Metabolic and Liver Benefits

VSG produces substantial and durable improvements in obesity-related comorbidities:

- *Type 2 diabetes and metabolic syndrome:*
  Weight loss and gut hormonal changes improve glycemic control and insulin sensitivity. In many patients, VSG achieves remission or marked improvement of type 2 diabetes, although in long-standing, insulinopenic diabetes RYGB may provide a stronger metabolic effect [1, 7, 19].
- *Obstructive sleep apnea, hypertension, and dyslipidemia:*
  These conditions usually improve in parallel with weight loss and are often sustained at mid- to long-term follow-up [7, 9, 19].
- *MASLD/MASH:*
  VSG, like other metabolic operations, is one of the few interventions capable of inducing resolution of MASH and regression of fibrosis in a meaningful proportion of patients [20–23]. This has important implications in the prevention of cirrhosis and hepatocellular carcinoma.

In patients with *compensated cirrhosis*, bariatric surgery can be safe in experienced centers and may even improve liver function and candidacy for transplantation. In this context, VSG is often preferred, as it avoids complex intestinal bypass and preserves anatomical orientation [24–28].

2.4.3 Super-Obesity and Staged Strategies

In patients with *BMI > 50–60 kg/m²* and high operative risk, VSG may be used as *the first step* of a staged approach:

1. Initial VSG to reduce weight and risk.
2. Potential second-stage conversion to RYGB or duodenal switch if weight loss or metabolic control proves insufficient.

Although high-quality randomized data are limited in this specific setting, observational series support this strategy [3, 4, 14].

2.4.4 Adolescents and Young Adults

Pediatric and adolescent metabolic surgery guidelines consider VSG a reference procedure in adolescents with severe obesity, provided it is performed in specialized centers with multidisciplinary support [16–18].

Common criteria include:

- *BMI ≥ 35 kg/m²* with a major comorbidity (such as type 2 diabetes, OSA, or severe MASLD/MASH), or *BMI ≥ 40 kg/m²*.
- Adequate *pubertal development* (Tanner stage IV–V).

- Demonstrated ability to adhere to long-term follow-up.
- Stable family or social support network.

In this age group, VSG offers strong weight loss and comorbidity remission with acceptable safety and nutritional profiles in the mid-term [17, 18].

2.4.5 Older and Frail Patients

In older or frail patients, the balance between benefit and risk is especially delicate. VSG may be an attractive option because it:

- Avoids major malabsorption.
- Is technically simpler and shorter than complex bypass procedures.

Nevertheless, the risk of sarcopenia and nutritional deficits remains and requires close monitoring [18, 29]. The decision to operate in this group should focus not only on survival but also on functional status and quality of life.

2.5 Contraindications to Vertical Sleeve Gastrectomy

Contraindications can be divided into *absolute*, *relative general,* and *VSG-specific*.

2.5.1 Absolute Contraindications to Bariatric–Metabolic Surgery

Although different guidelines use slightly different wording, there is broad agreement that metabolic surgery should *not* be offered when [1, 30]:

- The patient has a *prohibitive anesthetic or surgical risk* despite optimal medical management.
- There is *advanced terminal disease* with very limited life expectancy and minimal likelihood of meaningful benefit from surgery.
- There is *absolute inability to adhere* to follow-up and postoperative care, and no realistic support system to compensate for it.
- The patient is *pregnant* at the time of evaluation (surgery is deferred until postpartum and stabilization).

These situations are relatively straightforward: surgery does not address the main problem and adds unnecessary risk.

2.5.2 Relative General Contraindications

Many complex clinical situations fall into a gray area requiring individualized, multidisciplinary evaluation. Among the most relevant relative contraindications are [30–32]:

- *Severe psychiatric disorders not adequately treated.*
  - Active psychosis.
  - Severe major depression with suicidal ideation.
  - Severe eating disorders (e.g., uncontrolled binge eating, bulimia nervosa).
- *Active alcohol or substance use disorder*
  These conditions are associated with poorer postoperative outcomes, non-adherence, and a risk of "addiction transfer" after surgery.
- *Severe cardiopulmonary disease not optimized.*
  - Unstable coronary disease.
  - Advanced heart failure.
  - Severe COPD or pulmonary hypertension.
- *Cirrhosis with clinically significant portal hypertension or decompensation*
  In such cases, bariatric surgery should only be considered in transplant-capable centers and within carefully defined protocols [24–27].
- *Active malignant disease under treatment*, depending on type, stage, and expected prognosis.

Importantly, increasing data suggest that some patients with stable, well-managed psychiatric conditions can undergo bariatric surgery with outcomes comparable to those of the general bariatric population, provided there is close follow-up [31, 32].

2.5.3 VSG-Specific Contraindications

Here is where VSG clearly diverges from RYGB and other techniques.

2.5.3.1 Severe GERD and Barrett's Esophagus

Systematic reviews and long-term series consistently show an increased incidence of de novo GERD, esophagitis, and Barrett's esophagus after VSG [8–15]. While results are heterogeneous, a practical consensus has emerged:

- VSG is a *poor primary choice* in patients with:
  - Severe, medication-refractory GERD.
  - Los Angeles *grade C–D esophagitis*.
  - *Extensive Barrett's esophagus*, especially with dysplasia.

In these scenarios, *RYGB is generally preferred* because of its antireflux effect [8, 9].

2.5.3.2 Large Hiatal Hernia and Esophageal Motility Disorders

- In patients with *large hiatal hernia*, VSG alone is associated with worse reflux outcomes. If VSG is chosen, a proper hiatal repair is mandatory, and RYGB is often considered a better alternative, particularly in symptomatic GERD [9, 13].
- In *severe esophageal motility disorders* (achalasia, major spastic disorders), evidence is limited, but most experts avoid VSG because of the risk of dysphagia and persistent symptoms [8, 13].

2.5.3.3 High Risk of Malnutrition or Sarcopenia

Although VSG is not primarily malabsorptive, patients with:

- *Severe baseline malnutrition*,
- *Marked sarcopenia*, or.
- Conditions associated with poor oral intake,

may not tolerate the restrictive effect of the procedure. In these cases, careful preoperative nutritional optimization and, in some patients, non-surgical strategies may be more appropriate [18, 29].

2.6 Preoperative Evaluation and Shared Decision-Making

Beyond BMI and comorbidities, the indication for VSG is shaped by small but crucial clinical details and by an honest conversation with the patient.

Most international guidelines recommend that every candidate for bariatric surgery be assessed by a *multidisciplinary team* including, at minimum, a bariatric surgeon, endocrinologist, dietitian, psychologist or psychiatrist, and anesthesiologist [1, 7, 29–32].

Key elements of the evaluation include:

- A *detailed history of GERD* and upper gastrointestinal symptoms.
- *Upper endoscopy* before surgery, to detect esophagitis, Barrett's esophagus, or hiatal hernia.
- Comprehensive assessment of *metabolic and cardiovascular comorbidities*.
- *Psychological evaluation*, focusing on mood disorders, eating behavior, and coping mechanisms.
- Screening for *alcohol and substance use*.
- Discussion of *risks, benefits, alternatives* (including "no surgery yet"), and realistic postoperative expectations.

In practice, an essential part of this process is to align expectations: explaining that surgery is a powerful tool, not a magic solution; that for VSG to achieve its full potential, the patient must be prepared for permanent changes in diet, physical activity, and relationship with food.

2.7 Controversies and Future Directions

Despite its widespread use, several questions remain open regarding VSG:

- *VSG in patients with BMI 30–34.9 kg/m² and metabolic disease*:
  Guidelines now support metabolic surgery in this group [1, 7], but long-term data for VSG specifically are still limited [19].
- *True incidence and clinical impact of Barrett's esophagus and esophageal adenocarcinoma after VSG*:
  Reported rates of Barrett's vary across series; standardized surveillance programs are needed to clarify long-term risk [8–15].
- *"Sleeve-plus" techniques* (such as VSG with concomitant fundoplication or systematic hiatal repair):
  Early systematic reviews suggest improved reflux control in selected patients, but heterogeneity and limited follow-up preclude firm conclusions [28].
- *Neuropsychiatric and addiction-related outcomes*:
  Bariatric surgery, including VSG, may alter vulnerability to substance use and mood changes, underlining the importance of long-term psychosocial follow-up [31, 32].

These controversies do not undermine the value of VSG, but remind us that indications will likely continue to be refined as new data emerge.

2.8 Conclusions

Vertical sleeve gastrectomy has become a central component of modern metabolic surgery. Its advantages—relative technical simplicity, preserved anatomy, absence of major malabsorption, and strong weight-loss and metabolic outcomes—make it a very attractive option for many patients with severe obesity [1, 3, 12, 14].

However, VSG is *not* a one-size-fits-all solution. Its propensity to induce or worsen GERD, esophagitis, and Barrett's esophagus, as well as the particular needs of patients with advanced liver disease, complex psychiatric conditions, or frailty, demand a nuanced and individualized indication.

Ultimately, good results with VSG depend on:

- Careful *multidisciplinary selection*,
- Honest *expectation management*, and.
- A truly *shared decision-making process* that matches the characteristics of the procedure with the values, fears, and goals of each patient.

Used in this way—thoughtfully, not automatically—VSG is a powerful tool for improving health and quality of life in people living with severe obesity.

References

1. Eisenberg D, Shikora SA, Aarts EO, et al. ASMBS and IFSO indications for metabolic and bariatric surgery. Surg Obes Relat Dis. 2022;18(12):1345–56.
2. Salminen P, Grönroos S, Helmiö M, et al. Effect of laparoscopic sleeve gastrectomy vs roux-en-Y gastric bypass on weight loss, comorbidities, and reflux at 10 years: SLEEVEPASS trial. JAMA Surg. 2022;157(8):656–66.
3. Seeras K, et al. Sleeve gastrectomy. In: StatPearls [Internet]. Treasure Island: StatPearls Publishing; 2023.
4. Zhao H, et al. Long-term and midterm outcomes of sleeve vs Roux-en-Y gastric bypass: meta-analysis. Obes Surg. 2019;29(4):1251–60.
5. Cummings DE, et al. Gastric bypass and sleeve gastrectomy: mechanisms of action and metabolic effects. Nat Rev Endocrinol. 2022;18(2):131–46.
6. Shimizu H, et al. Endoscopic access after bariatric surgery: implications for procedure selection. Obes Surg. 2021;31(3):1150–8.
7. Courcoulas AP, et al. New indications for metabolic and bariatric surgery. Lancet Diabetes Endocrinol. 2023;11(5):329–40.
8. Genco A, Soricelli E, Casella G, et al. GERD and Barrett's esophagus after sleeve gastrectomy. Surg Obes Relat Dis. 2017;13(4):568–74.
9. Pavone G, et al. New onset GERD after sleeve gastrectomy: systematic review. Ann Med Surg (Lond). 2022;81:104541.
10. Biter LU, et al. Long-term effect of sleeve vs roux-en-Y on GERD: randomized trials. Lancet Reg Health Eur. 2024;3:100102.
11. Home S, et al. Bariatric surgery. Aust J Gen Pract. 2025;54(4):209–16.
12. Swei E, et al. Reflux and Barrett's esophagus after sleeve gastrectomy. Surg Obes Relat Dis. 2023;19(7):497–505.
13. Pratt JSA, Browne A, Browne NT, et al. ASMBS pediatric metabolic and bariatric surgery guidelines, 2018. Surg Obes Relat Dis. 2018;14(7):882–901.
14. Singhal V, et al. Use of sleeve gastrectomy in adolescents and young adults with severe obesity. Curr Obes Rep. 2020;9(3):326–35.
15. Stenberg E, et al. ERAS guidelines for perioperative care in bariatric surgery. World J Surg. 2022;46(7):1761–85.
16. Mingrone G, et al. Bariatric-metabolic surgery vs conventional medical therapy in type 2 diabetes: 10-year outcomes. N Engl J Med. 2021;384(10):895–907.
17. Theel WB, et al. Effect of bariatric surgery on MASLD/MASH: systematic review. Hepatol Commun. 2023;7(4):e1003–15.
18. Lassailly G, et al. Bariatric surgery provides long-term resolution of steatohepatitis and regression of fibrosis. Gastroenterology. 2020;159(4):1290–301.
19. Lee Y, et al. Resolution of fatty liver after bariatric surgery: systematic review and meta-analysis. Clin Gastroenterol Hepatol. 2019;17(6):1040–60.
20. Głuszyńska P, et al. MASLD and bariatric/metabolic surgery: an update. J Clin Med. 2021;10(24):5721.
21. Hanipah ZN, et al. Bariatric surgery in patients with cirrhosis and portal hypertension. Obes Surg. 2018;28(10):3332–41.
22. Mehdorn AS, et al. Bariatric surgery in liver cirrhosis. Front Surg. 2022;9:986297.
23. Temime V, et al. Outcomes of bariatric surgery in compensated cirrhosis with portal hypertension. Int J Surg. 2024;112:106082.
24. Manzano-Núñez R, et al. Bariatric surgery in severe obesity and cirrhosis with portal hypertension: systematic review. Obes Surg. 2023;33(4):1001–12.
25. Amorim-Cruz F, et al. Fundoplication sleeve gastrectomy vs sleeve alone: systematic review and meta-analysis. J Clin Med. 2025;14(21):7723.

26. Shilton H, et al. Bariatric surgery in older adults: outcomes and considerations. Aust J Gen Pract. 2023;52(9):645–52.
27. Fried M, et al. Interdisciplinary European guidelines on metabolic and bariatric surgery. Obes Facts. 2013;6(5):449–68.
28. Francois Z, et al. Psychiatric complications of bariatric surgery. In: StatPearls [Internet]. Treasure Island: StatPearls Publishing; 2024.
29. Kanji S, et al. Pre- and post-surgery substance use disorder in bariatric patients. Obes Med. 2019;15:100113.
30. Moizé V, et al. Bariatric surgery and alcohol and substance abuse disorder. Cir Esp. 2021;99(7):436–44.
31. Martinelli S, et al. New-onset substance use disorders after bariatric surgery: systematic review and meta-analysis. Obes Surg. 2024;34(3):1120–33.
32. Znamirowski P, et al. GERD as a complication of laparoscopic sleeve gastrectomy. J Clin Med. 2023;12(15):4887.

Nutritional Optimization

3

Marta González-Ramos

3.1 Introduction

Obesity is a serious public health problem worldwide. According to the World Health Organization (WHO), in 2022, more than 1 billion people worldwide were obese, equivalent to one in eight people. Of these, 890 million were adults, and 160 million were children and adolescents aged 5–19 [1, 2]. It is considered a chronic disease that can increase the risk of type 2 diabetes and heart disease, affect bone health and reproduction, and increase the risk of certain types of cancer. Obesity also affects other aspects of quality of life, such as sleep and mobility [1, 2].

Bariatric surgery (BS) has become the treatment of choice for many patients with morbid obesity. Among the most common procedures are sleeve gastrectomy (SG), which reduces the stomach's size, and Roux-en-Y gastric bypass, which creates a smaller stomach and bypasses parts of the small intestine [2]. These procedures lead to significant and sustained weight loss, improving or resolving many obesity-related health problems by changing appetite, satiety, and metabolism [2].

The success of this surgery treatment is not solely due to the type of surgery performed, but also to the combination of bariatric surgery with nutritional and dietary monitoring by a multidisciplinary team, both before and after the operation, which significantly improves initial weight loss and also helps to maintain it in the long term [2, 3]. Multidisciplinary care for patients undergoing bariatric surgery has gained importance in recent years. This interdisciplinary team should comprise medical, surgical, psychiatric, and nutritional experts. The core multidisciplinary bariatric team includes a bariatric/obesity specialist, a bariatric psychologist, a bariatric dietitian, a bariatric coordinator, and a bariatric surgeon. Additionally, other

M. González-Ramos (✉)
Health Sciences Department, San Juan de Dios School of Nursing and Physical Therapy, Comillas Pontifical University, Madrid, Spain
e-mail: mgonzalezr@comillas.edu

J. Ruiz-Tovar (ed.), *Multidisciplinary Management of Sleeve Gastrectomy*,
https://doi.org/10.1007/978-3-032-25644-7_3

professionals may provide support in specific cases, such as physiotherapists, cardiologists, pulmonologists, gastroenterologists, and plastic surgeons. The management of patients undergoing BS involves a multifaceted and holistic approach that is critical to the success and sustainability of surgical outcomes [3, 4].

In addition, in recent years, greater importance has been placed on preoperative nutritional optimization, as it has become a key factor in reducing postoperative risks and increasing postoperative recovery [2].

3.1.1 Micronutrient Deficiencies Pre-surgery

Unhealthy body weight has long been viewed as a consequence of excessive caloric intake; however, it has also been linked to an unexpected issue: malnutrition stemming from multiple nutrient deficiencies [2, 5–7]. Patients undergoing BS often present with micronutrient deficiencies even before surgery; approximately 20–30% of candidates exhibit micronutritional deficiencies [5], commonly including deficiencies in vitamin D, folate, vitamin B12, iron, and others [2, 5, 7]. A pre-surgery diet, which is high in energy but lacking in various nutrients, and the use of restrictive diets may contribute to exacerbating these deficiencies. Studies analyzing dietary intake in a sample of SG candidates revealed a non-variety, high-calorie, high-fat, and poor micronutrient content. The intakes for iron (46%), calcium (48%), folic acid (58%), vitamin B12 (14%), and vitamin B1 (34%) were below the dietary reference intake (DRI) recommendations [8]. Easy availability of inexpensive processed foods, increased consumption of calorie-rich but nutrient-poor products, sedentary lifestyles, metabolic alterations that hinder nutrient absorption, prolonged use of certain medications, individual dietary habits, and the inflammation commonly associated with an unhealthy body mass index (BMI) are the main related malnutrition causes in obesity [5]. Obesity itself may contribute to nutritional deficiencies prior to surgery, and surgery may exacerbate these deficiencies [7–9].

3.1.1.1 Vitamin B12

Preoperative vitamin B12 deficiency is a common deficiency in bariatric patients. Some studies identified a prevalence of 13.1% vitamin B12 deficiency before surgery. It is also one of the most common deficiencies following surgery in patients undergoing SG [10]. Current data indicate a 4.69% prevalence of this vitamin deficiency at 6 months and 0.93% at 12 months post-surgery. In their 2025 review, Agarwal and Sharma establish prevalence data for vitamin B12 deficiency in the range of 5–29% [5]. This highlights the importance of identifying and addressing these deficiencies both before and after surgery, as well as incorporating a dietary plan that complements them [7].

3.1.1.2 Vitamin D, Calcium, and Parathyroid Hormone

Although a study conducted in SG found that candidates' calcium levels were within normal values. The prevalence of preoperative hypovitaminosis D was considerably high [9]. Several studies have reported a high prevalence of vitamin D deficiency preoperatively, with values ranging from 74.24% to 99.4% in this patient group [4–7]. Recent reviews establish prevalence values for 25-OH-vitamin D deficiency before undergoing weight loss surgery at 40–68% and report that vitamin D deficiency affects approximately 85% [5].

Additionally, a disturbed bone metabolism with secondary hyperparathyroidism was found in more than one-fifth of the patients preoperatively, with elevated parathyroid hormone (PTH) levels in 40.9% of cases [7, 10].

Various factors may cause the high prevalence of hypovitaminosis D before surgery in obese individuals. On the one hand, the body storing lipid-soluble vitamins in adipose tissue, reduced sunlight exposure due to reduced physical activity, and the low intake of dairy products could contribute [7]. Additionally, impaired liver function due to fatty liver disease could decrease the synthesis of vitamin D by the liver, which is common among obese individuals. Finally, it can also be attributed to geographical, seasonal, and fortification policy differences [3]. Adequate monitoring and supplementation of this vitamin is highly recommended.

3.1.1.3 Iron, Anemia, and Folate

Low serum iron levels were observed in 47% of the patients before surgery, according to Ben-Porat et al. Additionally, before surgery, 15% of patients had anemia. Folate deficiencies were reported in 32% of cases [10]. In a study conducted by Vieira de Sousa et al., preoperative iron deficiency was observed in 12.69% of patients undergoing sleeve gastrectomy. Van Rutte et al. reported the following data: before surgery, 5% of patients were anemic, 7% had low serum ferritin levels, and 24% had low folic acid levels. Overall, anemia was observed in 6% of patients, while low ferritin was detected in 8% [9]. Recent reviews report that iron deficiency is observed in 14–43% of patients before BS. Iron deficiency in individuals with an abnormal BMI arises from multiple factors, including chronic inflammation caused by excess adipose tissue, dilution due to increased plasma volume, suboptimal dietary intake, limited access to iron-rich foods, and adherence to vegetarian diets. In overweight individuals, low iron levels may result from a combination of decreased absorption and increased sequestration [5].

Low levels of serum folate were already present in a quarter of the patients preoperatively. Recent reports indicate a prevalence of 24%. This deficiency is mainly associated with reduced intake of folate-rich foods, such as lettuce and vegetables [5, 9].

3.1.1.4 Vitamin B1

Vitamin B1 deficiency is prevalent, affecting between 15.5% and 29% of the population. Preoperative vitamin B1 (thiamine) deficiency is common among patients undergoing BS. Because of the heightened risk of thiamine deficiency after surgery—often due to recurrent vomiting and the potential for serious neurological complications—addressing this deficiency before surgery is essential [5].

3.1.1.5 Vitamin A, E, and K

Vitamin A deficiency is reported in 2–17% of cases. Screening for Vitamin E and K deficiencies is often overlooked in the bariatric population due to insufficient preoperative data [5].

3.1.1.6 Magnesium, Selenium, Zinc

Van Rutte et al. found a magnesium deficiency in 2% of the patients preoperatively, a deficiency also reported in more recent studies. The unvaried high-calorie diet of the obese patients often does not contain adequate amounts of magnesium. Also, hypomagnesemia has been linked to insulin resistance and metabolic syndrome. Several studies have shown that serum selenium levels are lower in populations with abnormal weight, particularly in patients who have undergone malabsorptive procedures. Studies indicate that zinc deficiency affects 28% of patients preoperatively [5, 7, 9].

3.1.2 Macronutrient Pre-surgery

Although obesity is often associated with overnutrition, bariatric surgery candidates frequently have significant macronutrient deficiencies, especially in protein, due to poor dietary quality, sedentary lifestyle, altered metabolism, and chronic inflammation. Protein is crucial for tissue repair, immune function, and the preservation of lean body mass, and deficiencies can impair wound healing, increase the risk of infection, and delay recovery. Prevalence of protein deficiency varies, with up to 27% of patients affected. Bariatric procedures further complicate protein intake due to reduced stomach capacity, altered gastrointestinal function, and postoperative intolerance to protein-rich foods. Preoperative nutritional counseling, tailored dietary strategies, and the use of protein supplements are essential to ensure adequate intake, optimize surgical outcomes, and support long-term recovery [2].

3.1.3 Preoperative Nutritional Evaluation

3.1.3.1 Screening Tools

Preoperative nutritional evaluation is crucial for patients undergoing weight-loss surgery, as described before, many of them present with multiple vitamin and mineral deficiencies. It is estimated that two-thirds of bariatric patients are malnourished before surgery. Detecting malnutrition and micronutrient deficiencies is crucial, as they have a significant impact on both short-term and long-term outcomes. Better nutritional status before surgery is associated with a lower risk of surgical wound infections, shorter hospital stays, lower mortality rates, and improved postoperative recovery [2].

There are multiple nutritional screening tools available; however, none have been validated specifically in patients undergoing SG. Many tools used to detect malnutrition in other clinical settings have also not yet been validated for this population.

Several instruments that may be of interest for assessing nutritional status in the context of bariatric surgery include the Nutritional Risk Index (NRI), a tool used to measure nutritional risk in hospitalized patients and applied in gastrointestinal surgery; the Geriatric Nutritional Risk Index (GNRI), which is used to assess the risk of malnutrition and mortality in elderly patients undergoing gastrectomy; and the Malnutrition Screening Tool (MST). The Malnutrition Universal Screening Tool (MUST) and Nutritional Risk Screening 2002 (NRS 2002) may be more effective for identifying nutritional problems in older adults. Finally, the Subjective Global Assessment (SGA) is recognized as a practical and feasible method for evaluating nutritional status in surgical patients [2, 11].

3.1.3.2 Biochemical Screening Pre-surgery

Several clinical practice guidelines recommend monitoring the nutritional status of patients undergoing SG both before and after the procedure. In the review conducted by Steenackers et al., an overview is provided of clinical practice guidelines from various scientific societies regarding nutritional screening in SG candidates. Nine clinical guidelines co-authored by 26 learned societies were analyzed [12].

In summary, this review informed that, before SG, most of them recommended screening for iron, vitamin B12, folate, and vitamin D levels. Five guidelines recommend assessing calcium status preoperatively, while three guidelines advise screening for vitamin A. Four guidelines also recommend performing a complete blood count, including hemoglobin, hematocrit, and mean corpuscular volume (MCV), before surgery. Finally, preoperative screening for vitamin B1, vitamin K, and magnesium was less commonly recommended [12].

Other reviews also included albumin and prealbumin as biomarkers. Albumin and prealbumin are key indicators used to assess protein stores. Because prealbumin has a shorter half-life, it is beneficial for identifying rapid or recent changes, while albumin is more indicative of long-term nutritional status. Together, these markers are crucial for evaluating protein–energy malnutrition. C-reactive protein (CRP) is also highly relevant, as it reflects inflammatory activity that can interfere with the interpretation of nutritional biomarkers such as albumin and prealbumin. When CRP levels are elevated, they signal the presence of inflammation that may mask underlying nutritional inadequacies [11].

3.1.4 Nutritional Interventions

3.1.4.1 Preoperative Dietary Plans

The preoperative period of bariatric surgery is a crucial stage for preparing patients to handle the metabolic and anatomical requirements of the procedure. Calorie-restricted diets are the most commonly used approach for optimizing the nutritional status of patients undergoing bariatric surgery. These dietary interventions not only support weight reduction but also help optimize metabolic conditions, contributing to greater surgical safety and improved long-term results [2, 13, 14].

The most commonly prescribed preoperative diet for bariatric patients before surgery is the low-calorie diet (LCD), the very low-calorie diet (VLCD), or the very low-calorie ketogenic diet (VLCKD), with variations in consistency (liquid or solid) and duration [2, 13, 14].

A low-energy diet (LCD) usually contains 800–1200 kcal/day for 2–4 weeks, and a very low energy diet (VLCD) provides 450–<800 kcal/day for 2–4 weeks. These eating plans are characterized by low carbohydrate intake (50-100 g/day, 35–40% of total calories), high protein content (1.2–1.5 g/kg/ideal body weight a day or 35–40% of total calories), and minimal fat (<30% of total calories, prioritizing healthy fats). Patients preparing for bariatric surgery are often advised to use commercially available high-protein shakes, which supply between 650 and 900 kcal per day during this phase. Evidence suggests that following a low-calorie, low-carbohydrate diet can reduce liver volume by up to 19% and decrease visceral fat by approximately 17% [13, 15, 16].

Frias-Toral et al. indicated in their review that very low-calorie diets (VLCDs) effectively reduce body weight and liver size before surgery. Although they can make the procedure technically easier for surgeons, they do not substantially lower intraoperative or postoperative complications. Some evidence indicates that following a 4-week VLCD may shorten hospital stays and enhance weight loss at 3 months and 1 year after surgery compared with no preoperative VLCD. In patients with severe obesity (BMI > 50 kg/m^2), reductions in liver volume and visceral fat can simplify the operation and lessen surgical risk [13].

On the other hand, the systematic review by Nilsen et al. concluded that LCD tends to produce total body weight loss comparable to that of VLCD. A 2–4 week LCD may also offer benefits by reducing liver volume and improving insulin sensitivity before surgery. Moreover, steering clear of overly restrictive calorie intakes and excessively long regimens may help preserve lean mass and reduce treatment dropout. For these reasons, clinicians and manufacturers should reconsider whether VLCDs are necessary or if LCDs provide a sufficient alternative [15].

As a conclusion, low-calorie diets effectively reduce liver size and visceral fat, helping to prepare patients for BS. While they may enhance surgical feasibility, evidence regarding their direct impact on operative safety remains mixed [2, 13, 15–19].

Recently, low-calorie ketogenic diets (LCKD) and very low-calorie ketogenic diets (VLCKD) have been proposed as effective interventions for reducing liver size and improving outcomes in BS [2, 14, 16]. Both rely on nutritional ketosis—triggered by severe carbohydrate restriction and reduced caloric intake—to promote rapid fat loss while preserving lean mass. Recent evidence suggests that VLCKD can lead to substantial weight reduction, reduction in volume and fat liver, reduction in visceral adipose tissue, and improved glycemic control and lipid profile in individuals with obesity and type 2 diabetes. This protocol typically provides 700–800 kcal per day, limits carbohydrates to 30–50 g/day, and includes moderate amounts of fats (20–40 g/day) and protein (about 1.2–1.5 g per kg of ideal body weight) [14].

In addition, patients who follow a 4-week preoperative ketogenic regimen with added micronutrient supplementation can experience notable decreases in body weight, reductions in the volume of the left hepatic lobe, and improvements in micronutrient status [13]. Ketosis reduces appetite, improves adherence, and helps preserve lean mass. Overall, current evidence supports VLCKD as an effective, safe, and rapid strategy to optimize patients before bariatric surgery [14].

Due to the limited current evidence, it is not possible to clearly assess how LCD, VLCD, or VLCKD influence the duration of surgery or length of hospitalization. More interventional research is needed to identify the most effective preoperative diet—one that is well-tolerated and accepted by patients, supports adherence, and leads to better surgical outcomes [20].

In conclusion, multiple systematic reviews and randomized trials consistently demonstrate that preparing for BS with short-term (2–4 weeks) very low-calorie diets—especially ketogenic variants—is the most supported approach for maximizing preoperative weight loss, liver shrinkage, and metabolic improvement, with potential benefits for surgical safety and recovery. Both VLCDs and VLCKDs should be implemented under medical supervision to ensure safety and nutritional adequacy [2, 11–13, 15–19, 21].

3.1.4.2 Micronutrient Supplementation

As previously noted, micronutrient deficiencies are common among patients scheduled for BS. Micronutrient supplementation is a crucial aspect of preoperative preparation. Correcting these deficiencies before the procedure is essential to minimize surgical risks and support optimal recovery [2, 22, 23].

Recent trials and systematic reviews have shown that specialized multivitamin supplementation before surgery significantly improves serum levels of key nutrients (iron, folic acid, vitamin D, zinc) and reduces the prevalence of deficiencies. Chronic oral supplementation is effective for vitamin D and folate, while iron status may require intravenous or higher-dose oral strategies for optimal correction. However, some nutrients (e.g., magnesium, phosphate) may not respond to treatment and require individualized management [11, 24, 25].

Recent reviews recommend regular monitoring of biochemical markers and the use of individualized supplementation strategies tailored to each patient's unique needs to ensure adequate repletion of these critical nutrients. Starting supplementation 8–10 weeks before surgery allows enough time to correct nutrient deficiencies and better prepare the body for the physiological demands of the procedure [11].

A summary published by Reytor-González et al. of the latest recommendations from preoperative micronutrient supplementation for bariatric surgery candidates is:

Vitamin D deficiency significantly impairs both bone health and immune function; low levels are associated with an increased susceptibility to infections and autoimmune diseases. Repletion is effectively achieved with high-dose cholecalciferol (4000–6000 IU/day), followed by a postoperative maintenance dose of 2000 IU/

day, often combined with calcium citrate (1200–1500 mg/day) to maintain adequate calcium levels and prevent secondary hyperparathyroidism [11].

Iron deficiency—frequently associated with anemia—requires 100–200 mg of elemental iron daily, accompanied by vitamin C (250–500 mg/day) to enhance absorption. Intravenous iron is recommended for patients who are unable to tolerate oral formulations [11].

Vitamin B12 deficiency, commonly caused by impaired absorption, is typically treated with intramuscular injections of 1000 μg every 2 weeks or with high-dose oral alternatives. Folate supplementation (2 mg/day) is also essential, particularly in patients presenting with anemia [11].

Thiamine (vitamin B1) supplementation at 100 mg/day is critical for individuals with poor intake or vomiting. Supplementation of fat-soluble vitamins (A, E, and K) should be tailored to specific deficiencies and closely monitored, especially in patients undergoing hypocaloric or hypocaloric procedures [11].

3.1.4.3 New Approach: Immunonutrition Pre-surgery

Immunonutrition (IMN) refers to the use of specific nutrients, such as arginine, omega-3 fatty acids, glutamine, nucleotides, and antioxidants, to modulate the immune response and improve outcomes in surgical patients. It is designed to reduce complications, such as infections, and promote faster recovery after surgery [26–30].

It is well established that surgery induces stress and inflammation, which can suppress the immune system and increase the risk of infection. Immunonutrition aims to counteract these effects by modulating immune and inflammatory responses, improving wound healing, and reducing susceptibility to infections. These nutrients could help enhance immune cell function, reduce inflammation, and support tissue repair [26–30].

Major nutrition societies recommend immunonutrition for high-risk or malnourished patients undergoing major surgery, especially in cancer and gastrointestinal procedures. While immunonutrition is well-studied in gastric cancer and gastrectomy, direct research specifically on immunonutrition in the context of SG is limited [26–29, 31–33].

Studies comparing SG and gastric bypass show that both procedures induce immunometabolic changes, including shifts in T and B lymphocyte populations and changes in immune gene expression, suggesting a reactivation of the immune response after surgery. However, these studies do not directly test immunonutrition interventions in SG patients [34, 35].

Other studies evaluated the effects of nutritional supplements, such as omega-3 polyunsaturated fatty acids (PUFA), in people with fatty liver disease. The results showed that omega-3 supplementation reduced liver fat and improved serum markers related to liver damage [36].

Although there are only a few studies evaluating the effectiveness of preoperative immunonutrition in bariatric surgery, some of them show quite promising results [37–40].

Bakker et al. conducted a clinical trial comparing two preoperative interventions before bariatric surgery: a very low-calorie diet (800 kcal/day) for 2 weeks and a standard diet (2000 kcal/day) for 4 weeks, supplemented with 2 g of omega-3 per day. Both approaches reduced total liver volume, left liver lobe volume, and visceral fat. The low-calorie diet achieved greater reductions in liver volumes but also caused significant loss of muscle mass and had poorer tolerance due to side effects. The authors concluded that omega-3 supplementation may represent a safer and more comfortable option for patients, although further studies are needed [40].

Another study was conducted on morbidly obese patients who were administered oral omega-3 PUFAs (1500 mg daily) for 4 weeks before undergoing the laparoscopic Roux-en-Y gastric bypass (LRYGBP) without any dietary restriction. The results indicated that the mean volume of the left hepatic lobe decreased by 20% after the treatment [38].

A prospective, randomized clinical trial conducted by Ruiz-Tovar et al. (2019) in patients undergoing laparoscopic Roux-en-Y gastric bypass evaluated the effect of pre-surgery omega-3 formula. Participants were assigned to one of two groups: a control group that received a balanced, high-protein preoperative formula, and an experimental group that received the same formula enriched with omega-3 fatty acids. Both groups followed a 900-kcal/day dietary regimen starting 10 days before surgery. As a main result, they indicated that the use of a nutritional supplement enriched with omega-3 was associated with greater preoperative weight loss, reduced postoperative pain, and decreased postoperative levels of C-reactive protein [41].

Another prospective randomized clinical trial, conducted by Ruiz-Tovar, evaluated patients undergoing laparoscopic SG who were assigned to three preoperative diets 2 weeks before surgery: a regular 900 kcal/day diet, a 900 kcal high-protein formula, and a 900 kcal IMN formula. IMN formula included glutamine, arginine, omega-3 fatty acids, and nucleic acids. Among the 60 patients included, the immunonutrition group achieved the most significant preoperative weight loss, the lowest postoperative pain, and significantly lower levels of C-reactive protein and liver enzymes compared to the other two groups, despite all diets having a similar caloric intake [42].

They discuss how IMN formulas, which contain glutamine, arginine, omega-3 fatty acids (EPA and DHA), and nucleotides, exert anti-inflammatory and immunomodulatory effects. Glutamine supports cell division and antioxidant defense, while arginine improves nitrogen balance, T-cell function, wound healing, and nitric oxide production. Additionally, omega-3 fatty acids reduce proinflammatory mediators. Nucleotides are crucial for a robust immune response. In the study, patients receiving IMN showed significantly lower postoperative CRP and liver enzyme (AST and ALT) levels compared to those on high-protein or regular diets, reflecting reduced inflammation and liver stress. These effects may relate to decreased postoperative pain and potential mitigation of liver injury, including non-alcoholic fatty liver disease. However, further studies are needed to confirm these mechanisms and clinical benefits [42].

3.2 Conclusion

In summary, patients undergoing SG frequently present with both macro- and micronutrient deficiencies, despite consuming excessive calories. Common deficiencies include protein, vitamins (B1, B12, D, A, E, K, folate), and minerals such as iron, magnesium, selenium, and zinc. These deficits are influenced by poor dietary quality, sedentary lifestyle, chronic inflammation, and altered metabolism associated with obesity. Preoperative nutritional assessment and individualized interventions, including low- or very-low-calorie diets, micronutrient supplementation, and emerging strategies such as immunonutrition, are crucial for correcting deficiencies, optimizing surgical outcomes, and supporting recovery. Evidence suggests that targeted preoperative nutrition can enhance weight loss, reduce liver volume, preserve lean body mass, mitigate inflammatory responses, and potentially decrease postoperative complications. Overall, a structured, multidisciplinary nutritional approach is a crucial component of bariatric surgery preparation, laying the groundwork for both short-term and long-term success.

References

1. Obesity and overweight [Internet]. [cited 2025 Nov 22]. Available from: https://www.who.int/news-room/fact-sheets/detail/obesity-and-overweight
2. Simancas-Racines D, Frias-Toral E, Campuzano-Donoso M, Ramos-Sarmiento D, Zambrano-Villacres R, Reytor-González C, et al. Preoperative nutrition in bariatric surgery: a narrative review on enhancing surgical success and patient outcomes. Nutrients. 2025;17(3):566.
3. Al-Sabah S, Aminian A, Angrisani L, Al Haddad E, Kow L, eds. Laparoscopic sleeve gastrectomy [internet]. Cham: Springer; 2021. [cited 2025 Nov 21]. Available from: https://link.springer.com/10.1007/978-3-030-57373-7
4. Budny A, Janczy A, Mika A. New approaches to the treatment of severe obesity—Prehabilitation as the key to success. Curr Nutr Rep. 2025;14(1):64.
5. Agarwal N, Sharma K. Optimizing micro and macro nutrients. Endocrinol Metab Clin N Am. 2025;54(1):135–47.
6. Deledda A, Pintus S, Loviselli A, Fosci M, Fantola G, Velluzzi F. Nutritional management in bariatric surgery patients. Int J Environ Res Public Health. 2021;18(22):12049.
7. Vieira De Sousa JP, Santos-Sousa H, Vieira S, Nunes R, Nogueiro J, Pereira A, et al. Assessing nutritional deficiencies in bariatric surgery patients: a comparative study of roux-en-Y gastric bypass versus sleeve gastrectomy. J Pers Med. 2024;14(6):650.
8. Dagan SS, Zelber-Sagi S, Webb M, Keidar A, Raziel A, Sakran N, et al. Nutritional status prior to laparoscopic sleeve gastrectomy surgery. Obes Surg. 2016;26(9):2119–26.
9. Van Rutte PWJ, Aarts EO, Smulders JF, Nienhuijs SW. Nutrient deficiencies before and after sleeve gastrectomy. Obes Surg. 2014;24(10):1639–46.
10. Ben-Porat T, Elazary R, Yuval JB, Wieder A, Khalaileh A, Weiss R. Nutritional deficiencies after sleeve gastrectomy: can they be predicted preoperatively? Surg Obes Relat Dis Off J Am Soc Bariatr Surg. 2015;11(5):1029–36.
11. Reytor-González C, Frias-Toral E, Nuñez-Vásquez C, Parise-Vasco JM, Zambrano-Villacres R, Simancas-Racines D, et al. Preventing and managing pre- and postoperative micronutrient deficiencies: a vital component of long-term success in bariatric surgery. Nutrients. 2025;17(5):741.

12. Steenackers N, De Boer L, Dekempeneer C, Deleus E, Lannoo M, Mertens A, et al. Current clinical practice guidelines for nutritional screening before and after sleeve gastrectomy and roux-En-Y gastric bypass: a scoping review. Curr Obes Rep. 2025;14(1):16.
13. Frias-Toral E, Chapela S, Gonzalez V, Martinuzzi A, Locatelli J, Llobera N, et al. Optimizing nutritional management before and after bariatric surgery: a comprehensive guide for sustained weight loss and metabolic health. Nutrients. 2025;17(4):688.
14. Barrea L, Verde L, Schiavo L, Sarno G, Camajani E, Iannelli A, et al. Very low-calorie ketogenic diet (VLCKD) as pre-operative first-line dietary therapy in patients with obesity who are candidates for bariatric surgery. Nutrients. 2023;15(8):1907.
15. Nilsen I, Andersson A, Laurenius A, Österberg J. Low-energy diets before metabolic bariatric surgery: a systematic review of the effect on total body weight, liver volume, glycemia and side effects. Obes Rev. 2025;26(4):e13876.
16. Bettini S, Belligoli A, Fabris R, Busetto L. Diet approach before and after bariatric surgery. Rev Endocr Metab Disord. 2020;21(3):297–306.
17. Holderbaum M, Casagrande DS, Sussenbach S, Buss C. Effects of very low calorie diets on liver size and weight loss in the preoperative period of bariatric surgery: a systematic review. Surg Obes Relat Dis. 2018;14(2):237–44.
18. Xu Y, Yang S, Luo R, Wu L, Lin Y, Xi Y, et al. Optimizing bariatric surgery outcomes: the dual benefits of preoperative very-low-calorie diets. Obes Surg. 2025;35(8):3057–63.
19. Yolsuriyanwong K, Thanavachirasin K, Sasso K, Zuro L, Bartfield J, Marcotte E, et al. Effectiveness, compliance, and acceptability of preoperative weight loss with a liquid very low-calorie diet before bariatric surgery in real practice. Obes Surg. 2019;29(1):54–60.
20. Khalooeifard R, Rahmani J, Ghoreishy SM, Tavakoli A, Najjari K, Talebpour M. Evaluate the effects of different types of preoperative restricted calorie diets on weight, body mass index, operation time and hospital stay in patients undergoing bariatric surgery: a systematic review and meta analysis study. Obes Surg. 2024;34(1):236–49.
21. Lange UG, Moulla Y, Schütz T, Blüher M, Peter V, Shang E, et al. Effectiveness and tolerability of a two-week hypocaloric protein-rich diet prior to obesity surgery with two different diet interventions: a prospective randomized trial. Obes Surg. 2022;32(9):2903–13.
22. Argyrakopoulou G, Konstantinidou SK, Dalamaga M, Kokkinos A. Nutritional deficiencies before and after bariatric surgery: prevention and treatment. Curr Nutr Rep. 2022;11(2):95–101.
23. Gasmi A, Bjørklund G, Mujawdiya PK, Semenova Y, Dosa A, Piscopo S, et al. Dietary supplements and bariatric surgery. Crit Rev Food Sci Nutr. 2023;63(25):7477–88.
24. Sander J, Torensma B, Siepe J, Schorp T, Schulte T, Schmeer C, et al. Assessment of preoperative multivitamin use on the impact on micronutrient deficiencies in patients with obesity prior to metabolic bariatric surgery. Obes Surg. 2025;35(5):1818–26.
25. Tang X, Reidlinger DP, Crichton M, Craggs-Dino L, Fayet-Moore F, Marshall S. Preoperative micronutrient repletion strategies in metabolic and bariatric surgery: a systematic review. J Acad Nutr Diet. 2025;125(6):761–784.e6.
26. Calder PC. Immunonutrition in surgical and critically ill patients. Br J Nutr. 2007;98(S1):S133–9.
27. Goyal A, Macias CA, Corzo MP, Vargas VPS, Mendoza M, Guarecuco Castillo JE, et al. Perioperative immunonutrition in gastrointestinal oncology: a comprehensive umbrella review and meta-analysis on behalf of TROGSS—the robotic global surgical society. Nutrients. 2025;17(14):2304.
28. García-Malpartida K, Aragón-Valera C, Botella-Romero F, Ocón-Bretón MJ, López-Gómez JJ. Effects of Immunonutrition on cancer patients undergoing surgery: a scoping review. Nutrients. 2023;15(7):1776.
29. Ham HJ, Kim J. Targeted nutritional strategies in postoperative care. Anesth Pain Med. 2025;20(1):34–45.
30. Shanmugasundaram Prema S, Ganapathy D, Shanmugamprema D. Prehabilitation strategies: enhancing surgical resilience with a focus on nutritional optimization and multimodal interventions. Adv Nutr. 2025;16(4):100392.

31. Buzquurz F, Bojesen RD, Grube C, Madsen MT, Gögenur I. Impact of oral preoperative and perioperative immunonutrition on postoperative infection and mortality in patients undergoing cancer surgery: systematic review and meta-analysis with trial sequential analysis. BJS Open. 2020;4(5):764–75.
32. Marik PE, Zaloga GP. Immunonutrition in high-risk surgical patients: a systematic review and analysis of the literature. J Parenter Enter Nutr. 2010;34(4):378–86.
33. D'Ignazio A, Kabata P, Ambrosio MR, Polom K, Marano L, Spagnoli L, et al. Preoperative oral immunonutrition in gastrointestinal surgical patients: how the tumour microenvironment can be modified. Clin Nutr ESPEN. 2020;38:153–9.
34. Rivera-Carranza T, Azaola-Espinosa A, Bojalil-Parra R, Zúñiga-León E, León-Téllez-Girón A, Rojano-Rodríguez ME, et al. Immunometabolic changes following gastric bypass and sleeve gastrectomy: a comparative study. Obes Surg. 2025;35(2):481–95.
35. Lazaro A, Tiago I, Mendes J, Ribeiro J, Bernardes A, Oliveira F, et al. Sleeve gastrectomy and gastric bypass impact in patient's metabolic, gut microbiome, and Immuno-inflammatory profiles—a comparative study. Obes Surg. 2025;35(3):733–45.
36. Jump DB, Lytle KA, Depner CM, Tripathy S. Omega-3 polyunsaturated fatty acids as a treatment strategy for nonalcoholic fatty liver disease. Pharmacol Ther. 2018;181:108–25.
37. Tabesh MR, Eghtesadi M, Abolhasani M, Maleklou F, Ejtehadi F, Alizadeh Z. Nutrition, physical activity, and prescription of supplements in pre- and post-bariatric surgery patients: an updated comprehensive practical guideline. Obes Surg. 2023;33(8):2557–72.
38. Iannelli A, Martini F, Schneck AS, Ghavami B, Baudin G, Anty R, et al. Preoperative 4-week supplementation with omega-3 polyunsaturated fatty acids reduces liver volume and facilitates bariatric surgery in morbidly obese patients. Obes Surg. 2013;23(11):1761–5.
39. Lewis MC, Phillips ML, Slavotinek JP, Kow L, Thompson CH, Toouli J. Change in liver size and fat content after treatment with Optifast very low calorie diet. Obes Surg. 2006;16(6):697–701.
40. Bakker N, van den Helder RS, Geenen RWF, Hunfeld MA, Cense HA, Demirkiran A, et al. Four weeks of preoperative Omega-3 fatty acids reduce liver volume: a randomised controlled trial. Obes Surg. 2019;29(7):2037–44.
41. Ruiz-Tovar J, Blanca M, Garcia A, Gonzalez J, Gutierrez S, Paniagua A, et al. Preoperative administration of Omega-3 fatty acids on postoperative pain and acute-phase reactants in patients undergoing roux-en-Y gastric bypass: a randomized clinical trial. Clin Nutr. 2019;38(4):1588–93.
42. OBELCHE Group, Ruiz-Tovar J, Zubiaga L, Diez M, Murcia A, Boix E, et al. Preoperative regular diet of 900 kcal/day vs balanced energy high-protein formula vs Immunonutrition formula: effect on preoperative weight loss and postoperative pain, complications and analytical acute phase reactants after laparoscopic sleeve gastrectomy. Obes Surg. 2016;26(6):1221–7.

Physical Prehabilitation

4

Carlos Cabrera-Vallejo

4.1 Introduction to Physical Prehabilitation in Bariatric Surgery

We define prehabilitation as a proactive and transformative strategy aimed at optimizing the patient's basal condition before surgical intervention [1, 2]. We conceive this process as a preventive and personalized intervention that integrates medical optimization, promotion of physical activity, and robust nutritional and psychological support [3]. Our main objective resides in amplifying the patient's physiological reserve and functional capacity to withstand the impact of surgical stress [1, 4–7], leveraging the preoperative phase as a critical window of opportunity to instigate positive and lasting lifestyle changes [1, 4, 8].

While we recognize that bariatric surgery, such as sleeve gastrectomy, constitutes the most effective long-term treatment for severe obesity [9, 10], we must address the fact that this population faces an elevated risk of complications and significant potential for functional deterioration [11, 12]. We base the clinical necessity of physical prehabilitation on three pathophysiological pillars. In the first instance, we observe that candidates often present with low physical fitness and reduced aerobic capacity [10], variables that directly correlate with adverse operative outcomes [13]. Secondly, we seek to actively counteract muscle atrophy and enhance preoperative strength [14, 15]; this is vital since the inevitable loss of lean body mass after the operation—which ranges between 17.5% and 31.3% of the weight loss—precipitates sarcopenia and functional deterioration if not mitigated through physical activity [16, 17]. Finally, we use exercise to expand the

C. Cabrera-Vallejo (✉)
San Juan de Dios University School of Nursing and Physiotherapy, Pontificia Comillas University, Madrid, Spain
e-mail: ccabrera@comillas.edu

J. Ruiz-Tovar (ed.), *Multidisciplinary Management of Sleeve Gastrectomy*,
https://doi.org/10.1007/978-3-032-25644-7_4

physiological and metabolic reserve, thereby attenuating the catabolic response and insulin resistance exacerbated by surgical stress [4, 7].

We understand prehabilitation as a concept that is complementary and, frequently, integral within Enhanced Recovery After Surgery (ERAS) protocols [1, 6, 18, 19]. While the multimodal ERAS system standardizes perioperative care to minimize the stress response [7, 20, 21], prehabilitation intervenes upstream to elevate the threshold of physiological reserve [5, 6]. We maintain that the synergistic integration of both approaches is the key to promoting surgical resilience [6], a stance validated by the ERAS Society formally including physical preparation in its guidelines for bariatric surgery [9, 22, 23].

4.2 Preoperative Assessment of Physical and Functional Condition

We consider the preoperative assessment not merely an administrative procedure, but the cornerstone for establishing a physiological baseline and, crucially, for isolating modifiable deficits that allow for risk stratification of postoperative complications [4, 6, 7]. We insist that this analysis must be rigorously objective and exhaustive [7], rejecting the reliability of purely subjective clinical judgment for complex decision-making [7, 8, 24].

For initial stratification, we employ validated risk and frailty classification tools—potent predictors of morbidity and mortality [24, 25]—such as the ASA-PS Classification [7, 18, 26] and phenotypic scales like Fried's or the FRAIL questionnaire [5, 25, 27]. Regarding aerobic fitness, we position the Cardiopulmonary Exercise Test (CPET) as the undeniable gold standard [4, 7, 18, 24, 28]. We focus on precise metrics such as maximal oxygen consumption (VO2max) and the Anaerobic Threshold (AT) [4, 6, 24]; we observe that VO2max values <15 mL/kg/min or an AT <11 mL/kg/min signal an unacceptably high surgical risk [4, 13, 24]. Given logistical limitations for CPET, we resort to validated submaximal alternatives such as the 6-Minute Walk Test (6MWT), evaluating its correlation with the demands of daily life [6, 9, 29]; we define a distance (6MWD) of less than 400 meters as the critical threshold for low functional capacity [4, 13]. Additionally, we use the Duke Activity Status Index (DASI) Questionnaire to estimate Metabolic Equivalents (METs), interpreting a score < 34 as a clear indicator of physical deterioration [4, 18, 24].

Given the hidden prevalence of sarcopenia in this population, the evaluation of strength and mobility is critical [2, 17]. We measure Handgrip Strength (HGS) using dynamometry—an independent predictor of complications [7, 17, 29, 30]—and triangulate it with lower extremity functional tests, such as the Sit-to-Stand Test [29, 30], and dynamic balance via the Timed Up and Go (TUG) [30–32]. Finally, we complete the physiological profile by evaluating respiratory function using Maximal Inspiratory Pressure (MIP) and spirometry (FVC, FEV1) [16, 33], and we monitor habitual activity using subjective tools (IPAQ, GPAQ) [9, 17, 30] or objective tools (accelerometry) [3, 29]. This integration of data is what allows us to abandon generic recommendations and precisely personalize exercise prescription [1, 4].

4.3 Components of Aerobic and Resistance Training

We structure the intervention regimen based on the physiological synergy derived from combining aerobic training (ET) with resistance training (RT) [4]. We position Aerobic Training (ET) as the cornerstone of prehabilitation [4, 31], with the explicit goal of expanding cardiorespiratory reserve [1, 7, 34]. We prioritize low-osteoarticular impact modalities—fast walking, cycling, or swimming— [1, 7], and insist that the dosage prescription (FITT) must be rigorously personalized [6, 26]. Our standard guideline advocates for a frequency of 3–5 sessions per week [1, 7, 28], with duration windows of 30–50 min [7, 31]. We modulate the intensity toward a moderate range, objectively defined as 50%–80% of the maximum heart rate [6, 7] or subjectively between 4 and 6 on the Borg scale [29, 35]; we recognize, however, the clinical utility of cumulative micro-sessions of at least 10 min [35].

In parallel, we consider Resistance Training (RT) imperative for enhancing contractile strength and shielding the patient against sarcopenia [1, 15, 17]. The protocol must recruit the main muscle groups [7, 28] through gravitational or body weight loads (squats, push-ups) [1, 29] and light external resistances such as elastic bands [1, 36]. We prescribe a frequency of 2–3 sessions per week [7, 15, 28], structured in blocks of 2–3 sets with a hypertrophy-resistance range of 8–15 repetitions [1, 7, 15, 31], calibrating the intensity between 60% and 80% of one repetition maximum (1RM) [15, 37].

We maintain that the effectiveness of the intervention depends on progressive overload, which demands gradual adjustments to intensity and volume [7, 29, 35], in addition to the incorporation of flexibility and balance exercises [6, 28, 35]. In scenarios of temporal restriction, we implement High-Intensity Interval Training (HIIT) as an efficient strategy for elevating aerobic capacity [7, 38], alternating 2-min bursts of high intensity (e.g., 70% of peak work rate) with 3 min of active recovery [26].

4.4 Preoperative Respiratory Physiotherapy

We identify preoperative respiratory physiotherapy as a critical component in bariatric management, given this population's high susceptibility to postoperative pulmonary complications (PPCs). The ventilatory mechanics of these patients are often severely compromised by anatomical restrictions that reduce both lung capacity and respiratory muscle strength [1, 16, 18, 33]. Therefore, our objective transcends mere functional improvement; we seek to aggressively optimize pulmonary function and equip the patient with technical skills for secretion management, a proven strategy for reducing the incidence of PPCs [1, 9, 39].

We position Inspiratory Muscle Training (IMT) as the central intervention of this approach. This resistive loading regimen specifically targets the diaphragm [1, 18], utilizing calibrated devices to generate resistance [9]. Our clinical guideline suggests executing daily or twice-daily sessions [1, 9, 40] with a duration of 10–15 min [1, 32], maintained during a preoperative window of 2–4 weeks [1, 24]. Typically, we set the initial intensity at 30% of Maximal Inspiratory Pressure (MIP) [9, 24]. Evidence strongly supports this strategy: according to Barbalho-Moulim et al. (2011) and Lloréns et al. (2015), preoperative IMT not only increases contractile strength but also significantly improves postoperative oxygenation in the obese cohort [1].

Complementarily, we integrate Incentive Spirometry (IS) to facilitate sustained maximal inspiration (SMI), emphasizing an air retention of 4–8 s [9]. We value the visual biofeedback provided by these devices for reaching target volumes and restoring pulmonary physiology [9, 20]; we prescribe its systematic use two to four times a day, with minimum blocks of 10 repetitions [9, 27]. Finally, we complete the prophylactic circle by educating the patient in deep breathing exercises—including the pursed-lip technique— and in assisted coughing maneuvers with wound protection, thus ensuring effective secretion management and abdominal wall integrity [9, 35, 41].

4.5 Specialized Physical Interventions and Program Design

We maintain that program design must radically move away from the "one-size-fits-all" approach; conversely, we demand a meticulous and personalized architecture [7, 26] that dynamically adapts to the patient's comorbidities and basal fitness [4, 42]. In terms of chronology, while the general literature places the optimal prehabilitation period between 4 and 8 weeks [28, 34], in the bariatric context, we validate extended regimens of 8–16 weeks to maximize the metabolic response [10, 31], establishing a minimum threshold of 3–6 weeks to obtain quantifiable functional gains [1, 15]. We stratify the intervention by prioritizing patients with compromised physiological reserve or manifest frailty [13, 18], specifically identifying the cohort with a 6-minute walk distance below 400 meters as the beneficiaries of the greatest clinical impact [13, 28].

In the prescription of functional exercises, we are not limited to brute strength; we integrate components that address specific biomechanical deficits such as mobility and balance, which are frequently deteriorated in the bariatric population [12, 17]. Our training matrix incorporates flexibility and stability exercises [6, 28, 35], with a particular emphasis on core stabilization, an intervention whose efficacy in obese patients is well-documented [43]. We emphasize that loading must be governed by the principle of progressivity, gradually increasing the difficulty by adding resistance or reducing the base of support [7, 25, 35].

When analyzing delivery modalities, we observe a clear dichotomy: direct hospital supervision guarantees the highest compliance rates [44, 45] thanks to the guidance of specialized physiotherapists [15, 26], whereas home-based programs

(Home-Based), although accessible, suffer from suboptimal adherence, hovering around 70% or less [1, 44, 46]. Given this, we advocate for hybrid models and tele-prehabilitation, which leverage digital tools for remote monitoring and coaching, merging the flexibility of the home environment with the rigor of clinical support [1, 3, 44].

Finally, we understand that the effectiveness of exercise is null without continuous monitoring of progression and adherence [3, 4]. We triangulate surveillance using subjective self-assessment tools such as the Borg Scale (RPE) [7, 44] and activity diaries [26, 29], contrasted with objective metrics derived from pedometers and accelerometers [3, 29], which serve a dual function of recording and motivation [7]. We reinforce this system with weekly motivational interviews, considering them crucial for overcoming psychological barriers and sustaining patient commitment [1, 13, 26].

4.6 Bridge to Postoperative Rehabilitation (Continuum of Physical Care)

We conceive of prehabilitation not as an isolated intervention, but as the inaugural link in a continuum of perioperative care [18, 34, 42], functioning as a strategic bridge that ensures faster and more complete recovery [1, 5]. This therapeutic continuity is fundamentally structured around Early Mobilization, a non-negotiable pillar of ERAS protocols [32, 47]. We establish that mobilization should ideally begin on the same day of surgery (POD 0) or, at the latest, on postoperative day 1 (POD 1) [32, 40, 47]. We categorically reject bed rest due to its iatrogenic nature; early mobilization is imperative to preserve muscle function and prevent the cascade of complications associated with immobility [47, 48]. In the bariatric context, we prescribe progressive physical activity beginning with short walks, escalating to a minimum frequency of four sessions per week of 30–45 min by the sixth week [49].

In parallel, we maintain that the respiratory physiotherapy initiated in the preoperative phase must be maintained without interruption to ensure prophylaxis against PPCs [1]. We validate the continuity of methods such as incentive spirometry [20, 27], along with deep breathing and effective coughing exercises [1, 9]. As Lloréns et al. (2015) suggests, it is notable that Inspiratory Muscle Training (IMT) has demonstrated a specific capacity to preserve respiratory muscle strength in the postoperative period of the obese cohort [1].

The clinical benefit of prehabilitation resides in the acceleration of functional recovery [5, 50]. We observe that prehabilitated patients tend to recover their basal functional capacity approximately 4 weeks postoperatively [13, 50]; moreover, the multimodal approach significantly attenuates the post-surgical erosion of lean body mass (LBM) [5, 7]. Accordingly, it can be stated that the most successful programs are those that extend the physical intervention into the postoperative period, frequently through structured home-based protocols during the 4 weeks following discharge [34, 36].

We project the final objective toward quality of life and effective social and occupational reintegration between 6 and 8 weeks after surgery [35], experiencing the preoperative period as a critical "teachable moment," using prehabilitation to instigate lasting behavioral modifications in lifestyle [8, 12, 16]. To ensure the sustainability of these results, we implement rigorous longitudinal surveillance (e.g., at 6 and 12 months) that evaluates adherence to exercise goals [12, 16, 36]. Ultimately, by raising the ceiling of functional capacity, prehabilitation not only optimizes adherence to postoperative rehabilitation but also catalyzes greater long-term functional independence [13, 51].

References

1. Ambulkar R, Kunte A, Solanki SL, Thakkar V, Deshmukh B, Rana PS. Impact of prehabilitation in major gastrointestinal oncological surgery: a systematic review. J Gastrointest Cancer. 2025;56(1):133.
2. Shakya P, Poudel S. Prehabilitation in patients before major surgery: a review article. JNMA J Nepal Med Assoc. 2022;60(254):909–15.
3. Barberan-Garcia A, Cano I, Bongers BC, Seyfried S, Ganslandt T, Herrle F, et al. Digital support to multimodal community-based prehabilitation: looking for optimization of health value generation. Front Oncol. 2021;11:662013.
4. Cho AR, Vongchaiudomchoke W, Balde D, Kim DJ, Carli F. Enhancing postoperative recovery with multimodal prehabilitation: the journey begins before surgery. Korean J Anesthesiol. 2025;78(5):401–17.
5. Gillis C, Ljungqvist O, Carli F. Prehabilitation, enhanced recovery after surgery, or both? A narrative review. Br J Anaesth. 2022;128(3):434–48.
6. Jirakulsawat A, Noocharoen N, Somnuke P. Prehabilitation in clinical practice: a review of concepts and implementation in enhancing postoperative outcomes. Siriraj Med J. 2024;76(9):646–54.
7. Popescu GA, Minca DG, Jafal NM, Toma CV, Alexandrescu ST, Costea RV, et al. Multimodal prehabilitation in major abdominal surgery—rationale, modalities, results and limitations. Medicina (Mex). 2025;61(5):908.
8. Sato M, Ida M, Nakatani S, Kawaguchi M. A cross-sectional survey of prehabilitation among surgeons and anesthesiologists. JA Clin Rep. 2024;10(1):66.
9. García-Delgado Y, López-Madrazo-Hernández MJ, Alvarado-Martel D, Miranda-Calderín G, Ugarte-Lopetegui A, González-Medina RA, et al. Prehabilitation for bariatric surgery: a randomized, controlled trial protocol and pilot study. Nutrients. 2021;13(9):2903.
10. Simancas-Racines D, Parise-Vasco JM, Angamarca-Iguago J, Cuzco-Macias AC, Soria C, Tramontano S, et al. Effects of preoperative exercise interventions in patients undergoing metabolic and bariatric surgery: a systematic review and meta-analysis. J Clin Med. 2025;14(17):6170.
11. Herrera-Santelices A, Argüello-Florencio G, Westphal G, Nardo Junior N, Zamunér AR. Effects of supervised physical exercise as prehabilitation on body composition, functional capacity and quality of life in bariatric surgery candidates: a systematic review and meta-analysis. J Clin Med. 2022;11(17):5091.
12. Suhaimi A, Saria Yuliawiratman B. From prehab to rehab: the functional restoration of a bariatric individual. Saiz-Sapena N, Miguel Oviedo J, eds. 27 de octubre de 2021 [citado 13 de noviembre de 2025]; Disponible en: https://www.intechopen.com/books/bariatric-surgery-from-the-non-surgical-approach-to-the-post-surgery-individual-care/from-prehab-to-rehab-the-functional-restoration-of-a-bariatric-individual

13. Minnella EM, Awasthi R, Gillis C, Fiore JF, Liberman AS, Charlebois P, et al. Patients with poor baseline walking capacity are most likely to improve their functional status with multimodal prehabilitation. Surgery. 2016;160(4):1070–9.
14. Ho C, Samwil SNM, Kahairudin Z, Jamhuri N, Abd Aziz A. Pre-habilitation with exercise and high whey-protein-based meal replacement therapy promotes weight loss and preserve muscle mass before bariatric surgery. Asian J Surg. 2023;46(9):3716–21.
15. Patel H, Le KDR, Wang AJ, Tay SBP. Integration of resistance exercise into a multimodal approach to prehabilitation for patients with sarcopenia prior to surgery: a narrative review. Front Rehabil Sci. 2025;6:1481233.
16. Abbasi M, Mohammadzadeh N, Shahi MHP, Soroush A, Eslamian R, Mir A, et al. The impact of sleeve gastrectomy on pulmonary function tests and physical activity one-year after surgery. BMC Surg. 2025;25(1):83.
17. Bullo V, Pavan D, Gobbo S, Bortoletto A, Cugusi L, Di Blasio A, et al. From surgery to functional capacity: muscle strength modifications in women post sleeve gastrectomy. BMC Sports Sci Med Rehabil. 2024;16(1):118.
18. Licker M, El Manser D, Bonnardel E, Massias S, Soualhi IM, Saint-Leger C, et al. Multimodal prehabilitation in thoracic surgery: from basic concepts to practical modalities. J Clin Med. 2024;13(10):2765.
19. Valenzano AA, Vasco P, D'Orsi G, Cassano T, Marzovillo R, Di Stasi A, et al. Impact of exercise therapy in ERAS prehabilitation for major surgery: a systematic review. Sports. 2025;13(9):315.
20. Aref H, Yunus T, Farghaly M, ElDahshan Y, Khan HJ, Alsaadi D, et al. Comparative outcomes of ERAS and conventional methods in laparoscopic sleeve gastrectomy: a 5-Year prospective cohort study in Saudi Arabia. BMC Gastroenterol. 2025;25(1):615.
21. Melnyk M, Casey RG, Black P, Koupparis AJ. Enhanced recovery after surgery (ERAS) protocols: time to change practice? Can Urol Assoc J. 2011:342–8.
22. Thorell A, MacCormick AD, Awad S, Reynolds N, Roulin D, Demartines N, et al. Guidelines for perioperative Care in Bariatric Surgery: enhanced recovery after surgery (ERAS) society recommendations. World J Surg. 2016;40(9):2065–83.
23. Stenberg E, Dos Reis Falcão LF, O'Kane M, Liem R, Pournaras DJ, Salminen P, et al. Guidelines for perioperative Care in Bariatric Surgery: enhanced recovery after surgery (ERAS) society recommendations: a 2021 update. World J Surg. 2022;46(4):729–51.
24. Bingül ES, Şentürk NM, Kaynar AM. Prehabilitation: a narrative review focused on exercise therapy for the prevention of postoperative pulmonary complications following lung resection. Front Med. 2023;10:1196981.
25. Schaller SJ, Kiselev J, Loidl V, Quentin W, Schmidt K, Mörgeli R, et al. Prehabilitation of elderly frail or pre-frail patients prior to elective surgery (PRAEP-GO): study protocol for a randomized, controlled, outcome assessor-blinded trial. Trials. 2022;23(1):468.
26. Barberan-Garcia A, Ubré M, Roca J, Lacy AM, Burgos F, Risco R, et al. Personalised prehabilitation in high-risk patients undergoing elective major abdominal surgery: a randomized blinded controlled trial. Ann Surg. 2018;267(1):50–6.
27. Chan KS, Junnarkar SP, Wang B, Tan YP, Low JK, Huey CWT, et al. Outcomes of an outpatient home-based prehabilitation program before pancreaticoduodenectomy: a retrospective cohort study. Ann Hepato-Biliary-Pancreat Surg. 2022;26(4):375–85.
28. Gonçalves CG, Groth AK. Pré-habilitação: como preparar nossos pacientes para cirurgias abdominais eletivas de maior porte? Rev Colégio Bras Cir. 2019;46(5):e20192267.
29. Suárez-Alcázar MP, Folch Ayora A, Muriach M, Recacha-Ponce P, Garcia-Roca ME, Coret-Franco A, et al. Multimodal prehabilitation in colorectal cancer: improving fitness, lifestyle, and post-surgery outcomes. Healthcare. 2025;13(9):1083.
30. Bausys A, Luksta M, Kuliavas J, Anglickiene G, Maneikiene V, Gedvilaite L, et al. Personalized trimodal prehabilitation for gastrectomy. Medicine (Baltimore). 2020;99(27):e20687.

31. Gierat-Haponiuk K, Wąż P, Haponiuk-Skwarlińska J, Wilczyński M, Haponiuk I. Physiotherapy in prehabilitation for bariatric surgery—analysis of its impact on functional capacity and original predictive models of functional status outcome. J Clin Med. 2025;14(15):5265.
32. Yang Q, Zhang S, Xu Z, Liu L, Fan S, Wu S, et al. The effectiveness of trigeminal nerve stimulation on traumatic brain injury. Neuromodulation Technol Neural Interface. 2022;25(8):1330–7.
33. Rossi D, Stedile NRDA, Silva EAD, Gasperi DD, Neto Santos L, Eibel B. Monitoring respiratory biomechanics, lung capacity and mobility in bariatric surgery: perioperative analysis. Arq Gastroenterol. 2024;61:e24066.
34. Shanmugasundaram Prema S, Ganapathy D, Shanmugamprema D. Prehabilitation strategies: enhancing surgical resilience with a focus on nutritional optimization and multimodal interventions. Adv Nutr. 2025;16(4):100392.
35. Carli F, Scheede-Bergdahl C. Prehabilitation to enhance perioperative care. Anesthesiol Clin. 2015;33(1):17–33.
36. Kumar S, Bhalerao AS, Prabhakar S, Verma K, Tandon V, Govil D. Optimising outcomes with prehabilitation before major abdominal surgery: a single-centre prospective study. Apollo Med. 2025, 09760016251367082;
37. Mao C, Rogers-Seeley M, Tay SB, Le KDR. Insights into contemporary practices in the prehabilitation of sarcopenic patients prior to surgery: an up-to-date review. Cureus [Internet]. 2025; [citado 13 de noviembre de 2025]; Disponible en: https://www.cureus.com/articles/387657-insights-into-contemporary-practices-in-the-prehabilitation-of-sarcopenic-patients-prior-to-surgery-an-up-to-date-review
38. Triguero-Cánovas D, López-Rodríguez-Arias F, Gómez-Martínez M, Sánchez-Guillén L, Peris-Castelló F, Alcaide-Quirós MJ, et al. Home-based prehabilitation improves physical conditions measured by ergospirometry and 6MWT in colorectal cancer patients: a randomized controlled pilot study. Support Care Cancer. 2023;31(12):673.
39. Ricci C, Alberici L, Serbassi F, Caraceni P, Domenicali M, Ingaldi C, et al. Physical prehabilitation in patients who underwent major abdominal surgery: a comprehensive systematic review and component network meta-analysis using GRADE and CINeMA approach. Ann Surg Oncol. 2024;31(3):1725–38.
40. Olsén MF, Andersson T, Nouh MA, Johnson E, Block L, Vakk M, et al. Development of and adherence to an ERAS® and prehabilitation protocol for patients undergoing pancreatic surgery: an observational study. Scand J Surg. 2023;112(4):235–45.
41. Zhang Y, Gao B, Zhang X, Zhao L, Han X, Zhang M, et al. The impact of prehabilitation strategies on psychological state, glucose metabolism, and postoperative outcomes in patients undergoing laparoscopic sleeve gastrectomy. BMC Surg. 2025;25(1):394.
42. Carli F, Silver JK, Feldman LS, McKee A, Gilman S, Gillis C, et al. Surgical prehabilitation in patients with cancer: state-of-the-science and recommendations for future research from a panel of subject matter experts. Phys Med Rehabil Clin N Am. 2017;28(1):49–64.
43. Shawkey OM, Al Sibai Mohamed A, Elkeblawy MM, Khalil ESW. Efficacy of balance training on balance performance in obese patients undergoing sleeve gastrectomy. Int J Health Sci. 2022:2143–51.
44. Franssen RFW, Bongers BC, Vogelaar FJ, Janssen-Heijnen MLG. Feasibility of a tele-prehabilitation program in high-risk patients with colon or rectal cancer undergoing elective surgery: a feasibility study. Perioper Med. 2022;11(1):28.
45. Hijazi Y, Gondal U, Aziz O. A systematic review of prehabilitation programs in abdominal cancer surgery. Int J Surg. 2017;39:156–62.
46. Sier MAT, Godina E, Mollema O, Cox MPPJ, Tweed TTT, Greve JW, et al. Participation and adherence to prehabilitation programs for colorectal cancer. Nutrients. 2025;17(11):1792.
47. Low DE, Allum W, De Manzoni G, Ferri L, Immanuel A, Kuppusamy M, et al. Guidelines for perioperative care in esophagectomy: Enhanced Recovery After Surgery (ERAS®) Society recommendations. World J Surg. 2019;43(2):299–330.

48. Patel BK, Hall JB. Perioperative physiotherapy. Curr Opin Anaesthesiol. 2013;26(2):152–6.
49. Rudiman R, Hanafi RV. Perioperative care for bariatric surgery. Diagnostics. 2024;14(18):2095.
50. Li C, Carli F, Lee L, Charlebois P, Stein B, Liberman AS, et al. Impact of a trimodal prehabilitation program on functional recovery after colorectal cancer surgery: a pilot study. Surg Endosc. 2013;27(4):1072–82.
51. Seyfried S, Herrle F, Téoule P, Betzler A, Reissfelder C. Patient-tailored approach for enhanced recovery after surgery. Visc Med. 2022;38(5):322–7.

Upper Digestive Endoscopy and Screening of Helicobacter Pylori Infection

5

Carlos Hermida and Marta Hermida-Lario

5.1 Introduction

Obesity and overweight are a major global public health problem, with recent publications showing a progressive increase in their worldwide prevalence, from 6.4 4% in 1990 to 16.06% in 2022, and projections suggesting that it may reach 38.96% by 2040 [1]. The most frequent comorbidities observed in patients with obesity are arterial hypertension (79.9%), joint disease (33.2%), diabetes mellitus (15.6%), and cardiovascular disease (10.5%) [2].

Bariatric surgery has become the most effective option for long-term sustained weight loss and improvement of associated diseases. Vertical sleeve gastrectomy has become one of the most common procedures due to its lower technical complexity and good clinical outcomes. As this technique modifies gastric anatomy, an adequate preoperative assessment of the digestive system is essential, with particular emphasis on performing an endoscopic examination of the esophagus, stomach, and duodenum and investigating the presence of Helicobacter pylori infection, with the aim of achieving a correct planning of the surgical procedure, preventing complications and improving the medium- and long-term prognosis, thus optimizing surgical outcomes and patient safety.

C. Hermida (✉)
Facultad de Ciencias Biomédicas y de la Salud, Universidad Alfonso X el Sabio, Madrid, Spain
e-mail: chermida@uax.es

M. Hermida-Lario
Hospital Universitario de la Princesa, Servicio de Aparato Digestivo, Madrid, Spain

J. Ruiz-Tovar (ed.), *Multidisciplinary Management of Sleeve Gastrectomy*,
https://doi.org/10.1007/978-3-032-25644-7_5

5.2 Role of Upper Digestive Endoscopy Before Bariatric Surgery

Upper digestive endoscopy (UDE) is a procedure that allows assessment of the mucosa of the upper digestive tract, identification of diseases that may require treatment before the surgical procedure and that may even modify the selected technique (reflux esophagitis, hiatal hernia, gastritis, peptic ulcer, etc.), and the collection of biopsies for microscopic evaluation and identification of Helicobacter pylori infection (urease test or microscopic identification).

5.2.1 Evidence from the International Federation for the Surgery of Obesity and Metabolic Disorders (IFSO)

The publication from the International Federation for the Surgery of Obesity and Metabolic Disorders [3], which includes the analysis of 63 published studies, described the following findings regarding upper digestive endoscopy (UDE) in patients with obesity:

1. The most frequent endoscopic findings were:
   - Gastritis: range 3–88.3% (mean 31.8%, pooled mean 19.3%).
   - Hiatal hernia: range 0.6–90.2% (mean 23.5%, pooled mean 19.6%).
   - Barrett's esophagus: range 0.1–9.9% (mean 2.3%, pooled mean 1%).
2. Endoscopic findings were analyzed in symptomatic patients, ranging from 12.1% to 59.6% (mean 32%, pooled mean 20.7%). In this group of symptomatic patients, at least one endoscopic finding was identified in 7.2–34.1% (mean 16%, pooled mean 15.2%). In the group of asymptomatic patients, findings ranged from 2.1% to 63.8% (mean 25.3%, pooled mean 15.4%).
3. A change in surgical intent (delay or modification of the technique) due to endoscopic findings occurred in 16.8% of patients, with gastritis, hiatal hernia, and Helicobacter pylori infection being the most common reasons for that decision.

The final recommendations of this publication include considering preoperative endoscopy in symptomatic patients, in asymptomatic patients given the high percentage of endoscopic findings in this group, and in patients from populations with a high incidence of esophageal and gastric pathology.

5.2.2 Evidence from the American Society for Metabolic and Bariatric Surgery (ASMBS)

The American Society for Metabolic and Bariatric Surgery (ASMBS) analyzed 28 published studies and reached the following conclusions [4]:

1. The most frequent endoscopic findings included:
    - Gastroesophageal reflux disease: 27.3%.
    - Hiatal hernia: 21%.
    - Erosive esophagitis: 16.4%.
    - Barrett's esophagus: 2.7%.
    - The percentage of malignant tumors in these studies ranged between 0 and 0.94%.
    - Other abnormal findings (gastritis, gastric polyps, ulcers, Helicobacter pylori infection, etc.): 34.6%.
2. The analysis showed that symptomatic patients had a higher frequency of endoscopic abnormalities, with findings in approximately 45–70% of cases. In the group of asymptomatic patients, between 20% and 40% had abnormal endoscopic findings, mainly mild gastritis, presence of H. pylori, or a small, previously undiagnosed hiatal hernia.
3. In the group of symptomatic patients, between 12% and 18% required modification or delay of the surgical procedure due to clinically significant findings, such as active ulcers or H. pylori infection. In the asymptomatic group, between 5% and 8% had endoscopic findings that led to changes in surgical planning, either due to the need for prior medical treatment or due to findings that altered the choice of technique, such as lesions suspicious for malignancy.

The final recommendations of this publication indicate that performing preoperative UDE, even in asymptomatic patients, can help treat modifiable conditions before bariatric surgery (such as duodenal ulcer, H. pylori infection, among others), allow identification of associated anatomical abnormalities that could be corrected during the bariatric procedure (e.g., a hiatal hernia), help adapt the choice of surgical approach, or even guide the decision not to proceed with surgery.

5.2.3 Other Studies

A recent meta-analysis [5] that reviewed 47 studies including 23,368 patients undergoing bariatric surgery showed the following findings on preoperative UDE:

- In 40.8% of patients, no abnormalities were found.
- Most frequent findings: gastritis 31%, hiatal hernia 19%. The rate of malignant tumors was 0.3%.
- In 39.7%, new findings were identified without impact on surgery.
- In 19.8%, findings modified surgical planning.
- Only 0.3% were considered unfit for surgery.

The final conclusions of the study state that preoperative UDE changes surgical planning in around 20% of patients undergoing bariatric surgery; most endoscopies do not modify medical or surgical management. A selective use of EGD is recommended, especially in patients with symptoms or risk factors, within a multidisciplinary team-based approach.

Similarly, a study analyzing how UDE impacts the management of a cohort of 897 bariatric patients [6] showed:

1. Prevalence of endoscopic findings
   62% of patients presented Some abnormality on endoscopy
   The most frequent findings were:
   - Gastritis or gastric erosions: 31%.
   - Hiatal hernia: 18%.
   - Reflux esophagitis: 12%.
   - Peptic ulcer: 3%.
   - Gastric polyps: 2%.
   - Helicobacter pylori infection: 24%.
2. Impact on surgery
   - In 18% of patients, endoscopic or radiological findings modified surgical planning.
   - In 8%, the decision was made to treat the detected pathology first (e.g., H. pylori eradication, ulcer or esophagitis treatment).
   - In 4%, surgery was delayed.
   - In 1%, surgery was canceled or the technique was changed (e.g., from sleeve gastrectomy to Roux-en-Y gastric bypass).

5.3 Role of Upper Digestive Endoscopy after Bariatric Surgery

5.3.1 Evaluation of Postoperative Symptoms

After sleeve gastrectomy, between 20% and 40% of patients may develop upper digestive symptoms [7, 8], such as:

- Gastroesophageal reflux (heartburn, regurgitation).
- Persistent nausea or vomiting.
- Epigastric pain or dysphagia.

UDE is the diagnostic tool of choice to investigate these symptoms, allowing the detection of:

- Reflux esophagitis (frequent after sleeve).
- Stenosis or torsion of the gastric tube.
- Ulcers on the staple line.
- Presence of undiagnosed or recurrent hiatal hernia.

In these cases, endoscopy guides treatment (e.g., endoscopic dilation, medical treatment with PPIs, or indication for conversion to gastric bypass).

5.3.2 Detection and Management of Gastroesophageal Reflux Disease (GERD)

Gastroesophageal reflux disease (GERD) is one of the most frequent complications after sleeve gastrectomy due to an increase in intragastric pressure, a decrease in the angle of His and the antireflux mechanism, or the presence of a hiatal hernia not corrected during surgery [8, 9].

In these cases, UDE allows the diagnosis of reflux esophagitis and classification of its severity (Los Angeles classification), as well as the detection and biopsy of Barrett's esophagus. The appearance of Barrett's esophagus or severe reflux symptoms may indicate conversion to gastric bypass, which usually improves GERD in more than 80% of cases [10, 11].

5.3.3 Evaluation of Mechanical Complications

UDE is also useful for detecting anatomical complications of the sleeve, such as stenosis of the gastric tube (usually in the middle third), leaks or fistulas at the staple line, and torsion or angulation of the gastric sleeve [12, 13]:

- These are serious but infrequent complications (1–6% after sleeve gastrectomy).
- Endoscopy enables early diagnosis through direct visualization and the application of non-surgical therapies such as:
  - Placement of self-expanding metal stents.
  - Large endoscopic clips.
  - Tissue sealants (such as cyanoacrylate or fibrin).
- In most cases, endoscopic management avoids surgical reintervention.

Stenosis or torsion of the gastric sleeve

- Usually presents with vomiting, food intolerance, or severe reflux.
- Endoscopic balloon dilation is the technique of choice, with clinical success rates of 85–95%.
- In refractory cases, temporary stent placement or even surgical conversion to gastric bypass may be required.

Marginal ulcers and postoperative bleeding

- Diagnostic endoscopy identifies ulcers at the anastomotic line or staple line.

- Treatment with proton pump inhibitors and H. pylori eradication is recommended.
- Endoscopic management of acute bleeding may include the application of hemostatic clips or thermal coagulation.

5.3.4 Long-Term Follow-Up

Although there is no universal consensus, several guidelines (IFSO [3], ASMBS [4], EAES [14]) suggest that UDE also has a role in long-term surveillance, especially in patients with persistent reflux symptoms, previously diagnosed esophagitis or Barrett's esophagus, and 3–5 years after surgery to detect early preneoplastic or inflammatory lesions in the distal esophagus or gastric remnant:

- IFSO [3]: suggests a surveillance endoscopy 3–5 years after surgery, even in asymptomatic patients, to assess changes in the esophageal and gastric mucosa.
- ASMBS [4]: recommends systematic UDE every 3–5 years after sleeve gastrectomy in the presence of symptoms or previous findings, and earlier if alarm signs (dysphagia, anemia, unexplained weight loss, or gastrointestinal bleeding) are present.
- EAES [14] recommends endoscopic surveillance in patients with persistent reflux symptoms, in those with previous esophagitis, or in those who develop new symptoms after the first postoperative year.

5.4 Helicobacter Pylori in Bariatric Surgery

Helicobacter pylori (H. pylori) infection remains one of the most relevant biological factors in the pathogenesis of various gastric diseases and, in recent years, has gained special importance in the context of bariatric surgery. It is a Gram-negative, microaerophilic, spiral-shaped, flagellated bacterium with a remarkable ability to survive in extreme conditions, such as the acidic environment of the human stomach, its main reservoir, and is transmitted mainly via the fecal–oral route. From a pathogenic perspective, H. pylori is classically associated with peptic ulcer, chronic gastritis, gastric carcinoma, and MALT lymphoma, but recent studies have broadened its spectrum, linking it to metabolic, hepatic, dermatologic and neurologic alterations, although the pathophysiologic mechanisms of these associations remain unclear [15].

Current data indicate that around 40–60% of the world's population is infected with H. pylori, with higher rates in low-income regions and among groups with unfavorable socioeconomic conditions. Although its prevalence has steadily decreased in recent decades, the infection continues to be a major public health problem [16, 17].

H. pylori infection affects approximately one-third of people with obesity worldwide, with wide geographic and socioeconomic variations. These findings underline the need to consider the regional context and development conditions when planning screening, diagnostic, and eradication strategies in this specific population [18].

The prevalence of H. pylori in patients undergoing bariatric surgery varies between series, although some studies based on histologic confirmation report relatively low figures (around 6.3%). In these studies, older age was identified as the main predictor of infection, while body mass index did not show a significant correlation. However, infection was associated with a higher frequency of hypertension and diabetes [19].

In patients with obesity, H. pylori infection acquires additional relevance due to its interaction with metabolism and systemic inflammation. Several studies have identified a higher prevalence of metabolic syndrome, insulin resistance, and hepatic steatosis in infected individuals, suggesting that bacterial eradication could have a positive effect on these disorders. It has been postulated that gastric inflammation induced by the bacterium alters hormonal mediators such as ghrelin and leptin, which are involved in appetite regulation and energy balance, thus contributing to obesity and metabolic dysfunction [20, 21].

Bariatric surgery, particularly vertical sleeve gastrectomy, provokes significant changes in gastrointestinal physiology: acceleration of gastric emptying, reduced acid secretion, and increased intestinal transit [22]. These transformations alter the gastric microenvironment and may modify the behavior and virulence of H. pylori. Since the impact of these changes on the course of infection is still uncertain, preoperative screening and eradication are recommended as preventive measures. In addition, prolonged use of proton pump inhibitors (PPIs) after this type of surgery may favor atrophic gastritis and the development of gastric neoplasia in the presence of the bacterium [23].

From a functional standpoint, H. pylori appears to influence the mechanical properties of the stomach. A retrospective study of 159 patients undergoing laparoscopic sleeve gastrectomy showed that those with active infection had significantly greater gastric compliance and volume, which could increase intake capacity and consequently hinder postoperative weight loss. It has been proposed that chronic inflammation induced by the bacterium alters the viscoelastic properties of gastric tissue, modifying its distensibility [22].

The consequences of infection are particularly relevant in the surgical setting. A systematic review and meta-analysis including more than 6000 patients undergoing laparoscopic sleeve gastrectomy showed a significant association between infection and an increase in postoperative complications, particularly staple-line leaks. This finding could be explained by the chronic inflammatory effect of H. pylori on the gastric mucosa, which compromises tissue healing and anastomotic integrity. Although no relevant differences were observed in the risk of bleeding, infection appears to contribute overall to postoperative morbidity [24].

Complementarily, another meta-analysis on the effect of preoperative eradication showed that H. pylori–positive patients had an almost sevenfold higher risk of developing postoperative gastric ulcers compared with negative patients, making infection an independent predictor of ulceration. Although evidence regarding bleeding or anastomotic leaks is not conclusive, prior antibiotic treatment is associated with better clinical outcomes and a lower incidence of severe complications. However, the methodological limitations of the studies—mainly their retrospective nature and lack of homogeneity in diagnostic methods—require cautious interpretation of these data [25].

Treatment should be administered using combination therapy based on proton pump inhibitors and antibiotics (amoxicillin, clarithromycin, metronidazole, tetracycline, or levofloxacin, depending on local resistance patterns), and its efficacy should be confirmed at least 4 weeks before surgery using a urea breath test or stool antigen test [26].

In patients already undergoing bariatric surgery, detection and eradication of H. pylori remain advisable in the presence of gastrointestinal symptoms, iron-deficiency anemia, or persistent nutritional deficiencies, as infection may contribute to poor absorption of iron and vitamin B12, thus exacerbating postoperative anemia.

Several studies have indicated that the presence of obesity, especially at advanced stages, may be associated with lower H. pylori eradication rates when standard therapeutic regimens are used. Although there is still no meta-analysis specifically designed to quantify the impact of body mass index (BMI) on treatment response, available evidence suggests that obesity is a risk factor for therapeutic failure.

The first data describing this association come from the study by Abdullahi et al., who observed that, after standard triple therapy, patients who were overweight or obese achieved an eradication rate of 55%, compared with 85.4% in normal-weight subjects. In their multivariate analysis, elevated BMI behaved as an independent predictor of therapeutic failure [27].

More recent studies confirm this trend even when using contemporary quadruple therapies. Laudanno et al. analyzed more than 200 patients treated with concomitant therapy for 14 days and found an eradication rate of 68.2% in people with obesity, significantly lower than the 88% documented in normal-weight individuals. Moreover, efficacy decreased progressively with increasing BMI, reaching just 51% in patients with class IV obesity [28]. These results support the hypothesis that morbid obesity alters the pharmacokinetics and pharmacodynamics of antibiotics and proton pump inhibitors, reducing effective intragastric concentrations.

On the other hand, it has been shown that this lower efficacy can be partially corrected by optimized strategies. In a prospective study, the same group compared a fixed-dose regimen versus a body-weight–adjusted regimen in patients with severe obesity. Eradication increased from 66.1% with standard dosing to 86.3% when adjusted by kg of body weight [29], reaching values comparable to those observed in the general population. This suggests that part of the problem lies in pharmacological underexposure when universal doses are administered to subjects with a high volume of distribution.

However, not all studies are completely consistent. Sayadishahraki et al. were unable to demonstrate a statistically significant association between BMI and therapeutic failure, although eradication rates varied according to the degree of obesity [30]. These discrepancies may be attributable to differences in adherence, prevalence of antibiotic resistance, strength of the regimen used, or sample size.

Available evidence suggests that obesity—especially morbid obesity—is associated with a higher risk of failure in H. pylori eradication when fixed-dose regimens or less potent treatments are used. Strategies that seem to improve response include 14-day quadruple therapies, use of high or optimized doses of proton pump inhibitors, and individualized antibiotic dosing according to body weight.

In summary, H. pylori infection plays a multifactorial role in bariatric surgery, affecting both gastric physiology and the risk of complications and metabolic outcomes. Although there is no absolute consensus, most data support the usefulness of preoperative screening and eradication as preventive measures. Beyond reducing the risk of ulcers and anastomotic leaks, H. pylori elimination may help optimize metabolic outcomes, decrease systemic inflammation, and reduce gastric carcinogenic potential, especially in procedures that leave gastric segments inaccessible after surgery.

References

1. Liu J, Fang Z, Lu Q, Wang Y, Zhang L. Projecting global trends and inequalities in adult overweight and obesity, 2023–2040: findings from the NCD-RisC database. Obesity (Silver Spring). 2025;33(10):1955–67.
2. Dicker D, Karpati T, Promislow S, Reges O. Implications of the European Association for the Study of obesity's new framework definition of obesity: prevalence and association with all-cause mortality. Ann Intern Med. 2025;178(8):1065–72.
3. Brown WA, Fisher OM, Johari Y, Au J, Stier C, Moore R, Parmar C, Dixon JB, Salminen P. International Federation for Surgery for Obesity and Metabolic Disorders Position Statement on the role of Upper Gastrointestinal Endoscopy Before and After Metabolic Bariatric Surgery. Obes Surg. 2025 Dec;35(12):4889–4916.
4. Campos GM, Mazzini GS, Altieri MS, Docimo S Jr, De Maria EJ, Rogers AM, et al. ASMBS position statement on the rationale for performance of upper gastrointestinal endoscopy before and after metabolic and bariatric surgery. Surg Obes Relat Dis. 2021;17(5):837–47.
5. Muir D, Choi B, Holden M, Clements C, Stevens J, Ratnasingham K, et al. Preoperative oesophagogastroduodenoscopy and the effect on bariatric surgery: a systematic review and meta-analysis. Obes Surg. 2023;33(8):2546–56.
6. Poljo A, Reichl JJ, Schneider R, Süsstrunk J, Klasen JM, Fourie L, et al. How preoperative upper gastrointestinal investigations affect the management of bariatric patients: results of a cohort study of 897 patients. Surg Endosc. 2025;39(1):153–61.
7. Genco A, Soricelli E, Casella G, Maselli R, Castagneto-Gissey L, Di Lorenzo N, et al. Gastroesophageal reflux disease and Barrett's esophagus after laparoscopic sleeve gastrectomy: a possible, underestimated long-term complication. Surg Obes Relat Dis. 2017;13(4):568–74.
8. Yeung KTD, Penney N, Ashrafian L, Darzi A, Ashrafian H. Does sleeve gastrectomy expose the distal esophagus to severe reflux?: a systematic review and meta-analysis. Ann Surg. 2020;271(2):257–65.
9. Quero G, Fiorillo C, Dallemagne B, Mascagni P, Curcic J, Fox M, et al. The causes of gastroesophageal reflux after laparoscopic sleeve gastrectomy: quantitative assessment of the structure and function of the esophagogastric junction by magnetic resonance imaging and high-resolution manometry. Obes Surg. 2020;30(6):2108–17.
10. Parmar CD, Mahawar KK, Boyle M, Schroeder N, Balupuri S, Small PK. Conversion of sleeve gastrectomy to roux-en-Y gastric bypass is effective for gastro-oesophageal reflux disease but not for further weight loss. Obes Surg. 2017;27(7):1651–8.

11. Matar R, Monzer N, Jaruvongvanich V, Abusaleh R, Vargas EJ, Maselli DB, et al. Indications and outcomes of conversion of sleeve gastrectomy to Roux-en-Y gastric bypass: a systematic review and a meta-analysis. Obes Surg. 2021;31(9):3936–46.
12. Eguchi M, Nogueira R, Balthazar da Silveira CA, Vidotto L, Kasakewitch JPG, Lech GE, et al. Endoscopic management of gastric stenosis after sleeve gastrectomy: a systematic review and single-arm meta-analysis. Surg Endosc. 2025;39(8):5324–47.
13. Shenoy A, Schulman AR. Endoscopic management of bariatric surgery complications: fistulas, leaks, and ulcers. Gastrointest Endosc Clin N Am. 2024;34(4):655–69.
14. Di Lorenzo N, Antoniou SA, Batterham RL, Busetto L, Godoroja D, Iossa A, et al. Clinical practice guidelines of the European Association for Endoscopic Surgery (EAES) on bariatric surgery: update 2020 endorsed by IFSO-EC, EASO and ESPCOP. Surg Endosc. 2020;34(6):2332–58.
15. Malfertheiner P, Camargo MC, El-Omar E, Liou JM, Peek R, Schulz C, et al. Helicobacter pylori infection. Nat Rev Dis Primers. 2023;9(1):19.
16. Hooi JKY, Lai WY, Ng WK, Suen MMY, Underwood FE, Tanyingoh D, et al. Global prevalence of helicobacter pylori infection: systematic review and meta-analysis. Gastroenterology. 2017;153(2):420–9.
17. Zamani M, Ebrahimtabar F, Zamani V, Miller WH, Alizadeh-Navaei R, Shokri-Shirvani J, et al. Systematic review with meta-analysis: the worldwide prevalence of helicobacter pylori infection. Aliment Pharmacol Ther. 2018;47(7):868–76.
18. Sadeghi A, Nouri F, Taherifard E, Shahlaee MA, Dehdari EN. Estimates of global and regional prevalence of helicobacter pylori infection among individuals with obesity: a systematic review and meta-analysis. Infection. 2024;52(4):1223–34.
19. Baillargeon D, Greenblatt M, Côté M, Nadeau M, Couture CY, Hould FS, et al. Prevalence of helicobacter pylori infection in bariatric surgery patients. Obes Surg. 2023;33(7):2132–8.
20. Baradaran A, Dehghanbanadaki H, Naderpour S, Pirkashani LM, Rajabi A, Rashti R, et al. The association between helicobacter pylori and obesity: a systematic review and meta-analysis of case-control studies. Clin Diabetes Endocrinol. 2021;7(1):15.
21. Zhang D, Wang Q, Bai F. Bidirectional relationship between helicobacter pylori infection and nonalcoholic fatty liver disease: insights from a comprehensive meta-analysis. Front Nutr. 2024;11:1410543.
22. Kaplan K, Turgut E, Okut G, Bag YM, Sumer F, Kayaalp C. Helicobacter pylori increases gastric compliance on resected stomach after laparoscopic sleeve gastrectomy. Obes Surg. 2021;31(11):4776–80.
23. Emile SH. Should we test for and eradicate helicobacter pylori before bariatric surgery? Obes Surg. 2021;31(2):847–9.
24. Marcolin P, Machado Berleze M, Polettini J, Marchesan Rodrigues MA, Augustin SD. The impact of helicobacter pylori on laparoscopic sleeve gastrectomy postoperative complications: a systematic review and meta-analysis. Obes Surg. 2023;33(11):3649–57.
25. Kermansaravi M, Valizadeh R, ShahabiShahmiri S, Zakeri R, Safari S, Eghbali F, et al. Effect of helicobacter pylori infection on metabolic and bariatric surgical complications: a systematic review and meta-analysis. Updat Surg. 2025;77(7):2121–34.
26. Malfertheiner P, Megraud F, Rokkas T, Gisbert JP, Liou JM, Schulz C, et al. Management of Helicobacter pylori infection: the Maastricht VI/Florence consensus report. Gut. 2022;71(9):1724–62.
27. Abdullahi M, Annibale B, Capoccia D, Di Giulio E, Lahner E, Passi S, et al. Implications of obesity for the eradication of helicobacter pylori infection. Obes Surg. 2008;18(11):1450–4.
28. Laudanno O, Ahumarán G, Thomé M, Gollo P, Gonzalez P, Khoury M. Relationship between obesity severity and helicobacter pylori eradication in patients undergoing bariatric and metabolic surgery: a post hoc analysis. Obes Surg. 2024;34(10):3790–5.
29. Laudanno O, González M, Veiga MJ, et al. Helicobacter pylori eradication in obese patients: comparison between standard fixed-dose therapy and weight-adjusted regimens. Rev Esp Enferm Dig. 2020;112(10):743–50.
30. Sayadishahraki M, Fathi M, Norouzi M, et al. Helicobacter pylori eradication rates and their association with BMI in patients undergoing bariatric surgery. Ann Bariatr Surg. 2021;10(2):76–83.

Pneumological Evaluation

6

Rafael Martín-Holguera

6.1 Introduction

Sleeve gastrectomy is considered a fundamental and highly effective surgical technique in the management of severe obesity, offering substantial benefits that go beyond mere weight loss. It also facilitates the improvement or resolution of various metabolic comorbidities and, ultimately, contributes to a longer life expectancy for patients. However, the morbidly obese population has a high prevalence of respiratory disorders inherent to their condition, which can significantly complicate the perioperative course and impact the long-term outcomes of the surgery [1].

The presence of respiratory alterations in patients who are candidates for sleeve gastrectomy and other bariatric surgical techniques is a known risk factor for an increased number of perioperative and postoperative complications, such as atelectasis, pneumonia, and pulmonary thromboembolisms, in addition to being directly associated with a prolonged hospital stay [2]. Therefore, an exhaustive preoperative pneumological evaluation of the patient who is going to undergo this surgery is essential. Once the evaluation is complete, therapeutic strategies should be implemented to optimise the patient's pulmonary function before the surgical procedure. This will not only reduce perioperative risks but could also decrease the technical difficulty of the surgery itself and improve its short-term results. These therapeutic strategies should not be limited to correcting or improving the respiratory disorders detected during the evaluation but should seek to strengthen the patient's overall physiological capacity to cope with the surgical and anaesthetic stress. This will translate into greater resilience, more efficient recovery, and, in short, better overall results throughout the entire perioperative process [3].

The most prevalent respiratory disorders in morbidly obese patients that require special attention in the preoperative context of bariatric surgery are the following:

R. Martín-Holguera (✉)
Faculty of Health Sciences, Pontifical University of Salamanca, Salamanca, Spain

J. Ruiz-Tovar (ed.), *Multidisciplinary Management of Sleeve Gastrectomy*,
https://doi.org/10.1007/978-3-032-25644-7_6

6.1.1 Obstructive Sleep Apnoea (OSA)

OSA is extraordinarily prevalent in patients with morbid obesity, with a reported incidence ranging from 76% to 96% [3]. It is estimated that approximately 6 out of 10 bariatric surgery candidates have OSA. However, various studies estimate that this condition is underdiagnosed in this group of patients, and that only 15–20% of them are diagnosed before the surgical procedure [4–7].

Patients with OSA have a significantly higher risk of developing respiratory and cardiovascular complications during surgical procedures that require general anaesthesia, sedation, and/or analgesia. This risk is directly proportional to the Apnoea/Hypopnoea Index (AHÍ) and the degree of daytime or nocturnal hypoxaemia [8].

The collapse and total or partial occlusion of the upper airway that occurs during sleep is fundamental to the pathophysiology of OSA. This upper airway instability is exacerbated by the administration of anaesthetic drugs and opioid analgesics. These medications can attenuate the protective arousal mechanisms or act as muscle relaxants, further compromising airway patency. In addition, the patient's supine position, which is common during surgery and in the postoperative period, and the frequent airway oedema also contribute to respiratory collapse [8].

6.1.2 Obesity Hypoventilation Syndrome (OHS)

OHS is diagnosed by the coexistence of obesity (BMI > 30 kg/m^2) and daytime hypercapnia (arterial pressure of carbon dioxide, pCO_2, greater than 45 mmHg) in the absence of other concurrent causes of hypoventilation. It is a high-risk disorder that requires extremely careful surgical management, including the consideration of non-invasive mechanical ventilation in the perioperative period [9]. The overlap of OSA and OHS is detected relatively frequently in obese patients. Obesity aggravates OSA, which in turn can progress to OHS. Both conditions, whether isolated or combined, increase susceptibility to anaesthetic and surgical complications. The recognition of this overlap and the active search for OHS, beyond the mere detection of OSA, by performing an arterial blood gas analysis or determining serum bicarbonate levels are crucial for identifying patients who are candidates for sleeve gastrectomy with a higher risk, who will require more intensive interventions and an adapted perioperative plan [9].

6.1.3 Chronic Obstructive Pulmonary Disease (COPD)

COPD is also a common disease in obese individuals. The obstructive ventilatory alteration that this disorder causes can aggravate the daytime and nocturnal alveolar hypoventilation characteristic of patients with morbid obesity. The coexistence of obesity, COPD, and OSA has been called "triple O" (obstructive, obstruction, obesity), and it significantly increases the need for ventilatory support in various situations, such as in the perioperative period of bariatric surgery [10].

6.1.4 Bronchial Asthma

Although it is not a direct aetiological factor of bronchial asthma, obesity is a common comorbidity in asthmatic patients and is a factor that increases the incidence and severity of the disease, making asthma more difficult to control and less sensitive to usual treatments. Morbid obesity intensifies the inflammation and mechanical difficulties that make asthma more severe and resistant to treatments, while severe asthma limits physical activity, which facilitates weight gain [11].

6.2 Preoperative Pneumological Evaluation

The pneumological evaluation of a patient who is a candidate for sleeve gastrectomy should begin with an appropriate patient history and physical examination, searching for symptoms and signs that suggest respiratory alterations. Based on these findings, different complementary tests will then be requested.

6.2.1 Patient History and Physical Examination

The patient history and physical examination must be exhaustive, actively looking for symptoms that suggest respiratory pathology, especially the presence of OSA and/or OHS. The most characteristic are fatigue, daytime sleepiness, and a family member's observation of loud snoring and apnoea episodes during the patient's sleep. Other symptoms and signs are dyspnoea, nocturia, and oedema in the lower limbs [3].

During the examination, arterial oxygen saturation (SaO_2) should be measured with a pulse oximeter. An SaO2 below 92% during wakefulness and below 90% during sleep should raise suspicion of OHS, especially if it is accompanied by elevated serum bicarbonate values in the blood test (equal to or greater than 27 mmol/l). These findings indicate the need to perform an arterial blood gas analysis to confirm hypoventilation [3].

Likewise, the patient's upper airway should be examined and assessed, in anticipation that it may be a "difficult" airway for intubation. In this case, an established action protocol should be in place before the surgery, which includes endoscope-assisted intubation if necessary [3].

6.2.2 Population-Based OSA Screening Questionnaires

Nocturnal polysomnography (NPSG) is currently the gold standard for diagnosing OSA. This test has limited accessibility, requires expensive infrastructure, and, to be carried out, the patient must stay overnight in a specialised clinic or laboratory. All this implies the need to carry out population-based screening tests for the disease to detect individuals at risk of suffering from it, who will be the ones who have an indication to undergo NPSG. Training for family doctors should be encouraged in the recognition of the cardinal symptoms of the disease, especially in patients with a high BMI. Likewise, the application of the different screening methods that have been developed for the population-based diagnosis of OSA should be generalised in the field of primary health care, among which the Berlin Questionnaire and the STOP-Bang questionnaire stand out [13, 14].

The Berlin Questionnaire is one of the most widespread and used screening methods in primary care, and some studies have validated it as a predictor of OSA and an indicator of the need to perform an NPSG [15, 16].

Different studies have also shown the usefulness of the STOP-Bang questionnaire as a screening method for moderate/severe OSA [17]. Some authors consider that it has advantages over the Berlin for use in primary care, as it consists of dichotomous questions, with only the possibility of answering "yes" or "no", which makes it simpler than the Berlin questionnaire, which consists of questions that allow up to 5 response categories. A score of 3 or higher on the STOP-Bang questionnaire is a clear indication to proceed with polysomnography [3].

Recently, attempts have been made to validate an artificial intelligence tool, Machine Learning, to detect patients with possible OSA. This computer tool creates recognition patterns and makes predictions based on the data from patients' clinical histories, without having been explicitly programmed for it beforehand [12].

6.2.3 Complementary Tests

The main specific diagnostic tests that should be performed on bariatric surgery candidates to rule out or confirm suspected respiratory pathologies after the patient history and examination are the following:

6.2.3.1 Forced Spirometry

Forced spirometry is a simple, non-invasive, and low-cost technique that evaluates patient ventilation. It not only determines whether or not a ventilatory alteration exists but also indicates what type it is, obstructive or restrictive [18]. It is highly recommended that all obese patients who are candidates for any surgical procedure that requires general anaesthesia undergo an acceptable and reproducible spirometry within 3 months prior, with an adequate clinical interpretation [3]. Any spirometric alteration detected must be assessed by a pneumologist and treated appropriately before the surgery, especially in the context of bariatric surgery [3]. The recommendation that it be "acceptable and reproducible" and that the alterations be "interpreted by a pneumologist and treated" before surgery demonstrates that spirometry is a dynamic management and optimisation tool, not just a static diagnosis. Its results directly guide pre-surgical interventions, which are essential for patient safety.

Spirometry not only detects ventilatory alterations but also quantifies their severity, which is directly correlated with surgical risk. The two most important parameters for its interpretation are forced vital capacity (FVC), an alteration of which suggests the existence of a restrictive ventilatory problem, and forced expiratory volume in the first second (FEV1), an alteration of which suggests an obstructive problem. The severity of the obstructive alteration is determined based on the percentage of the reference value of the FEV1, according to the ATS/ERS guidelines [18]. Table 6.1 presents a basic interpretation guide for spirometry results, which provides bariatric surgeons with a quick and standardised reference that facilitates clinical decision-making and improves multidisciplinary communication, allowing them to quickly identify patients who require more intensive care or more aggressive optimisation before surgery.

In addition to the basal forced spirometry, a "bronchodilator test" should be performed on all patients. This consists of repeating the spirometry a few minutes after administering a bronchodilator drug to the patient, observing if there is a certain improvement in the absolute FEV1 value compared to the value observed in the basal spirometry. A positive result in this test indicates that the ventilatory obstruction is reversible, which suggests the existence of hypersensitivity and/or bronchial asthma.

6.2.3.2 Arterial Blood Gas (ABG) Analysis

ABG analysis is the fundamental test for the diagnosis of respiratory failure. It consists of measuring the arterial pressure of oxygen (pO_2) and the arterial pressure of carbon dioxide (pCO_2). The coexistence in the ABG of hypoxaemia (decrease in pO_2) and hypercapnia (increase in pCO_2) indicates that the patient has global respiratory failure and, therefore, hypoventilation. However, the ABG analysis should not be a routine test in the preoperative evaluation of all obese patients who are candidates for bariatric surgery. It should only be performed on those patients who present certain clinical histories and circumstances and to confirm the existence of OHS when suspected [3].

The criteria for the indication of preoperative ABG analysis include [3]:

- History or background of ventilatory failure in previous surgery.
- BMI > 40 kg/m^2 with an SaO_2 in the consultation of less than 93%, which suggests a risk of hypercapnia.
- Serum bicarbonate levels greater than or equal to 27 meq/l without another apparent justification, which indicates a high probability of nocturnal hypoventilation and OHS, and therefore, requires a pCO_2 determination for confirmation.

Table 6.1 Basic interpretation of spirometry results

FEV1/FVC	FVC	Suggested pattern	Severity (FEV1% predicted)
Normal	Normal	Normal	Normal
Normal	Decreased	Restrictive	Mild: > 70%
Decreased	Normal	Obstructive	Moderate: 60–69%
Decreased	Decreased	Mixed	Moderately severe: 50–59%
			Severe: 35–49%
			Very severe: < 35%

- Observation, in sleep studies, of an SaO_2 below 90% for more than 30% of the recording time. This data indicates significant nocturnal hypoxaemia and suggests nocturnal hypoventilation.
- Patients with a previous diagnosis of OSA with marked desaturation and excessive sleepiness, which implies a high suspicion of OHS.
- Patients with the "triple O" (OSA, Obesity, and COPD), which entails a high probability of nocturnal hypoventilation.
- Obese patients diagnosed with bronchial asthma, which implies a risk of hypoxaemia and hypercapnia.

Table 6.2 summarises the criteria for indicating an ABG analysis for obese patients who are candidates for bariatric surgery. This table systematises the decision of when to request an ABG analysis, helping to identify patients with a higher risk of hypoventilation, hypercapnia, and OHS, which allows the surgical and anaesthetic team to prepare a much safer and adapted perioperative management plan.

6.2.3.3 Nocturnal Polysomnography (NPSG)

NPSG is currently the gold standard for diagnosing OSA. Given the high prevalence of this disease in bariatric surgery candidates, and to avoid underdiagnosis, it seems advisable that all of them routinely undergo NPSG as part of the preoperative pneumological evaluation, even if they do not report the characteristic symptoms of the disease [5, 6]. In addition to confirming the diagnosis of OSA, NPSG allows for determining the degree of severity of the disease and assessing the need to initiate treatment with continuous positive airway pressure (CPAP) devices or other specific therapies. The AHI is the main parameter of NPSG. A polysomnographic diagnosis of OSA is considered when one of the following criteria is met [19]:

Table 6.2 Indications for preoperative ABG analysis

Clinical criterion	Justification/associated risk
History or background of ventilatory failure in previous surgery	Evaluation of the risk of hypoventilation and hypoxaemia
BMI > 40 kg/m^2 with basal SaO_2 in the consulting room <93%	Risk of hypercapnia
Venous bicarbonate ≥27 meq/l without other justification	High probability of nocturnal hypoventilation/OHS
SaO2 < 90% in sleep study oximetry for more than 30% of the recording time	Nocturnal hypoxaemia/suggestion of nocturnal hypoventilation
Nocturnal desaturation in a sleep study without obvious apnoeas	Nocturnal hypoxaemia/suggestion of nocturnal hypoventilation
OSA with marked desaturation and sleepiness	Risk of OHS
Overlap of OSA-obesity-COPD	High probability of nocturnal hypoventilation
Overlap of asthma-obesity	Risk of hypoxaemia and hypercapnia

- Presence of an AHI $\geq$ 5/h, accompanied by one or more of the following factors: excessive daytime sleepiness (quantified with the Epworth test), non-restorative sleep, excessive fatigue, and/or a deterioration in sleep-related quality of life, not justifiable by other causes.
- Presence of an AHI $\geq$ 15/h, with a predominance of obstructive apnoeas, without the apparent existence of symptoms.

The degree of OSA severity is determined by the magnitude of the AHI and the intensity and duration of desaturations during the polysomnographic recording [19]:

- Mild OSA: AHI of 5 to 14.9 events per hour.
- Moderate OSA: AHI of 15 to 29.9 events per hour.
- Severe OSA: AHI of 30 or more events per hour.

In the context of preoperative evaluation, NPSG studies, reviewed by a specialist, performed within the 3 months prior to the date of surgery are considered acceptable. Those of a greater age should be discarded, as OSA is a dynamic condition that can progress or vary in its intensity depending on circumstances such as weight changes. An alternative to NPSG in the detection of OSA in the morbidly obese could be respiratory polygraphy performed at the patient's home. Although the diagnostic capacity of polygraphy is lower than that of NPSG, and it may not detect cases of mild OSA, various studies have demonstrated its validity for detecting clinically relevant cases of OSA in obese patients [5, 6, 20].

If a sleep study is not possible (e.g., in non-elective surgeries), patients with a presumptive clinical diagnosis of OSA should be managed with the same perioperative and postoperative precautions as those with confirmed OSA [3].

6.3 Therapeutic Strategies for Preoperative Respiratory Optimisation

Once the evaluation is complete, therapeutic strategies should be carried out to optimise the patient's pulmonary function before the surgical procedure. In addition to correcting or improving the respiratory disorders detected in the evaluation, these strategies should seek to strengthen the patient's overall physiological capacity to cope with the surgical and anaesthetic stress with the best possible guarantees. The main respiratory optimisation strategies in the preoperative period for patients who are candidates for bariatric surgery are the following:

6.3.1 Smoking Cessation

Quitting smoking is an absolute recommendation for all patients undergoing bariatric surgery, especially for those diagnosed with COPD. It is advised that they stop smoking as soon as possible, ideally a year before the surgery, but at a minimum,

6 weeks before the bariatric procedure. This abstinence must also be maintained in the postoperative period, given the increased risk of delayed healing, anastomotic ulcer, and general deterioration of health associated with smoking. Given the difficulty of achieving this goal in many of the patients, the action should not be limited to generally advising the individual, and a regulated smoking cessation treatment under the supervision of a pneumologist is preferable [3].

6.3.2 Respiratory Physiotherapy

Respiratory physiotherapy is fundamentally based on training the inspiratory muscles in order to improve their strength and endurance. It is recommended that it be carried out not only in the preoperative period but also in the postoperative period to prevent the deterioration of pulmonary function after bariatric surgery [3]. It should not be limited to the patient's isolated use of an incentive spirometer, but rather comprehensive preoperative and postoperative respiratory physiotherapy is recommended. Techniques include deep breathing exercises, incentivised spirometry, early mobilisation, mobility and strengthening exercises, and bronchial hygiene techniques for airway clearance, such as postural drainage [3].

6.3.3 General Improvement of Physical Condition

Patients with morbid obesity often lead sedentary lifestyles that lead to poor physical condition. Preoperative diets, although effective in reducing fat mass, can lead to a decrease in lean mass, which can be prevented through strength training. If the patient's functional capacity allows, it is advised to implement an exercise programme focused on improving physical condition, maximising fat mass loss, and reducing lean mass loss. It is recommended to start the programme 3–6 months before the surgery, combining cardiorespiratory and strength training. It should be carried out 2 days a week, later increasing to four. The intensity should initially be moderate (40–50% of maximum oxygen consumption for cardiorespiratory training and ~50% of one repetition maximum for strength training), and then progress to higher intensities according to the patient's tolerance. For patients who are not in a condition to follow the programme, it is advised to increase the number of daily steps, starting with 5000 steps/day and progressing up to 10,000 [3].

6.3.4 Treatment of OSA and OHS

In many of the patients diagnosed with OSA, the application of CPAP devices should be initiated. CPAP is a very effective treatment for reducing the severity of OSA, and it currently remains the treatment of choice for the disease. The indication for CPAP is considered in patients with an AHI $\geq$ 15/h who also have a score greater than 10 on the Epworth Sleepiness Scale, sleep-related quality of life alterations, and/or HTA. In patients with an AHI of less than 15/h but who are very symptomatic or have significant cardiovascular or metabolic morbidity, a CPAP treatment trial could also be indicated [21].

CPAP treatment should begin at least 4 weeks before the date of surgery. In addition, this therapy should be continued as soon as possible in the post-anaesthetic care unit to minimise the risk of apnoea, hypoxaemia, or other pulmonary complications. The use of CPAP in the immediate postoperative period is safe and is not associated with an increased risk of anastomotic fistulas or dehiscences [1].

It is essential to ensure compliance and adherence to CPAP treatment for bariatric surgery candidates with OSA. Good compliance is considered to be the use of CPAP for at least 6 h per night, on a minimum of 70% of nights, which has been shown to have positive effects on neurocognitive and cardiovascular health. In addition, it must be objectively verified that the treatment is effective. According to current criteria, the goal of CPAP treatment is to achieve an Apnoea-Hypopnoea Index (AHI) of less than 10 per hour, and ideally, below 5 per hour [22].

The treatment of patients with OHS has the objectives of eliminating obstructive apnoeas and hypopnoeas and correcting nocturnal hypoxaemia and daytime hypercapnia. The recommended initial treatment is CPAP, especially if OHS is associated with OSA, as occurs in many of the patients. The titration of a CPAP as a treatment for OHS follows the same principles and protocols as in the case of OSA. If CPAP is not well tolerated or if it fails to normalise pCO_2 levels, treatment with non-invasive mechanical ventilation (NIMV) with pressure support modes, such as BiPAP or pressure support ventilation, will be initiated. It will also be used in patients with pure OHS (without significant OSA) [23].

Although weight loss after bariatric surgery usually significantly improves the symptoms of OSA and OHS, some patients may continue to have moderate, even severe, OSA. Therefore, symptomatic improvement alone is not sufficient to discontinue treatment after bariatric surgery. A new NPSG should be performed after a 10–15% body weight loss to determine the need to continue therapy and/or adjust the parameters. Clinical guidelines suggest continuing CPAP/NIMV for at least 3–6 months after surgery [1].

6.3.5 Treatment of Bronchial Asthma and COPD

In patients with bronchial asthma and/or COPD who are candidates for sleeve gastrectomy, it is essential to optimise the control of these conditions before surgery. This involves ensuring that the patient is stable in terms of their symptoms with the appropriate use of medication and, if necessary, consulting with a pneumologist to adjust the treatment.

6.4 Perioperative and Postoperative Respiratory Considerations

The management of the bariatric patient in the perioperative and postoperative setting requires specific strategies to minimise respiratory complications [1]:

- During anaesthetic induction, pre-oxygenation with 100% oxygen is advisable.
- Short-acting and easily reversible anaesthetic agents and muscle relaxants should be selected to facilitate early and safe extubation.
- It is crucial to maximise efforts to control the risk of gastro-oesophageal reflux and pulmonary aspiration, a serious complication in this population.
- To optimise oxygenation and pulmonary mechanics, the reverse Trendelenburg position (raising the head and upper part of the chest 20–30° above the horizontal plane) is recommended.
- During anaesthetic induction in patients with OSA, the use of CPAP can help maintain functional residual capacity and reduce desaturation time.
- Benzodiazepines should be avoided and low doses of short-acting opioids should be used, as patients with OSA are particularly sensitive to these drugs.
- Continuous monitoring of oxygenation by oximetry, and of PCO_2 levels with capnography, is recommended.
- Extubation should be performed when spontaneous ventilation and oxygenation are adequate, with the patient in a semi-seated position, ensuring that airway reflexes are preserved and that the effects of neuromuscular blockers have been completely reversed.
- It is important to note that atelectasis persists for a longer time in obese patients, which increases the risk of postoperative hypoxaemia.
- In the early postoperative period, the use of sedatives and opioids should be minimised and a semi-seated position is recommended to reduce postoperative hypoxaemia, diaphragmatic dysfunction, and obstructive events.
- Patients who require supplemental oxygen should be administered the lowest oxygen flow that maintains adequate saturation and PCO_2 levels should be monitored with capnography or ABG analysis, as in patients with OSA, oxygen administration without CPAP can worsen CO_2 retention and decrease protective micro-arousals.

References

1. Stenberg E, Dos Reis Falcão LF, O'Kane M, Liem R, Pournaras DJ, Salminen P, et al. Guidelines for perioperative care in bariatric surgery: enhanced recovery after surgery (ERAS) society recommendations: a 2021 update. World J Surg. 2022;46(4):729–51.
2. Ruiz-Tovar J, Martínez R, Bonete JM, et al. Long-term weight and metabolic effects of laparoscopic sleeve gastrectomy calibrated with a 50-Fr bougie. Obes Surg. 2016;26(1):32–7.

3. Mechanick JI, Apovian C, Brethauer S, Garvey WT, Joffe AM, Kim J, et al. Clinical practice guidelines for the perioperative nutrition, metabolic, and nonsurgical support of patients undergoing bariatric procedures—2019 update: cosponsored by American Association of Clinical Endocrinologists/American College of Endocrinology, the Obesity Society, American Society for Metabolic & Bariatric Surgery, Obesity Medicine Association, and American Society of Anesthesiologists - executive summary. Endocr Pract. 2019;25(12):1346–59.
4. Ribeiro JP, Araújo A, Vieira C, Vasconcelos F, Pinto PM, Seixas B, et al. Undiagnosed risk of obstructive sleep apnea in obese individuals in a primary health care context. Acta Medica Port. 2020;33(3):161–5.
5. Van Veldhuisen SL, Nijland LMG, Ravesloot MJL, de Vries N, van Veen RN, Hazebroek EJ, et al. Preoperative assessment of obstructive sleep apnea in bariatric patients using polysomnography or polygraphy. Obes Surg. 2022;32(6):1814–21.
6. Khan A, King WC, Patterson EJ, Laut J, Raum W, Courcoulas AP, et al. Assessment of obstructive sleep apnea in adults undergoing bariatric surgery in the longitudinal assessment of bariatric surgery-2 (LABS-2) study. J Clin Sleep Med. 2013;9(1):21–9.
7. Loo GH, Rajan R, Mohd Tamil A, Ritza KN. Prevalence of obstructive sleep apnea in an Asian bariatric population: an underdiagnosed dilemma. Surg Obes Relat Dis. 2020;16(6):778–83.
8. Ruiz-Tovar J, Sanchez-Santos R, Martín-García-Almenta E, García Villabona E, Hernandez AM, Hernández-Matías A, et al. Enhanced recovery after bariatric surgery. Cir Esp (Engl Ed). 2019;97(10):551–9.
9. Bjork S, Jain D, Marliere MH, Predescu SA, Mokhlesi B. Obstructive sleep apnea, obesity hypoventilation syndrome, and pulmonary hypertension: a state-of-the-art review. Sleep Med Clin. 2024;19(2):307–25.
10. Hanson C, Rutten EP, Wouters EF, Rennard S. Influence of diet and obesity on COPD development and outcomes. Int J Chron Obstruct Pulmon Dis. 2014;9:723–33.
11. Moitra S, et al. Long-term effect of asthma on the development of obesity among adults: an international cohort study, ECRHS. Thorax. 2022;77(1):5–12.
12. Aiyer I, Shaik L, Sheta A, Surani S. Review of application of machine learning as a screening tool for diagnosis of obstructive sleep apnea. Medicina (Kaunas). 2022;58(11):1574.
13. Chung F, Abdullah H, Liao P. STOP-Bang questionnaire: a practical approach to screen for obstructive sleep apnea. Chest. 2016;149:631–8.
14. Ramachandran SK, Josephs LA. A meta-analysis of clinical screening tests for obstructive sleep apnea. Anesthesiology. 2009;110(4):928–39.
15. Netzer NC, Stoohs RA, Netzer CM, Clark K, Strohl KP. Using the Berlin questionnaire to identify patients at risk for the sleep apnea syndrome. Ann Intern Med. 1999;131(7):485–91.
16. Chung F, Yegneswaran B, Liao P, et al. Validation of the Berlin questionnaire and American Society of Anesthesiologists checklist as screening tools for obstructive sleep apnea in surgical patients. Anesthesiology. 2008;108(5):822–30.
17. Muñoz-Gómez R, Navarrete-Martínez E, Serrano-Merino J, Silva-Gil F, Roldán-Villalobos A, Martín-Rioboó E, et al. The usefulness of the Spanish version of the STOP-Bang questionnaire for screening for moderate or severe sleep apnea syndrome in primary care. Front Public Health. 2022;10:975114.
18. Bhakta NR, McGowan A, Ramsey KA, Borg B, Kivastik J, Knight SL, et al. European Respiratory Society/American Thoracic Society technical statement: standardisation of the measurement of lung volumes, 2023 update. Eur Respir J. 2023;62(4):2201519.
19. Ito E, Inoue Y. The international classification of sleep disorders, third edition. American Academy of Sleep Medicine. Nihon Rinsho. 2015;73(6):916–23.
20. de Raaff CAL, Gorter-Stam MAW, de Vries N, Sinha AC, Jaap Bonjer H, Chung F, et al. Perioperative management of obstructive sleep apnea in bariatric surgery: a consensus guideline. Surg Obes Relat Dis. 2017;13(7):1095–109.
21. Mediano O, González Mangado N, Montserrat JM, et al. Documento internacional de consenso sobre apnea obstructiva del sueño. Arch Bronconeumol. 2022;58:3–41.

22. Kapur VK, Auckley DH, Chowdhuri S, Kuhlmann DC, Mehra R, Ramar K, et al. Clinical practice guideline for diagnostic testing for adult obstructive sleep apnea: an American Academy of Sleep Medicine clinical practice guideline. J Clin Sleep Med. 2017;13(3):479–504.
23. Mokhlesi B, Masa JF, Brozek JL, Gurubhagavatula I, Murphy PB, Piper AJ, et al. Evaluation and management of obesity hypoventilation syndrome. An official American Thoracic Society clinical practice guideline. Am J Respir Crit Care Med. 2019;200(3):e6–e24.

Preoperative Nursing Evaluation 7

Maria-Cruz Signoret-Romero-De-Avila

7.1 Introduction

Preoperative nursing assessment in gastric sleeve surgery is fundamental for managing comorbidities [1–3] commonly present in patients with morbid obesity, enabling their identification, control, and stabilization to prevent intraoperative and postoperative complications, thereby contributing to patient safety.

The main comorbidities observed in patients with morbid obesity include type 2 diabetes, arterial hypertension, obstructive sleep apnea syndrome, and dyslipidemia.

7.1.1 Type 2 Diabetes

Poor glycemic control can lead to metabolic disturbances during surgery, impair wound healing, and increase the risk of postoperative infection [4–6].

A thorough nursing assessment can address these aspects by performing an exhaustive record of blood glucose monitoring, evaluating the presence of hyperglycemia or significant variability in glucose levels [4–6]. Treatment adherence, whether with oral antidiabetic agents or insulin, must be assessed. Finally, patients should be educated on preventing hypoglycemia during the preoperative fasting period by adjusting basal insulin and discontinuing oral antidiabetic medications before surgery.

M.-C. Signoret-Romero-De-Avila (✉)
Alcala de Henares University, Madrid, Spain

J. Ruiz-Tovar (ed.), *Multidisciplinary Management of Sleeve Gastrectomy*,
https://doi.org/10.1007/978-3-032-25644-7_7

7.1.2 Arterial Hypertension

Poorly controlled blood pressure for a prolonged period before surgery may pose intraoperative risks such as bleeding, hemodynamic instability, arrhythmias, or cerebrovascular events during the procedure.

The nurse should monitor blood pressure at different times of the day to obtain accurate readings, verify adherence to pharmacological treatment and lifestyle recommendations, and review laboratory data to assess potential renal or cardiac damage related to hypertension. Patients should be educated on the importance of not discontinuing antihypertensive medication prior to surgery [7].

7.1.3 Obstructive Sleep Apnea Syndrome

Obstructive sleep apnea is one of the most hazardous comorbidities for anesthesia. It increases the risk of hypoxia during anesthesia, reintubation, and opioid-induced respiratory depression in the postoperative period [8].

Through assessment, nurses can detect undiagnosed cases by asking about snoring, breathing pauses, daytime sleepiness (Epworth scale) [8], nocturnal sweating, and morning headaches. If the patient is already diagnosed and uses a Continuous Positive Airway Pressure (CPAP) device, proper device use should be verified and the patient should be instructed to bring it on the day of surgery. Neck circumference should be measured in all patients, with risk indicators being greater than (>) 40–43 cm in men and 35–38 cm in women. Finally, respiratory patterns should be assessed, including thoracic expansion, functional capacity, and respiratory effort.

7.1.4 Dyslipidemia

Altered triglyceride and cholesterol levels are common in obese patients. Dyslipidemia leads to atherosclerosis, hypertension, and cardiovascular disease, increasing intraoperative risk for arrhythmias, ischemic events, and reduced tolerance to surgical stress [9]. Additionally, fatty liver may complicate laparoscopic access, increasing bleeding risk and sometimes prolonging surgery.

The nurse should review laboratory data on cholesterol and triglycerides, assess adherence to pharmacological treatment, and explain the need for a preoperative diet low in carbohydrates and fats. Alcohol consumption should be strongly discouraged [9].

7.2 Nutritional Education

Proper nutritional education prior to gastric sleeve surgery is essential for the success of the surgical intervention, as well as for reducing or preventing complications and optimizing postoperative outcomes.

Through assessment, nurses can identify behavioral patterns that may compromise the success of the procedure. These include binge eating with loss of control, using food to manage anxiety or stress, continuous snacking, overeating after restrictive diets, or using certain foods as rewards [12, 13]. A thorough evaluation may lead to referral to psychology before surgery to improve the patient's relationship with food. The following scales can be used: BES, EDE-Q, DEBQ, PHQ-9, GAD-7, and emotional eating questionnaires [12].

7.3 Dietary Recommendations

It is highly recommended that patients follow a hypocaloric, high-protein diet for 1–4 weeks before surgery, not only to reduce weight but also to promote metabolic changes that facilitate postoperative recovery. Guidelines aim for a diet of 800–1200 kcal/day, depending on patient characteristics, with 60–100 g of protein per day, low in carbohydrates (especially simple sugars), and completely limiting saturated fats while allowing small amounts of unsaturated fats. Water intake should be 1.5–2 liters per day [10, 11].

7.4 Beneficial Effects of Preoperative Weight Loss

Preoperative weight reduction offers multiple benefits. Surgically, reducing liver size makes the procedure safer, and decreased visceral fat facilitates laparoscopic access, reducing bleeding risk and shortening operative time [10]. Regarding anesthesia, weight loss improves respiratory function, minimizing intubation difficulties and reducing cardiac and thrombotic complications. Psychologically, it reinforces patient motivation and helps to establish habits that will be crucial during the postoperative period.

7.5 Training in Fractionated and Mindful Eating Techniques

The success of gastric sleeve surgery is not solely due to reducing stomach capacity by 70–80%; a change in the patient's relationship with food is necessary for satisfactory and lasting results.

Mindful eating refers to all recommendations aimed at teaching patients to eat attentively, without haste or automatic behaviors. Patients should be instructed on the importance of eating without distractions, avoiding screens during meals, eating slowly (20–30 min per meal), chewing each bite 20–30 times, and taking pauses.

Additionally, after bariatric surgery, the stomach has much less capacity; without fractionated eating, patients may experience pain, regurgitation, and vomiting. Therefore, patients should eat 5–6 small meals throughout the day, avoid skipping meals, start each meal with protein, and refrain from drinking fluids 30 min before and after eating [12].

7.6 Barriers to Dietary Adherence

Patients often experience feelings of loss of control, anxiety, and low self-esteem, leading to emotional and uncontrolled eating.

Social barriers may include uncooperative family members, social pressure to eat certain foods, frequent social events, and long work hours that hinder meal planning.

Economic barriers may involve the higher cost of healthy foods or protein supplements, and lack of time for weekly meal planning and cooking can be a significant obstacle to following dietary recommendations.

Nursing assessment can identify these barriers using standardized questionnaires such as BES and EDE-Q, conducting thorough nutritional interviews, analyzing usual eating patterns, maintaining food records, and involving family and social support in the process [12].

To help patients overcome these challenges, psychological support should be provided, participation in support groups encouraged, and guidance offered on weekly meal planning and affordable healthy food alternatives.

7.7 Patient Motivation for Dietary Adherence

Patient motivation is a key factor in adhering to dietary recommendations, preventing postoperative complications, and avoiding future weight regain.

Low motivation may stem from low self-esteem, frustration from previous failed attempts, anxiety, or unrealistic expectations about the procedure, such as believing surgery alone guarantees weight loss [12].

To address this, it is essential to establish a trusting relationship with the bariatric surgery team, explaining preoperative recommendations clearly so the patient understands their purpose and health benefits. This approach promotes active patient involvement throughout the process and increases motivation.

7.8 Promotion of Healthy Lifestyle Habits

One of the main recommendations for patients is to establish a routine of regular physical exercise before bariatric surgery. This helps with preoperative weight loss, improves cardiovascular and respiratory function, enhances physical condition for recovery, fosters adherence to healthy lifestyle habits, boosts self-esteem, and reduces stress and anxiety [14, 15].

Exercise should be personalized, gradual, and safe according to the patient's functional limitations. High-impact activities are discouraged; instead, patients should progressively increase daily walks until reaching 20–30 min per day. If physical condition allows, cycling or swimming 2–3 times per week can be recommended, alternating with 30-min walks. To prevent muscle loss during a hypocaloric diet, simple strength exercises adapted to each patient should be indicated.

Smoking cessation and alcohol abstinence are essential for preparing patients before bariatric surgery [2, 3]. These habits increase anesthetic risk, respiratory complications, likelihood of leaks, impaired wound healing, and overall poorer long-term outcomes. Nurses should conduct a detailed assessment of both habits to provide effective guidance and support for cessation prior to surgery. Initially, patients should be educated on the impact of these habits on surgical outcomes. A multidisciplinary approach may involve referral to support groups or psychological therapy, and pharmacological interventions may be considered if necessary. The most critical recommendations include quitting smoking at least 4 weeks before surgery (ideally 8 weeks) and abstaining from alcohol for 4 weeks prior to surgery, although heavy drinkers should aim for 3 months and undergo psychiatric evaluation.

Other important factors include sleep hygiene and stress management, as both negatively affect preoperative and postoperative outcomes. Stress and poor sleep increase blood pressure, irritability, reduce adherence to preoperative recommendations, perpetuate binge eating, and make healthy decision-making more difficult [12].

For sleep hygiene, patients should maintain a regular sleep schedule, avoid long naps and electronic devices before bedtime, and establish a bedtime routine. Heavy meals should be avoided before sleep, with no food intake 2–3 h before bedtime, and large amounts of water should not be consumed before sleeping. Energy drinks, coffee, and tea should be avoided from mid-afternoon onward.

For stress control, simple relaxation exercises, distraction techniques to shift focus away from stress triggers, and deep breathing exercises, as emotional regulation therapy, can be recommended.

7.9 Surgical Preparation and Perioperative Planning

Patients should approach bariatric surgery with clear information about the process. They should understand that the stomach will have a capacity of 100–150 ml without causing malabsorption issues. This will result in a 60–70% excess body weight loss, improving quality of life and controlling chronic diseases prevalent in this population [1, 2].

The surgical procedure, performed via minimally invasive laparoscopic access, typically takes about one to one and a half hours. Hospital stay generally does not exceed 2 days. Depending on their occupation, patients can usually return to work within 1 month.

In addition to the preoperative hypocaloric, high-protein diet, patients should follow a liquid diet for 1 or 2 days before surgery. A 6-h fasting period must be respected, with the last meal being light. Clear liquids are allowed up to 2 h before surgery.

Patients may take antihypertensive medications (except ACE inhibitors/ARBs), antidepressants, anxiolytics, levothyroxine, and statins before surgery. Insulin doses should be adjusted the night before and the morning of surgery. Medications that must be discontinued include metformin and anticoagulants. Patients should be advised to avoid non-steroidal anti-inflammatory drugs (NSAIDs) days before surgery due to the risk of ulcers and bleeding [10].

Although gastric sleeve surgery is generally safe, it is not free from risks and complications, which largely depend on surgical technique, the patient's preoperative health status, and adherence to preoperative recommendations.

The most serious early complication is leakage, which occurs when the stomach does not heal properly and gastric contents leak, potentially causing abscesses, peritonitis, or sepsis, significantly prolonging hospital stay. Other early risks include hemorrhage (internal or external), infection, pulmonary thromboembolism, especially in patients with severe obesity and smoking history, and respiratory complications such as pneumonia, particularly in untreated sleep apnea patients. Other complications may include gastroesophageal reflux (common due to the tubular shape of the stomach), nausea, and vomiting [16].

Late complications may include sleeve stenosis or obstruction, leading to persistent vomiting, pain after eating, and inability to progress the diet; nutritional deficiencies (vitamin B12, iron, vitamin D, calcium, and protein); and weight regain within 2–3 years due to noncompliance with the nutritional plan.

7.10 Postoperative Care and Organization of Resources at Discharge

Postoperative care for this type of surgery aims to protect the suture line, ensure adequate hydration and nutrition, and promote the acquisition of new eating and behavioral habits.

Initially, pain management is a priority. Nurses should use pain assessment scales such as the Visual Analog Scale (VAS). Pain is usually associated with residual gas from laparoscopic access and typically does not last more than 5–7 days. To alleviate it, patients will be instructed to use analgesics (paracetamol and mild opioids), avoiding NSAIDs due to bleeding risk.

To protect the suture line, omeprazole will be prescribed for 2–3 months. Nausea should be controlled, as it increases intragastric pressure and may pose a leakage risk; patients should be advised to seek medical attention if nausea persists.

Regarding diet, only clear liquids (water, infusions, sugar-free gelatine, fat-free broth…) are allowed during the first 2 days, and patients should sip slowly rather than drink large gulps. The goal is to reach 600–800 ml per day initially and gradually increase to 1.5–2 liters by one-month post-surgery. During the following 1–2 weeks, full liquids will be introduced, including protein shakes, liquid yogurt, skim milk, and soups. From the second week to the first month, pureed foods (soft vegetables, chicken, and fish) can be added. If the patient experiences pressure, hiccups, or nausea, they should return to previously tolerated foods. After the first month, soft solids can be introduced, progressing to full chewing (shredded chicken, tender meat, fish, tuna, peeled ripe fruits, steamed vegetables, etc.) [17]. Patients must be instructed to eat slowly and chew each bite 20–30 times. From 6 weeks onward, a complete diet based on lifelong healthy habits should be followed, prioritizing protein, vegetables, soluble fiber, healthy fats, and limiting complex carbohydrates. Carbonated drinks and drinking with a straw should be avoided due to increased intragastric pressure.

Patients will require lifelong vitamin supplementation, including complete multivitamins, vitamin B12, iron, calcium, and vitamin D3 according to laboratory results [17].

Wound care consists of keeping incisions clean and dry, using soap and water, avoiding creams, and leaving wounds uncovered from the second day onward. Patients should monitor incision sites for color changes or discharge. Sutures are typically removed about 10 days after surgery.

Early mobilization should be encouraged from the first postoperative day to promote bowel function and prevent thromboembolism. If thrombotic risk is present, anticoagulants will be prescribed for 1–2 weeks. Physical activity should gradually increase until normal activity resumes within the first month, avoiding heavy lifting to protect the abdominal wall. From the second month, strength training, swimming, and cycling are recommended [15].

As part of a multidisciplinary approach, patients will have outpatient follow-up appointments with various professionals after discharge.

- The surgeon will review the patient 15 days post-surgery, then monthly during the first trimester, followed by visits every 3–6 months until annual check-ups.
- The nurse will monitor surgical wounds, watch for signs of infection, and remove sutures as scheduled.
- The nutritionist will oversee progressive dietary phases during the first year.
- The primary care physician will continue managing comorbidities (hypertension, diabetes, sleep apnea, etc.).
- The psychologist and psychiatrist will address anxiety management and adaptation to the new situation.

All professionals involved should assess family support, especially during the first days after discharge, ensuring the patient has help with meals, shopping, and household tasks. Patients should be informed about support groups to help them cope with lifestyle changes and provide reassurance through interaction with others in similar situations.

References

1. Angrisani L, Santonicola A, Iovino P, Formisano G, Buchwald H, Scopinaro N. Bariatric surgery worldwide 2019. Obes Surg. 2021;31:2471–82.
2. Sociedad Española de Cirugía de la Obesidad (SECO). Guía de práctica clínica para el manejo de la obesidad mórbida. Madrid: SECO; 2022.
3. American Society for Metabolic and Bariatric Surgery (ASMBS). ASMBS clinical guidelines. ASMBS; 2020.
4. Alfaro-LeFevre R. Aplicación del proceso enfermero. 8th ed. Barcelona: Elsevier; 2014.

5. Carpenito LJ. Diagnósticos enfermeros: aplicación a la práctica clínica. 15th ed. Madrid: Wolters Kluwer; 2019.
6. American Diabetes Association. Standards of medical Care in Diabetes—2023. Diabetes Care. 2023;46(Suppl 1):S1–290.
7. Williams B, Mancia G, Spiering W, et al. ESH guidelines for the management of arterial hypertension. J Hypertens. 2023;41:187–300.
8. Epstein LJ, Kristo D, Strollo PJ Jr, et al. Clinical guideline for the evaluation, management and long-term care of obstructive sleep apnea in adults. J Clin Sleep Med. 2009;5(3):263–76.
9. Grundy SM, Stone NJ, Bailey AL, et al. 2018 AHA/ACC guideline on the management of blood cholesterol. Circulation. 2019;139:e1082–143.
10. Mechanick JI, Youdim A, Jones DB, et al. Clinical practice guidelines for the perioperative nutrition, metabolic, and nonsurgical support of patients undergoing bariatric procedures. Obesity (Silver Spring). 2020;28(4):O1–58.
11. Sociedad Española de Endocrinología y Nutrición (SEEN). Protocolo nutricional en cirugía bariátrica. Madrid: SEEN; 2022.
12. Fairburn CG. Cognitive behavior therapy and eating disorders. New York: Guilford Press; 2008.
13. Kroenke K, Spitzer RL, Williams JBW. The PHQ-9: validity of a brief depression severity measure. J Gen Intern Med. 2001;16:606–13.
14. American College of Sports Medicine (ACSM). ACSM'S guidelines for exercise testing and prescription. 11th ed. Philadelphia: Lippincott Williams & Wilkins; 2021.
15. World Health Organization. WHO guidelines on physical activity and sedentary behaviour. Geneva: WHO; 2020.
16. Busetto L, Dicker D, Azran C, et al. Practical recommendations of the obesity management task force of the European Association for the Study of obesity for the post-bariatric surgery medical management. Obes Facts. 2017;10:597–632.
17. Sociedad Española de Cirugía de la Obesidad (SECO), Sociedad Española de Endocrinología y Nutrición (SEEN). Seguimiento multidisciplinar tras cirugía bariátrica. Madrid: SECO-SEEN; 2021.

Part II

Intraoperative Procedure

Surgical Technique

8

Arturo Cruz-Cidoncha

8.1 Introduction

Since its origin as a partial sleeve gastrectomy performed by Doug Hess in 1988 as an intermediate step in duodenal switches, it has been demonstrated to have good functionality as a unique procedure. It has evolved from open to laparoscopic techniques, and is currently the most frequently performed bariatric surgery technique due to its effectiveness in weight loss and improvement of comorbidities. It is considered the most widespread bariatric surgical procedure worldwide. In recent years, the high efficacy of this procedure has been proven, both associated with the restrictive component and with the modifications of hormonal control that occur in these patients.

According to the American Gastroenterological Association and The Obesity Society, sleeve gastrectomy is a first-line surgical option in the global management of obesity, yielding excellent results regarding metabolic improvement and weight loss compared to other surgical procedures. Likewise, it is a procedure that presents a lower percentage of complications compared to other surgical interventions for the management of obesity [1, 2].

In order to minimize the risks of morbidity and mortality associated with the procedure, it is essential to be meticulous with every step. A wrong decision, an incorrect measurement, or undue traction could imply a complication or an undesired outcome. Therefore, it is important to know the technical details of the surgical intervention and the possible complications.

A. Cruz-Cidoncha (✉)
Department of General and Digestive Surgery, Henares University Hospital, Madrid, Spain

Alfonso X El Sabio University, Madrid, Spain

J. Ruiz-Tovar (ed.), *Multidisciplinary Management of Sleeve Gastrectomy*,
https://doi.org/10.1007/978-3-032-25644-7_8

8.2 Most Frequent Complications Associated with the Surgical Technique

8.2.1 Hemorrhage

Bleeding is associated with up to a tenfold increase in the risk of mortality. Therefore, extreme care must be taken during the surgical technique, especially regarding aspects related to effective hemostasis. This complication can fundamentally be associated with trocar placement or intraluminal bleeding, although intraperitoneal hemorrhages can also occur due to other causes. Several patient factors are more frequently associated with bleeding, such as advanced age, prior cardiac surgery, arterial hypertension, chronic kidney failure, use of anticoagulant therapy, diabetes mellitus, and obstructive sleep apnea. Conversely, staple-line reinforcement and over-sewing or an elevated body mass index are protective factors against bleeding. Postoperative bleeding following sleeve gastrectomy occurs in slightly above 15% of cases [3, 4].

8.2.2 Staple Line Leak

Leaks in the sleeve gastrectomy suture line occur between 0% and 5.5% according to the literature. Although it does not involve an anastomosis, it is more frequent than in other bariatric procedures because it requires a long staple line for the creation of the gastric sleeve. Moreover, the gastric remnant, after resection of a large part of the stomach, located between the pylorus and the lower esophageal sphincter, harbors high pressures. On the other hand, the staple line can present areas of ischemia, hematoma, and staple failure, which favors leaks [5, 6].

8.2.3 Stenosis

Stenoses of the gastric sleeve are reported between 0.26% and 4%. Less than 1% are symptomatic and require endoscopic or surgical treatment. The causes of stenosis include the use of excessively thin bougies or the creation of a torsional sleeve. Functional stenoses can occur transiently due to edema or hematomas that typically resolve with conservative treatment [7].

8.2.4 Gastroesophageal Reflux (GER)

One of the frequent problems in sleeve gastrectomy is the appearance of gastroesophageal reflux or the worsening of pre-existing GER. Pre-existing esophagitis and Barrett's esophagus may appear or worsen, and a small percentage of patients may require conversion to Roux-en-Y gastric bypass (RYGB). Increased reflux risk has been associated with an altered reservoir morphology, a narrow reservoir (due to the use of small-caliber bougies), and a greater distance from the start of the resection to the pylorus [8].

8.2.5 Portomesenteric Thrombosis

A small percentage of patients undergoing bariatric surgery, and especially sleeve gastrectomy, may present with portomesenteric thrombosis. To prevent thrombotic complications, compression devices on the limbs and low-molecular-weight heparin prophylaxis are employed. Clinically, portomesenteric thrombosis usually presents with epigastric pain and is typically diagnosed via abdominal CT scan. Stable patients with non-occlusive disease will require anticoagulation for 3–6 months, whereas patients presenting with occlusive disease require thrombolysis and/or thrombectomy with subsequent anticoagulation.

8.3 Surgical Procedure

8.3.1 Patient Positioning

The patient is placed in the supine position with French legs (abducted legs), which facilitates the placement of the surgeon and access to the abdominal cavity. Some surgeons advocate for other positions, placing themselves to the left of the patient, although the French position remains the most commonly used worldwide. Pressure areas must be padded. Fixation devices using a vacuum mattress or straps should be used to prevent displacement during the intervention. A pneumatic anti-thrombotic prophylaxis device must be applied to minimize the possible risks of deep venous thrombosis in the lower limbs. The surgeon stands between the legs, the camera assistant stands to the patient's right, and the first assistant and instrument nurse stand to the patient's left [1].

8.3.2 Trocar Placement and Surgical Field Exposure

The most accepted arrangement is a reverse trapezoid pattern with a predominance on the left side of the abdomen, which facilitates the exposure and manipulation of the stomach. An anesthetic is administered locally with lidocaine or mepivacaine at the trocar insertion sites. Specific trocars with lengths up to 15 cm must be used for trocar placement in bariatric surgery procedures. Among the various trocar optic locations, the supraumbilical level is the most frequent. Additional trocars will be placed under direct vision. A 5 mm trocar is placed at the subxiphoid level for the hepatic separator. In the anterior axillary line of the upper left quadrant, a 5 mm trocar is placed at the level of the twelfth rib for the assistant. Accessory 12 mm trocars for endostapler insertion are placed in the upper right quadrant, epigastrium, upper left quadrant, or right paramedian line for endostapler placement.

It is advisable to use a hepatic separator to minimize the risk of hepatic lacerations. The Nathanson liver retractor or a similar one can be used.

8.4 Surgical Fundamentals

The surgical procedure carries several risks. Early complications, common to many surgeries, include hemorrhage, thrombus formation, staple line leaks, or infection. Late complications may include nutritional deficiencies, such as vitamin B12 or iron deficiency, weight regain, or the onset or worsening of gastroesophageal reflux. To prevent these, technical details associated with postoperative complications must be considered.

8.4.1 Reservoir Creation. Size, and Shape

Sleeve gastrectomy is a restrictive bariatric procedure that involves the creation of a reduced gastric reservoir (ranging from 90 to 220 ml according to various authors) by resecting the majority of the greater gastric curvature (70–80%) while maintaining a reduced tubular structure along the lesser curvature, which exhibits less distensibility. A minimum volume threshold for the reservoir exists to induce sustained weight loss; therefore, a significant reduction in the volume of the gastric remnant is crucial for procedural success. The tubular configuration presents superior outcomes compared to others.

8.4.2 Pressure and Weight Loss Correlation

Due to the increase in pressure generated within the reservoir at larger volumes, weight loss is lower with greater safety for the staple line, whereas at smaller volumes, initial weight loss is greater, albeit with an increased risk at the staple line. This inverse correlation tends to equalize over time [9, 10].

The significant reduction in gastric capacity induces the development of early satiety and limitation of intake in patients, potentially leading to vomiting in cases of copious consumption.

8.4.3 Bougie Insertion

The role of a bougie is to serve as a calibrating guide to define the diameter and shape of the gastric sleeve during resection. The majority of experts in obesity surgery agree on the need to calibrate the gastric sleeve. For this, a bougie must be inserted transorally by an experienced anesthetist, given the risk of esophageal injury. This operator must position the bougie alongside the lesser curvature, under direct visualization of the pylorus. The optimal bougie caliber remains debated, although most surgeons utilize a 36 French size. With larger calibers, there is a risk of insufficient restriction, resulting in very limited weight loss or excessively early weight regain. Calibers smaller than 32 French could create an overly narrow sleeve with elevated pressures, increasing the risk of stenosis or staple line leak. Regarding bleeding from the staple line, larger-sized bougies and a prolonged duration of the intervention increase the risk [11].

Following the placement of the trocars and hepatic retraction, the entire lesser gastric curvature is fully exposed, from the right crus of the diaphragm down to the pylorus. The surgeon must identify the pylorus by visualizing the pre-pyloric vein of Mayo and by laparoscopic palpation. Furthermore, the presence of hiatal diaphragmatic hernias must be evaluated during the procedure. Significant hernias should be repaired using standard techniques [12].

8.4.4 Gastric Mobilization

Once the location of the gastric transection is identified, the greater curvature is devascularized using an advanced vascular sealing device, proceeding from the pyloric region to the fundic region, including the division and sealing of the short gastric vessels. During the mobilization of the greater curvature and the gastric portion to be resected, the posterior gastric adhesions must be released, including the posterior gastric vessels, until the left crus of the diaphragmatic esophageal hiatus is identified. Bleeding in the short gastric vessels may occasionally occur; to prevent this, careful ligation using specific sealing devices is essential. Hemorrhage of the splenic surface may also occur at this level due to small lacerations of the capsule, which are usually controllable with compression or hemostatic agents. Exceptionally, in the presence of major bleeding, a splenectomy is necessary. To prevent splenic hemorrhage, adequate exposure of the upper left quadrant of the abdomen during the intervention is advised. It is important to note that the vascular supply of the lesser curvature via the left gastric artery must be preserved, as this alone will guarantee the vascularity of the gastric sleeve.

8.4.5 Distance to the Pylorus and Antral Resection

Following gastric mobilization, resection must proceed. A technical detail of importance is the distance of the staple line to the pylorus. During the procedure, the stomach is vertically divided along the lesser curvature, typically starting between 2 and 6 cm proximal to the pylorus, leaving the pyloric sphincter intact and a viable portion of the antrum. There is debate regarding whether the staple line should be positioned closer to or further from the pylorus. Following the division of the greater gastric curvature vessels, the mechanical stapling most commonly begins in an intermediate position, approximately 4 centimeters from the pylorus. The distance of the staple line from the pylorus dictates the extent of antral resection, which directly affects the surgical outcomes. Greater distances may reduce risks but yield poorer results, while distances closer to the pylorus may improve functional results despite higher risks. A retrospective study from the American College of Surgeons (ACS) Metabolic and Bariatric Surgery Accreditation and Quality Improvement Program (MBSAQIP) database found that the combination of a staple line distance of 4 centimeters or more from the pylorus associated with a bougie calibration smaller than 36 French presented a lower probability of developing dehydration [13] (Fig. 8.1).

Conversely, the gastric sleeve alters pyloric physiology. Several studies show an increase in postoperative pyloric distensibility, which contributes to changes in gastric emptying and the worsening of gastroesophageal reflux. The pylorus maintains functional gastric emptying, regulating it and preventing rapid emptying into the duodenum, which distinguishes the gastric sleeve from the Roux-en-Y Gastric Bypass. In cases where the section begins further from the pylorus, there would be partial preservation of the antrum, which, according to some authors, could accelerate gastric emptying. However, controversy remains as to whether greater antral preservation would imply faster gastric emptying, while other authors argue the opposite. Various studies comparing antral resection versus preservation demonstrate that, although there is greater initial weight loss in patients with antral resection, this equalizes 1 year after the intervention [14–16].

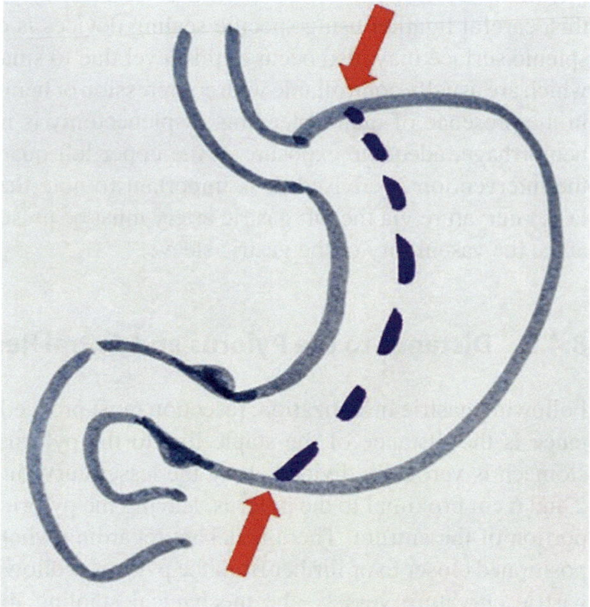

Fig. 8.1 There are two critical points in the formation of the gastric sleeve. One is at the antral level, where an appropriate distance from the pylorus must be chosen, and the other is at the angle of His, where the gastric resection is completed

8.4.6 Tubular Configuration

The stapling line proceeds up to the angle of His, adjusting the transection to the bougie. Among the staple cartridges available for the endo-stapler, those whose staple height corresponds to the thickness of the gastric wall should be selected. The majority of leaks occur in the proximal staple line, near the gastroesophageal junction, within the first 15 days post-surgery. Hence, the proper selection of the staple cartridge based on the tissue characteristics, particularly its thickness, is of great importance. The management of leaks is individualized per case, following recommendations from the 2011 expert consensus panel and the American Society for Metabolic and Bariatric Surgery. Treatment modalities include conservative management, the use of stents, surgical re-intervention, or even conversion of the procedure to RYGB (Roux-en-Y Gastric Bypass).

A technical detail of great importance is that during the gastric section, twisting of the sleeve should be avoided, as this can lead to the formation of a stenosis zone. Special care should be taken in the area of the incisura angularis, as this is often the point of origin of stenosis or twisting. Both twisting and stenosis can be associated with distal sleeve obstruction, which is the cause of most leaks and their persistence in the most proximal part of the staple line during the postoperative period. To avoid both stenosis and twisting, it is important that during the gastric transection procedure, the assistant maintains constant and balanced contralateral traction.

Another technical detail to consider is to avoid cutting too close to the esophagogastric junction, which could induce ischemia and therefore leakage at the suture site (Fig. 8.1).

8.4.7 Reinforcement of the Stapling Line

A common complication can be bleeding in the staple line. This can be intraluminal or intra-abdominal. Intra-abdominal bleeding is easier to detect as it is visible during the procedure and can be easily controlled with clips, sutures, or some type of glue. However, intraluminal bleeding usually manifests indirectly in the postoperative period through hematemesis, melena, or anemia in laboratory tests. An endoscopic study can then confirm the diagnosis, although the bleeding will often have stopped spontaneously. Many experts recommend reinforcing the suture, which can be done either with reinforced sutures or by performing oversutures. If oversutures are chosen, they should be performed with the bougie still in place to avoid further narrowing. Reinforced mechanical sutures can use a sheet of resorbable polymer material. Sealants or biological materials such as bovine pericardium strips have also been used for reinforcement [17].

Reinforcement of the staple line has been associated with a decrease in bleeding, but not in postoperative leaks. A study of more than 200,000 laparoscopic sleeve gastrectomies from the Metabolic and Bariatric Surgery Accreditation and Quality Improvement Programme (MBSAQIP) database between 2015 and 2016 showed that reinforcing the staple line significantly reduced bleeding and readmissions, although not leaks in the suture line [18].

8.4.8 Intraoperative Test

After gastric resection, an intraoperative test should be performed to check for possible leaks. However, many surgeons do not support this practice, as there are studies showing that a negative test result does not predict postoperative leakage. Postoperative leaks in the staple line are no longer common in centers where suture leak tests are not performed. Therefore, based on current evidence, this practice is only beneficial for the surgeon's peace of mind.

8.4.9 Management of Wall Wounds and Completion of Surgery

The gastric segment is removed through the umbilical incision using a specific bag, enlarging it if necessary, and then closed to complete the surgical procedure. Prior to completing the procedure, hemostasis must be checked at the trocar insertion sites under direct visualization. Trocar bleeding can be immediate or insidious. Immediate bleeding is easy to visualize and can be resolved without difficulty. Delayed bleeding becomes apparent after evacuating the pneumoperitoneum as intra-abdominal pressures decrease. It usually presents with the formation of a hematoma at the trocar site. At the end of the surgical procedure, to minimize the risk of trocar bleeding, evisceration, or incisional hernias, specific conical suture anchors can be used for trocar fascial closure primarily for 12 mm trocars.

8.5 Conclusions

Gastric sleeve surgery is a first-line procedure in the surgical treatment of obesity. Among the procedures that address obesity from a surgical point of view, gastric sleeve surgery is one of the least complex. However, there are some critical points that require great care in order to minimize possible complications such as bleeding or leaks in the suture line. All surgeons dedicated to bariatric surgery must be aware of these points in order to achieve the best possible results.

References

1. Brethauer SA. Sleeve gastrectomy. Surg Clin North Am. 2011;91(6):1265–79.
2. Gagner M, Hutchinson C, Rosenthal R. Fifth international consensus conference: current status of sleeve gastrectomy. Surg Obes Relat Dis. 2016;12(4):750–6.
3. De Angelis F, Abdelgawad M, Rizzello M, Mattia C, Silecchia G. Perioperative hemorrhagic complications after laparoscopic sleeve gastrectomy: four-year experience of a bariatric center of excellence. Surg Endosc. 2017;31(9):3547–51.

4. Sermet M, Ekinci O, Alimoglu O. Late complications of bleeding in the first 24 H after laparoscopic sleeve gastrectomy: a retrospective cohort study. Obes Surg. 2025;35(8):3141–8.
5. American Society for Metabolic and Bariatric Surgery (ASMBS). ASMBS Position Statement on Prevention, Detection & Treatment of Gastrointestinal Leak. Available at: https://asmbs.org/resources/prevention-and-detection-of-gastrointestinal-leak
6. Clapp B, Corbett J, Ahmad M, Vivar A, Sharma I, Hage K, Ghanem OM. When do leaks occur? An analysis of the metabolic and bariatric surgery accreditation and quality improvement program. Surg Obes Relat Dis. 2023;19(10):1128–33.
7. Binda A, Jaworski P, Tarnowski W. Stenosis after sleeve gastrectomy—cause, diagnosis and management strategy. Pol Przegl Chir. 2013;85(12):730–6.
8. Lyyjynen HS, Andersen JR, Liem RSL, Mala T, Nienhuijs SW, Ottosson J, Sundbom M, Thorell A, Våge V. Surgical aspects of sleeve gastrectomy are related to weight loss and gastroesophageal reflux symptoms. Obes Surg. 2024;34(3):902–10.
9. Yehoshua RT, Eidelman LA, Stein M, Fichman S, Mazor A, Chen J, Bernstine H, Singer P, Dickman R, Beglaibter N, Shikora SA, Rosenthal RJ, Rubin M. Laparoscopic sleeve gastrectomy—volume and pressure assessment. Obes Surg. 2008;18(9):1083–8. https://doi.org/10.1007/s11695-008-9576-x. Epub 2008 Jun 6. Erratum in: Obes Surg. 2009;19(1):134
10. Pañella C, Busto M, González A, Serra C, Goday A, Grande L, Pera M, Ramón JM. Correlation of gastric volume and weight loss 5 years following sleeve gastrectomy. Obes Surg. 2020;30(6):2199–205.
11. Jumaev N, Teshaev O, Lim I, Kurbanov G. Calibration Bougie size selection in sleeve gastrectomy: a systematic review and meta-analysis. Obes Surg. 2025;35(8):3221–7.
12. Crawford C, Gibbens K, Lomelin D, Krause C, Simorov A, Oleynikov D. Sleeve gastrectomy and anti-reflux procedures. Surg Endosc. 2017;31(3):1012–21.
13. Yu Q, Saeed K, Okida LF, Gutierrez Blanco DA, Lo Menzo E, Szomstein S, Rosenthal R. Outcomes of laparoscopic sleeve gastrectomy with and without antrectomy in severely obese subjects. Evidence from randomized controlled trials. Surg Obes Relat Dis. 2022;18(3):404–12.
14. Gagner M, Kemmeter P. Comparison of laparoscopic sleeve gastrectomy leak rates in five staple-line reinforcement options: a systematic review. Surg Endosc. 2020;34(1):396–407.
15. Steenackers N, Vanuytsel T, Augustijns P, Tack J, Mertens A, Lannoo M, Van der Schueren B, Matthys C. Adaptations in gastrointestinal physiology after sleeve gastrectomy and Roux-en-Y gastric bypass. Lancet Gastroenterol Hepatol. 2021;6(3):225–37.
16. Hsu JL, Ismail S, Hodges MM, Agala CB, Farrell TM. Bariatric surgery: trends in utilization, complications, conversions and revisions. Surg Endosc. 2024;38(8):4613–23.
17. Demeusy A, Sill A, Averbach A. Current role of staple line reinforcement in 30-day outcomes of primary laparoscopic sleeve gastrectomy: an analysis of MBSAQIP data, 2015-2016 PUF. Surg Obes Relat Dis. 2018;14(10):1454–61.
18. Mocanu V, Dang J, Ladak F, Switzer N, Birch DW, Karmali S. Predictors and outcomes of bleed after sleeve gastrectomy: an analysis of the MBSAQIP data registry. Surg Obes Relat Dis. 2019;15(10):1675–81.

Anesthetic Considerations for Patients Undergoing Sleeve Gastrectomy

9

Carolina Llavero and Jaime Ruiz-Tovar

9.1 Introduction

All individuals with severe obesity who are being considered for bariatric surgery must undergo a comprehensive preoperative assessment to identify any uncontrolled comorbidities that could contraindicate the procedure. Patients with severe obesity are frequently classified as high-risk for both anesthesia and surgery—not solely due to their excess weight, but also because of associated comorbid conditions, which may be undiagnosed or poorly managed. These factors carry significant implications during the perioperative period and must be carefully evaluated when planning a sleeve gastrectomy [1].

9.2 Obesity-Related Health Conditions

9.2.1 Respiratory Alterations in Obesity

Obesity induces a range of respiratory changes, primarily affecting lung volumes, thoracic compliance, and the ventilation/perfusion (V/Q) ratio. These alterations often result in chronic hypoxemia due to inefficient respiratory mechanics. Expiratory reserve volume (ERV) decreases in proportion to excess body weight, while residual volume may remain stable or increase, leading to a reduction in functional residual capacity (FRC) and a heightened risk of atelectasis [2].

C. Llavero (✉)
Department of Nursery, Hospital del Henares, Madrid, Spain

J. Ruiz-Tovar
Department of Biomedicine and Health Sciences, Alfonso X University, Madrid, Spain
e-mail: jruiztovar@gmail.com

J. Ruiz-Tovar (ed.), *Multidisciplinary Management of Sleeve Gastrectomy*,
https://doi.org/10.1007/978-3-032-25644-7_9

Thoracic compliance is diminished, increasing the work of breathing and limiting the ability to meet elevated ventilatory demands. These changes stem from fat accumulation around the costal margins, below the diaphragm, and within the abdominal cavity. Pulmonary compliance typically remains unaffected unless obesity is prolonged, at which point it may decline due to increased pulmonary blood volume and reduced FRC.

Gas exchange is further compromised by two mechanisms:

- Dead space ventilation (elevated V/Q ratio) arises from circulatory disturbances and hypoxemic pulmonary vasoconstriction.
- Shunt-like effects (reduced V/Q ratio) result from alveolar collapse linked to decreased FRC and increased pulmonary blood flow.

Despite these challenges, hyperventilation often compensates to maintain normocapnia, driven by the elevated metabolic demands of obesity, which increase both oxygen consumption and carbon dioxide production [3].

Two respiratory conditions commonly associated with obesity are alveolar hypoventilation syndrome (AHS) and sleep apnea-hypopnea syndrome (SAHS). SAHS is an uncommon disorder marked by the coexistence of hypoxemia and hypercapnia, often presenting alongside features of Pickwickian syndrome—characterized by obesity, excessive daytime sleepiness, cyclical breathing patterns, chronic hypoventilation, polycythemia, and right ventricular hypertrophy. Affected individuals typically exhibit increased pulmonary blood volume and may develop pulmonary hypertension [4].

In obese individuals, hypoventilation is frequently driven by central hypoxia and hypercapnia resulting from intrinsic ventilatory dysfunction, compounded by the mechanical limitations imposed by excess body weight. When these respiratory disturbances lead to repeated episodes of apnea—lasting at least 10 s—during sleep, the condition is classified as sleep apnea-hypopnea syndrome (SAHS). Obesity is the primary risk factor, with a prevalence of approximately 5% among obese individuals, predominantly affecting males. SAHS manifests as excessive daytime sleepiness, cognitive impairment, and emotional instability. When the frequency of apneic episodes surpasses 20 per hour of sleep, it is considered a significant contributor to mortality. A definitive diagnosis is established through polysomnographic evaluation [5].

The respiratory impairments seen in obesity are further exacerbated when transitioning from a seated to a supine position. This shift causes upward displacement of the diaphragm, leading to a reduction in functional residual capacity (FRC). In obese individuals, FRC often approaches the closing capacity (CC), resulting in portions of the respiratory cycle occurring within the closing volume (CV), which promotes airway closure and increases the risk of atelectasis.

Closing capacity refers to the lung volume below which airway closure begins during a slow maximal expiration, while closing volume is defined as the difference between CC and FRC. The likelihood of hypoxemia rises as the alveolar-arterial oxygen gradient narrows, a change directly linked to the reduction in the FRC–CC differential.

Additionally, the supine posture increases venous return to the thoracic cavity, overloading the pulmonary vasculature and reducing pulmonary compliance—further impairing gas exchange. These effects are intensified in the Trendelenburg position, which accentuates diaphragmatic displacement and vascular congestion.

Conversely, the anti-Trendelenburg position offers respiratory benefits: it enhances lung compliance, allows for lower pressure at equivalent lung volumes, promotes alveolar recruitment, and increases FRC. Hemodynamically, this posture reduces venous return and cardiac output, yet improves arterial oxygenation (PaO_2) due to more efficient pulmonary mechanics [6].

9.2.2 Cardiovascular Alterations in Obesity

In obese individuals, cardiac changes arise as adaptive responses to excess body weight and elevated metabolic demands. As body mass increases—encompassing fat and muscle tissue—there is a corresponding rise in blood volume and oxygen consumption. This volume expansion is further influenced by heightened activity of the renin-angiotensin system. However, despite the absolute increase in blood volume, the volume-to-weight ratio remains lower than in individuals of normal weight.

To meet these demands, cardiac output increases primarily through an elevated stroke volume, while heart rate remains relatively stable. This leads to increased preload, left ventricular dilation, and elevated afterload—exacerbated by the frequent coexistence of arterial hypertension in obesity. Over time, these hemodynamic stresses contribute to the development of hypertrophic cardiomyopathy, impairing ventricular relaxation and ultimately progressing to congestive heart failure [7].

While most regional blood flows remain stable, splanchnic circulation increases by approximately 20%. Additionally, pulmonary hypertension may develop due to increased pulmonary blood volume and hypoxic vasoconstriction. Left ventricular dysfunction further elevates pulmonary pressures, which in turn strain the right ventricle, leading to its hypertrophy and dilation [8].

Hypertension is notably more prevalent among individuals with obesity, affecting approximately 50–60% with moderate forms and 5–10% with severe presentations. This association is particularly pronounced in women, individuals under the age of 60, and those with a familial predisposition to hypertension. Multiple physiological mechanisms contribute to this condition, including activation of the renin-angiotensin system, expansion of vascular volume, and heightened sympathetic activity—often driven by hyperinsulinemia. Hypertension in this context is strongly linked to increased mortality, as it initiates a cascade of hemodynamic alterations that elevate cardiac workload and significantly raise the risk of cardiogenic failure [9].

Individuals with obesity face an elevated risk of developing cardiac arrhythmias, which may be linked to sudden cardiac death. This vulnerability arises from a combination of contributing factors, including left ventricular hypertrophy, chronic hypoxemia, and hypokalemia—often secondary to frequent diuretic use. Additional contributors include underlying coronary artery disease, elevated circulating catecholamines, bradycardia associated with sleep apnea-hypopnea syndrome (SAHS), and fatty infiltration of both the myocardium and the cardiac conduction system [10].

9.2.3 Gastrointestinal Disorders in Obesity

Obesity is associated with a higher incidence of hiatal hernia and elevated intra-abdominal pressure, both of which contribute to an increased risk of acid aspiration syndrome (AAS). Additionally, obese individuals typically exhibit a gastric volume approximately 75% greater than that of non-obese individuals, resulting in higher residual gastric content and accelerated gastric emptying. These alterations may be partially reversed with weight loss. The presence of hiatal hernia and increased intra-abdominal pressure also predisposes patients to gastroesophageal reflux disease (GERD). Growing evidence underscores the importance of identifying GERD preoperatively to guide the selection of the most appropriate bariatric procedure. GERD is considered by many experts to be a relative contraindication for restrictive techniques such as sleeve gastrectomy, due to the potential for exacerbating reflux symptoms. In cases where GERD is present, Roux-en-Y gastric bypass remains the preferred surgical approach. However, emerging studies suggest that sleeve gastrectomy may improve GERD symptoms in some patients, likely due to the reduction in intra-abdominal pressure following weight loss. In response to this, some surgeons have introduced the Nissen-sleeve—a modified technique combining fundoplication with sleeve gastrectomy—to mitigate reflux while preserving the benefits of restriction [11].

Biliary disorders are frequently observed in morbidly obese individuals, particularly among women, largely due to delayed gallbladder emptying and increased biliary cholesterol saturation. Histological liver changes are present in approximately 90% of obese patients, with about one-third exhibiting hepatic steatosis—typically without significant functional impairment. The degree of fatty infiltration correlates more strongly with the duration of obesity than with its severity. The most common biochemical abnormality is elevated alanine aminotransferase (GPT), which tends to normalize following bariatric surgery, in proportion to the amount of weight lost [12].

9.2.4 Endocrine Disorders in Obesity

In individuals with obesity, excessive caloric intake leads to persistently elevated blood glucose levels, which in turn heightens insulin demand and increases the risk of pancreatic dysfunction and the development of type 2 diabetes mellitus. Chronic hyperglycemia also elevates circulating triglyceride concentrations, stimulating lipolysis and hepatic cholesterol synthesis. The excess cholesterol is excreted via bile, contributing to gallstone formation. Simultaneously, levels of HDL-cholesterol tend to decline, further amplifying the risk of coronary artery disease [13].

Morbidly obese women often experience hormonal imbalances, primarily driven by elevated androgen levels. These changes manifest as hirsutism, acne, androgenic alopecia, and disruptions in estrogen regulation, which contribute to menstrual irregularities such as dysmenorrhea, infertility, and the development of polycystic ovarian morphology. In men, obesity may lead to a reduction in total testosterone levels, with hypogonadism occurring infrequently but notably in more advanced cases [14].

Subclinical hypothyroidism affects approximately 20% of individuals with morbid obesity. While the overall requirement for thyroid hormone replacement therapy is similar to that of non-obese patients, this condition warrants attention in the surgical setting, as perioperative management may necessitate temporary or adjusted treatment to ensure metabolic stability [15].

9.2.5 Metabolic Syndrome

Individuals with severe obesity often exhibit a distinct metabolic profile shaped by a constellation of interrelated pathologies. This synergistic effect elevates their overall health risk beyond what would be expected from each condition in isolation—a phenomenon referred to as metabolic syndrome or syndrome X.

Metabolic syndrome is primarily driven by insulin resistance, which serves as a central mechanism in the development of multiple chronic diseases. Visceral adiposity, particularly brown and intra-abdominal fat located in the omentum and mesentery, is believed to play a key role in promoting this resistance.

According to the International Diabetes Federation (IDF) criteria, a diagnosis of metabolic syndrome requires:

- Central (abdominal) obesity, defined by waist circumference exceeding 94 cm in men and 80 cm in women (based on regional standards), plus at least two of the following metabolic abnormalities:
  - Dyslipidemia: Triglycerides >150 mg/dL and/or HDL cholesterol <40 mg/dL in men or < 50 mg/dL in women.
  - Hypertension: Blood pressure > 135/85 mmHg.
  - Type 2 diabetes mellitus: Fasting glucose >100 mg/dL.

Metabolic syndrome is recognized as an independent predictor of morbidity and mortality, largely due to its strong association with cardiovascular disease. In patients undergoing malabsorptive bariatric procedures, the prevalence of metabolic syndrome is notably higher, necessitating careful preoperative assessment and tailored perioperative management [16].

9.3 Intraoperative Factors

9.3.1 Operating Theatre Preparation

All equipment within the operating theatre must be appropriately scaled and reinforced to safely accommodate the patient's body weight, ensuring structural integrity and patient safety. Transfers to and from the operating table should be performed using mechanical lifting devices rather than relying on manual handling by staff, to prevent injury and ensure proper positioning. Patient posture must be meticulously assessed and maintained, as excessive adipose tissue—particularly around the knees—can obscure harmful joint hyperextensions or flexions, posing risks to peripheral nerves and joint structures. Additionally, all pressure-prone areas should be adequately padded, as patients with severe obesity are at increased risk for pressure injuries and decubitus ulcers due to compromised adipose tissue perfusion [17].

9.3.2 Upper Airway Anatomical Alterations in Obesity

Obesity induces several structural changes in the upper airway that complicate airway management:

- Cervicothoracic adipose deposits restrict cervical flexion and extension.
- Submental fat accumulation limits mouth opening.
- Hypertrophy of soft tissues—including the cheeks, tongue, soft palate, pharynx, and supralaryngeal structures—reduces airway diameter and increases the risk of obstruction, particularly during sleep.
- The glottis tends to be positioned more anteriorly and superiorly.

These anatomical modifications contribute to a significantly higher incidence of difficult orotracheal intubation in obese patients. Therefore, airway management must be meticulously planned, with access to specialized equipment such as intubation guides, appropriately sized masks and tubes, and advanced laryngoscopes. In certain cases, awake intubation using a flexible fiberoptic scope may be the safest approach [18].

9.3.3 Anesthetic Challenges in Obese Patients

Obesity significantly increases the complexity and risk associated with anesthetic management. It introduces technical challenges and physiological vulnerabilities that place obese patients at a distinct disadvantage compared to individuals of normal weight. These disadvantages span multiple domains:

- Medical: Altered physiology complicates drug pharmacokinetics and respiratory mechanics.
- Diagnostic: Imaging modalities such as X-ray and ultrasound often yield suboptimal results, delaying accurate diagnosis.
- Practical: Patient transfers, positioning, and early mobilization are more difficult and resource-intensive.

Given these factors, anesthetic planning must be exceptionally thorough to anticipate and mitigate potential complications. The perioperative risk, including the risk of mortality, is markedly elevated in this population and demands heightened vigilance throughout the surgical process [19].

9.4 Main Early Postoperative Complications

9.4.1 Thromboembolism

Thromboembolic events represent the leading cause of mortality following sleeve gastrectomy, with reported fatality rates ranging from 20% to 30%. The overall incidence of thromboembolic disease in this patient population is estimated between 2.4% and 4.5%, reflecting the strong correlation with obesity-related alterations in coagulation dynamics—namely, reduced levels of circulating antithrombin III and diminished fibrinolytic activity. These risks are compounded by postoperative hypercoagulability and limited mobility. Pulmonary embolism, occurring in approximately 1–2% of cases, is further exacerbated by the increased blood volume and polycythemia commonly seen in morbidly obese individuals, often secondary to chronic hypoxemia [20].

The laparoscopic approach can heighten the risk of thromboembolic events. The creation of pneumoperitoneum exerts pressure on the inferior vena cava, leading to reduced venous return, increased stasis, and a prothrombotic environment that favors platelet aggregation and clot formation. To mitigate this risk, early postoperative mobilization, the use of intermittent pneumatic compression devices, and prophylactic administration of low molecular weight heparins are essential components of perioperative care [21].

9.4.2 Pulmonary Complications

The postoperative phase is often marked by a deterioration in pulmonary function, with increased hypoxemia—typically peaking between postoperative days 1 and 4—and a heightened risk of atelectasis. The incidence of these complications varies widely, ranging from 6% in patients with normal preoperative respiratory function to as high as 70% in those with impaired pulmonary tests. Contributing factors include the supine position, the residual effects of anesthesia, surgical trauma, and postoperative immobility.

Supine positioning promotes cephalad displacement of the diaphragm and venous shift from the abdominal to the thoracic cavity, both of which compromise respiratory mechanics and contribute to respiratory insufficiency. During anesthetic induction, functional residual capacity (FRC) is further reduced, exacerbating the risk of hypoventilation.

Surgical factors such as intra-abdominal manipulation, use of subdiaphragmatic retractors, and the nature of the incision also influence pulmonary outcomes. Incisions located near the diaphragm—particularly transverse, supra-umbilical laparotomies and thoracotomies—have the most pronounced impact on respiratory function.

Laparoscopic surgery offers several postoperative advantages, including reduced pain and lower opioid requirements, which facilitate respiratory physiotherapy and decrease the incidence of pulmonary complications. These benefits contribute to faster recovery and shorter hospital stays. However, laparoscopic procedures may pose greater intraoperative respiratory and cardiovascular challenges compared to open surgery.

Additional postoperative factors—such as patient positioning, limited mobility, pain, and restrictive abdominal dressings—can further impair pulmonary function and oxygenation. Moreover, pre-existing conditions unrelated to the surgical intervention, such as bronchiectasis (with increased secretions), elevated closing volume in smokers or patients with COPD, and dehydration, may also predispose patients to respiratory complications.

To mitigate these risks, early initiation of spontaneous breathing, semi-upright positioning, and rigorous respiratory physiotherapy are strongly recommended to promote lung expansion, prevent atelectasis, and improve oxygenation [22].

9.4.3 Incisional Surgical Site Infection

Surgical site infection (SSI) remains the leading cause of postoperative morbidity in individuals with obesity. The reduced vascular supply within extensive adipose tissue, combined with the tendency for serous fluid accumulation, creates an environment conducive to bacterial colonization and infection. The adoption of laparoscopic techniques—with smaller incisions and reduced tissue disruption—has significantly lowered the incidence of this complication [23].

9.4.4 Staple Line Leak

Gastric leak is one of the most serious and feared complications following sleeve gastrectomy, with an average incidence of approximately 1%. When leakage of gastric contents occurs, it can trigger a wide range of clinical manifestations—from localized abscess formation to diffuse peritonitis, septic shock, multi-organ failure, and potentially death. Due to its high morbidity and mortality risk, prompt recognition and early diagnosis are critical to initiate timely and appropriate therapeutic intervention [24].

9.5 Conclusions

Patients with severe obesity present a heightened anesthetic and surgical risk due to the constellation of comorbidities commonly associated with obesity. This complexity makes perioperative management particularly challenging. In the immediate postoperative period, the most frequent and serious complications include thromboembolic events, respiratory compromise, and surgical site infections. Therefore, comprehensive preventive strategies must be implemented to mitigate these risks and ensure patient safety.

References

1. Stenberg E, Bruze G, Sundström J, Marcus C, Näslund I, Ottosson J, Neovius M. Comparison of sleeve gastrectomy vs intensive lifestyle modification in patients with a BMI of 30 to less than 35. JAMA Netw Open. 2022;5(7):e2223927.
2. Steier J, Lunt A, Hart N, Polkey MI, Moxham J. Observational study of the effect of obesity on lung volumes. Thorax. 2014;69(8):752–9.
3. De Jong A, Chanques G, Jaber S. Mechanical ventilation in obese ICU patients: from intubation to extubation. Crit Care. 2017;21(1):63.
4. Lee CH, Sethi R, Li R, Ho HH, Hein T, Jim MH, Loo G, Koo CY, et al. Obstructive sleep apnea and cardiovascular events after percutaneous coronary intervention. Circulation. 2016;133(21):2008–17.
5. Masa JF, Pépin JL, Borel JC, Mokhlesi B, Murphy PB, Sánchez-Quiroga MÁ. Obesity hypoventilation syndrome. Eur Respir Rev. 2019;28(151):180097.
6. Couture EJ, Carrier-Boucher A, Provencher S, Tanoubi I, Marceau S, Bussières JS. Effect of reverse Trendelenburg position and positive pressure ventilation on safe non-hypoxic apnea period in obese, a randomized-control trial. BMC Anesthesiol. 2023;23(1):198.
7. Ren J, Wu NN, Wang S, Sowers JR, Zhang Y. Obesity cardiomyopathy: evidence, mechanisms, and therapeutic implications. Physiol Rev. 2021;101(4):1745–807.
8. Ayinapudi K, Singh T, Motwani A, Le Jemtel TH, Oparil S. Obesity and pulmonary hypertension. Curr Hypertens Rep. 2018;20(12):99.
9. Parvanova A, Reseghetti E, Abbate M, Ruggenenti P. Mechanisms and treatment of obesity-related hypertension-part 1: mechanisms. Clin Kidney J. 2023;17(1):sfad282.
10. Yao Y, Xue J, Li B. Obesity and sudden cardiac death: prevalence, pathogenesis, prevention and intervention. Front Cell Dev Biol. 2022;10:1044923.
11. Greenwald D. Preoperative gastrointestinal assessment before bariatric surgery. Gastroenterol Clin N Am. 2010;39(1):81–6.
12. Theel WB, Boxma-de Klerk BM, Dirksmeier-Harinck F, van Rossum EF, Kanhai DA, Apers JA, van Dalen BM, De Knegt RJ, et al. Effect of bariatric surgery on NAFLD/NASH: a single-centre observational prospective cohort study. BMJ Open. 2023;13(7):e070431.
13. Ilyas S, Al-Refai R, Maharjan R, Diaz Bustamante L, Ghattas KN, Khan S. Bariatric surgery and type 2 diabetes mellitus: assessing factors leading to remission. A systematic review. Cureus. 2020;12(8):e9973.
14. Eng PC, Phylactou M, Qayum A, Woods C, Lee H, Aziz S, Moore B, Miras AD, Comninos AN, Tan T, Franks S, Dhillo WS, Abbara A. Obesity-related hypogonadism in women. Endocr Rev. 2024;45(2):171–89.
15. Biondi B. Subclinical hypothyroidism in patients with obesity and metabolic syndrome: a narrative review. Nutrients. 2023;16(1):87.
16. Alberti KG, Zimmet P, Shaw J. Metabolic syndrome--a new world-wide definition. A Consensus Statement from the International Diabetes Federation. Diabet Med. 2006;23(5):469–80.
17. Sanford JA, Kadry B, Brodsky JB, Macario A. Bariatric surgery operating room time—size matters. Obes Surg. 2015;25(6):1078–85.
18. De Jong A, Molinari N, Pouzeratte Y, Verzilli D, Chanques G, Jung B, Futier E, Perrigault PF, et al. Difficult intubation in obese patients: incidence, risk factors, and complications in the operating theatre and in intensive care units. Br J Anaesth. 2015;114(2):297–306.
19. Pouwels S, Buise MP, Twardowski P, Stepaniak PS, Proczko M. Obesity surgery and anesthesiology risks: a review of key concepts and related physiology. Obes Surg. 2019;29(8):2670–7.

20. Liu C, Han Z, Zhang N, Peng J, Zhu B, Amin B, Du D, Yan W, Zhang D, Gong K. Laparoscopic sleeve gastrectomy affects coagulation system of obese patients. Obes Surg. 2020;30(10):3989–96.
21. Thaher O, Wendt E, Hukauf M, Croner RS, Stroh C. Thromboembolic prophylaxis in bariatric and metabolic surgery: state-of-the-art according to the results of a nationwide registry study. Updat Surg. 2025; https://doi.org/10.1007/s13304-025-02073-9.
22. Gupta PK, Gupta H, Kaushik M, Fang X, Miller WJ, Morrow LE, Armour-Forse R. Predictors of pulmonary complications after bariatric surgery. Surg Obes Relat Dis. 2012;8(5):574–81.
23. Meijs AP, Koek MBG, Vos MC, Geerlings SE, Vogely HC, de Greeff SC. The effect of body mass index on the risk of surgical site infection. Infect Control Hosp Epidemiol. 2019;40(9):991–6.
24. Iossa A, Martini L, De Angelis F, Micalizzi A, Watkins BM, Silecchia G, Cavallaro G. Leaks after laparoscopic sleeve gastrectomy: 2024 update on risk factors. Langenbeck's Arch Surg. 2024;409(1):249.

Revisional Surgery

10

Adriana Avilés-Oliveros

10.1 Introduction

Sleeve gastrectomy has surpassed all other metabolic procedures in global frequency, largely due to its relative technical simplicity, low perioperative morbidity, absence of intestinal bypass, and robust early metabolic effect [1]. However, long-term follow-up has revealed limitations related to weight durability, reflux physiology, and anatomical changes of the gastric tube [2]. As the global number of SGs increases, revisional surgery is now one of the fastest-growing domains in bariatric practice. GERD—both de novo and exacerbated pre-existing disease—has emerged as one of the most important long-term complications of SG [3].

These findings have transformed the landscape of bariatric surgery, leading to a steady increase in revisional operations.

10.2 Definitions and Mechanisms of Failure

Failure after SG represents a heterogeneous spectrum of anatomical and physiological conditions. Insufficient weight loss, defined conventionally as less than 50% excess weight loss (EWL) at 18–24 months, frequently results from a combination of inadequate gastric restriction and insufficient metabolic effect. Many patients initially achieve a reasonable weight reduction but subsequently experience weight regain, typically defined as a $\geq$ 10–15% increase from nadir weight [2].

GERD constitutes another major category of failure. The SG alters the geometry of the gastroesophageal junction, potentially impairing lower esophageal sphincter (LES) competency, reducing gastric compliance, increasing intragastric pressure, and creating a predisposition to reflux. Additionally, sleeve torsion, incisural

A. Avilés-Oliveros (✉)
General Surgery Department, Hospital Universitario del Henares, Madrid, Spain

J. Ruiz-Tovar (ed.), *Multidisciplinary Management of Sleeve Gastrectomy*, https://doi.org/10.1007/978-3-032-25644-7_10

stenosis, and de novo hiatal hernia may exacerbate symptoms. Long-term complications include erosive esophagitis and Barrett's esophagus, both of which require prompt evaluation and intervention [3].

10.3 Indications for Revisional Surgery

Revisional surgery is indicated when patients have failed to achieve or maintain adequate weight loss, develop severe or refractory GERD, or experience SG-related anatomical complications [4, 5].

Weight failure represents the most frequent indication and SG is multifactorial, including:

- Progressive dilation of the gastric tube.
- Retained or incompletely resected fundus.
- Adaptive eating behavior.
- Increased ghrelin-independent appetite signaling.
- High-calorie dietary patterns.

Most criteria define failure as <50% excess weight loss (EWL) **or** weight regain after reaching nadir resulting in BMI >35–40 kg/m^2 [2]. In these patients, endoscopy or radiographic imaging commonly reveals sleeve dilation or retained fundus, both of which diminish the restrictive effect of the operation and reduce satiety. Revisional procedures in this context aim to restore restriction, enhance malabsorption, or both [6].

Patients who develop **GERD** after SG often present with severe or persistent symptoms despite maximal proton pump inhibitor therapy [3].

SG is associated with a high incidence of de novo or worsened GERD. Mechanisms include:

- Loss of angle of His.
- Disruption of sling fibers.
- Decreased gastric compliance.
- Increased intragastric pressure.
- Occult or untreated hiatal hernia.
- "Neofundus" dilation producing stasis and acid pooling.

Endoscopy may reveal moderate-to-severe esophagitis or Barrett's esophagus, while contrast studies may demonstrate a hiatal hernia or sleeve torsion. These individuals benefit most consistently from conversion to RYGB, which reliably reduces both acid and bile exposure [3, 4, 7].

Complications necessitating revision include sleeve stenosis, which may manifest with progressive intolerance to solids, chronic vomiting, or weight loss beyond intended goals. Chronic leaks or gastro-bronchial fistulae present particularly complex scenarios, requiring individualized surgical reconstruction, often with omental patches, fistula tract excision, or conversion to bypass [6].

Patient-centered factors also influence procedural selection. Individuals with severe or recurrent diabetes may require procedures with greater metabolic potency, such as SADI-S or BPD-DS [6, 8]. Conversely, patients with limited ability to adhere to long-term nutritional follow-up may be better suited to RYGB.

10.4 Revisional Options for Weight Failure (Table 10.1)

10.4.1 Conversion to Roux-en-Y Gastric Bypass (RYGB)

RYGB remains the most widely performed revisional operation after SG [4, 5, 7]. Its combination of moderate restriction, reliable metabolic effect, and superior reflux control makes it a versatile choice.

10.4.1.1 Indications

- Refractory GERD (gold standard revisional procedure) [3]
- Weight regain or inadequate weight loss.
- Chronic leak or sleeve stricture.
- Complex foregut pathologies.

10.4.1.2 Technical Principles

Revision typically starts with careful adhesiolysis around the angle of His and upper sleeve. A small gastric pouch is created proximal to the incisura. Standard limb lengths include:

- Biliopancreatic limb: 50 cm.
- Roux limb: 100–150 cm, adjustable depending on metabolic goals.

Table 10.1 Comparative characteristics of revisional procedures after SG

Procedure	Expected weight loss	GERD control	Nutritional risk	Main indications
RYGB	++ to +++	+++ (best)	+	GERD, complications, weight failure
OAGB	+++	+	++	Weight regain, metabolic relapse
SADI-S	++++	+	+++	Severe obesity, diabetes
BDP-DS	+++++	+	++++	Super-obesity, maximal metabolic need
Re-SG	+	–	+	Sleeve dilation without reflux
Hiatal repair	–	+	–	Hernia-related reflux
Endoscopic revision	+	+/–	–	Early dilation, leaks, mild WR

The gastrojejunostomy must be tension-free and well perfused. In chronic leaks, pouch creation must avoid the fistulous area, sometimes requiring partial gastrectomy. Hiatal hernias should be repaired concurrently.

10.4.1.3 Advantages

- Best control of GERD.
- Solid metabolic effect and durable weight control.
- Effective management of strictures or fistulas.

10.4.1.4 Limitations

- Technically demanding due to scarring.
- Higher risk of leaks and internal hernias than primary RYGB.
- Potential for marginal ulcers.

10.4.2 Conversion to One-Anastomosis Gastric Bypass (OAGB/MGB)

OAGB has emerged as an effective alternative, particularly for patients with predominant weight failure. Its longer biliopancreatic limb provides greater malabsorptive effect than RYGB, translating into 60–80% EWL in revisional settings [9]. However, the potential risk of bile reflux, particularly in patients with pre-existing GERD, warrants careful patient selection. The revisional OAGB involves creation of a long, narrow gastric pouch along the lesser curvature, with a 150–200 cm biliopancreatic limb.

10.4.2.1 Indications

- Weight regain (most frequent).
- Insufficient metabolic response.
- Selected patients with GERD (if sleeve shape and hiatal anatomy permit).

10.4.2.2 Technical Features

The sleeve is transformed into a longer, narrow pouch along the lesser curvature. A gastrojejunostomy is created 150–200 cm from the ligament of Treitz.

Critical steps include avoiding excessive pouch length, ensuring alignment to prevent twisting, and maintaining a low-pressure anastomosis.

10.4.2.3 Advantages

- Excellent weight loss outcomes, often superior to RYGB.
- Single anastomosis and shorter operative time.
- Favorable metabolic effect.

10.4.2.4 Limitations

- Risk of bile reflux (controversial but documented).
- Potential for malnutrition with long biliopancreatic limb lengths.

10.4.3 Conversion to Biliopancreatic Diversion with Duodenal Switch (BDP-DS) or Single-Anastomosis Duodeno-Ileal Bypass (SADI-S)

SADI-S represents a powerful metabolic procedure with excellent weight loss and diabetes remission outcomes. It preserves pyloric function while introducing significant malabsorption through a single duodeno-ileal anastomosis. In revisional contexts, SADI-S can achieve 70–90% EWL with high rates of diabetes remission; however, the risk of protein–calorie malnutrition and micronutrient deficiencies necessitates rigorous long-term follow-up [10].

BPD-DS remains the most powerful procedure but is also the most nutritionally demanding [6]. For this reason, its use is generally reserved for super-obese patients or those with severe metabolic relapse.

10.4.3.1 Indications

- Severe obesity, BMI >50–60 kg/m^2.
- Inadequate metabolic control of diabetes.
- Patients who tolerated the sleeve and require stronger metabolic power.

10.4.3.2 Technical Details

Both procedures involve division of the duodenum just distal to the pylorus:

- **Classical DS**: Two anastomoses; common limb typically 75–150 cm.
- **SADI-S**: One duodeno-ileostomy; ileal anastomosis usually 250–300 cm from ileocecal valve.

Revisional BDP-DS/SADI-S is technically challenging due to scarring around the hiatus and pylorus.

10.4.3.3 Pros

- Most powerful metabolic and weight-loss effect.
- Low risk of dumping due to pylorus preservation.

10.4.3.4 Cons

- Higher nutritional deficiency rates.
- GERD persists if present pre-conversion.
- Requires experienced units with intensive nutritional follow-up.

10.4.4 Re-Sleeve Gastrectomy (ReSG)

Re-sleeve gastrectomy has a limited role and is best suited for patients with clear evidence of sleeve dilation without coexisting reflux. While it can restore restriction, long-term durability remains inferior to bypass procedures, and it does not address the underlying limitations of SG in patients with metabolic failure [6].

10.4.4.1 Indications

- Dilation of the gastric tube (neofundus or globally enlarged sleeve).
- Retained fundus from primary procedure.
- Weight regain without reflux.

10.4.4.2 Technique

Re-SG requires meticulous identification of the true angle of His and careful dissection of adhesions. Resection aims to restore a uniform, narrow gastric sleeve while avoiding stenosis at the incisura. Overlapping staple lines increase leak risk, and buttressing is often recommended.

10.4.4.3 Advantages

- Anatomical preservation without malabsorption.
- Shorter operative time compared with bypass conversion.

10.4.4.4 Limitations

- Not indicated in GERD; symptoms may worsen.
- Leak risk increased due to ischemia of re-stapled tissue.
- Weight loss less predictable and less durable.

10.4.5 Endoscopic Revisional Approaches

10.4.5.1 Indications

- Mild–moderate sleeve dilation.
- Functional stenosis or twists.
- Chronic leaks and fistulas.
- Patients unfit for surgery.

10.4.5.2 Techniques

- **Endoluminal plication (ESG-type)** to reduce gastric volume.
- **Endoscopic stricturotomy** with or without balloon dilation.
- **Septotomy + stenting + OverStitch** for chronic leaks/fistulas.
- **Endoluminal fundoplication (TIF/MASE)** for selected reflux cases.

10.4.5.3 Advantages

- Minimally invasive.
- Low morbidity, short recovery.
- Preserves surgical options.

10.4.5.4 Limitations

- Less durable weight-loss effect.
- Requires high endoscopic expertise.
- Limited evidence compared with surgical revisions.

10.5 Revisional Surgery for GERD

The management of GERD after SG is a distinct and increasingly recognized challenge. Evidence overwhelmingly supports conversion to RYGB as the most effective intervention in this context. RYGB diverts both acid and bile away from the esophagus, reduces intragastric pressure, and permits concurrent hiatal hernia repair. In multiple prospective and retrospective series, 80–90% of patients report significant improvement or complete resolution of reflux symptoms, with parallel healing of esophagitis in the majority [3]. Furthermore, RYGB reduces the progression of Barrett's esophagus and may even induce regression in a subset of cases.

OAGB and SADI-S are generally not indicated as revisional procedures for reflux, given the potential for bile reflux and the lack of robust antireflux mechanisms. Re-sleeve gastrectomy is specifically contraindicated in reflux-predominant patients.

10.6 Technical Considerations

Revisional bariatric surgery demands advanced surgical expertise due to the dense adhesions that typically surround the gastroesophageal junction and along the staple line. Identifying the correct anatomical planes is essential to minimize the risk of perforation or devascularization. Chronic inflammation may obscure the angle of His or distort the hiatal anatomy, requiring careful dissection to avoid injury to the esophagus or vagal nerves.

Intraoperative endoscopy is highly recommended in complex cases, particularly when the anatomy is uncertain or when leak testing is necessary. Fluorescence angiography with indocyanine green may assist in confirming optimal perfusion to anastomotic sites. Anastomoses should be constructed in a tension-free manner, with adequate length and mobility of the mesentery to reduce the risk of ischemia.

Limb lengths in bypass procedures may be tailored based on the patient's metabolic profile, BMI, and previous weight trajectory. However, the potential benefits of longer limbs must always be balanced against the increased risk of malnutrition, particularly in revisional cases.

10.7 Comparative Outcomes and Complications

The outcomes of revisional procedures vary, reflecting differences in metabolic effect, anatomic reconstruction, and patient selection. RYGB consistently provides the best outcomes for GERD and good weight loss, with a complication profile that is well characterized. OAGB and SADI-S offer greater metabolic potency, although they carry higher risks of nutritional deficiencies. BPD-DS yields the most profound weight reduction but also the highest long-term malnutrition burden.

Complications after revisional surgery remain higher than after primary procedures. Leak rates range from 2% to 6%, reflecting the complexity of repeat dissection and altered blood supply. Bleeding, strictures, and internal hernias also occur with varying frequency depending on the procedure. Long-term follow-up is essential for monitoring nutritional status, particularly after malabsorptive operations.

10.8 Conclusion

Revisional surgery after sleeve gastrectomy has become an essential component of modern bariatric practice. Success requires a careful and structured approach, beginning with a clear understanding of the mechanism of failure, followed by detailed preoperative evaluation and tailored choice of revisional procedure. With appropriate patient selection and meticulous operative technique, revisional surgery can provide significant improvements in weight, metabolic health, and GERD symptoms. However, it also demands a lifelong commitment to nutritional monitoring and multidisciplinary follow-up.

References

1. Gagner M, Hutchinson C, Rosenthal R. Fifth international consensus conference: current status of sleeve gastrectomy. Surg Obes Relat Dis. 2016;12(4):750–6.
2. O'Brien PE, MacDonald L, Anderson M, Brennan L, Brown WA. Long-term outcomes after bariatric surgery: a systematic review and meta-analysis. Surg Obes Relat Dis. 2018;
3. Parmar CD, Mahawar KK, Boyle M, Schroeder N, Balupuri S, Small PK. Conversion of sleeve gastrectomy to roux-en-Y gastric bypass is effective for gastro-oesophageal reflux disease but not for further weight loss. Obes Surg. 2017;27:1651–8. https://doi.org/10.1007/s11695-017-2542-8.
4. Dang JT, Vaughan T, Mocanu V, Mubashir H, Barajas-Gamboa JS, Corcelles R, Rodriguez J, Karmali S, Kroh M. Conversion of sleeve gastrectomy to roux-en-Y gastric bypass: indications, prevalence, and safety. Obes Surg. 2023;33(5):1486–93. https://doi.org/10.1007/s11695-023-06546-x.
5. Diaz G, Del Gobbo G, Mahmoud N, Barajas-Gamboa JS, Klingler M, Barrios P, Abril C, Raza J, Aminian A, Rosenthal RJ, Corcelles R, Kroh MD. Conversion of sleeve gastrectomy to roux-en-Y gastric bypass to enhance weight loss: single enterprise mid-term outcomes and literature review. Bariatr Surg Pract Patient Care. 2022;17(4):197–205. https://doi.org/10.1089/bari.2021.0096.
6. Andalib A, Alamri H, Almuhanna Y, Bouchard P, Demyttenaere S, Court O. Short-term outcomes of revisional surgery after sleeve gastrectomy: comparative analysis of re-sleeve, RYGB, and duodenal switch (roux-en-Y and single-anastomosis). Surg Endosc. 2021;35:4644–52. https://doi.org/10.1007/s00464-020-07891-z.
7. Landreneau JP, Strong AT, Rodriguez JH, Aleassa EM, Aminian A, Brethauer S, et al. Conversion of sleeve gastrectomy to roux-en-Y gastric bypass. Obes Surg. 2018;28:3843–50. https://doi.org/10.1007/s11695-018-3435-1.

8. Dijkhorst PJ, Al Nawas M, Heusschen L, Hazebroek EJ, Swank DJ, Wiezer RMJ, et al. Single anastomosis duodeno-ileal bypass or roux-en-Y gastric bypass after failed sleeve gastrectomy: medium-term outcomes. Obes Surg. 2021;31:4708–16. https://doi.org/10.1007/s11695-021-05609-1.
9. Robert M, Espalieu P, Pelascini E, et al. Efficacy and safety of one-anastomosis gastric bypass versus roux-en-Y gastric bypass for obesity (YOMEGA). Lancet. 2019;393:1299–309.
10. Thomopoulos T, Mantziari S, Joliat GR. Long-term results of roux-en-Y gastric bypass (RYGB) versus single anastomosis duodeno-ileal bypass (SADI) as revisional procedures after failed sleeve gastrectomy: a systematic literature review and pooled analysis. Langenbeck's Arch Surg. 2024;409:354.

Part III

Postoperative Course

Early Postoperative Complications 11

Ana Sánchez-Gollarte, Carlos Guijarro-Moreno,
Victor Vaello-Jodra, and Sara Jiménez-Blanco

11.1 Introduction

Laparoscopic sleeve gastrectomy (LSG) has emerged as one of the most frequently performed bariatric procedures globally, both as a standalone intervention and as the first stage of a two-step surgical approach in high-risk or super-obese patients. LSG popularity stems from several advantages, including a relatively straightforward surgical technique, preservation of the gastrointestinal continuity, acceptable weight loss outcomes, and significant improvement in obesity-related comorbidities such as type 2 diabetes, hypertension, and obstructive sleep apnea.

In spite of its feasibility, LSG is not free of complications which eventually become a diagnostic and management challenge. Early postoperative complications, defined as those occurring within the first 30 days following surgery, represent a critical period that requires high index of suspicion and prompt intervention to minimize morbidity and mortality. The most concerning early postoperative complications include staple-line leaks, postoperative bleeding, intra-abdominal abscesses, gastric pouch necrosis, wound complications, and thromboembolic events. Other issues such as sleeve stenosis, ileus, or cardiopulmonary complications are less common but also contribute to the early postoperative risk profile.

Postoperative LGS complications can be divided into surgical and medical complications. This chapter aims to detail the most relevant early postoperative complications associated with LSG, emphasizing their pathophysiology, clinical features,

A. Sánchez-Gollarte (✉) · C. Guijarro-Moreno · V. Vaello-Jodra
Department of General and Visceral Surgery, Henares University Hospital, Madrid, Spain
e-mail: carlos.guijarro@salud.madrid.org; victor.vaello@salud.madrid.org

S. Jiménez-Blanco
Department of Endocrinology and Nutrition, La Princesa University Hospital, Madrid, Spain
e-mail: sara.jimenez@salud.madrid.org

J. Ruiz-Tovar (ed.), *Multidisciplinary Management of Sleeve Gastrectomy*,
https://doi.org/10.1007/978-3-032-25644-7_11

diagnostic approaches, and current strategies for prevention and treatment when they appear.

11.2 Early Surgical Complications of Sleeve Gastrectomy

11.2.1 Staple-Line Leak

Staple-line leak is one of the most feared complications following a LSG due to its association with significant clinical deterioration, sepsis, and prolonged hospital stays. The incidence varies from 1% to 3% for primary procedures and up to 10% in revision procedures [1]. The majority of leaks occur at the proximal third staple line, near the gastroesophageal junction, in an area known as His angle.

11.2.1.1 Definition and Classification

Staple-line leak can be defined as the effluent of gastrointestinal content through a suture line, which may collect near the stapled line or exit through the abdominal cavity or the drain.

Leaks can be classified based on either the time of onset, clinical presentation, site of leak, radiological appearance, or mixed factors (Table 11.1). Csendes et al. classified leakage as early when appearing within the first four postoperative days, intermediate when appearing in postoperative days 5–9 and late when occurring in or after the tenth postoperative days. By clinical presentation and extent of dissemination, type I or subclinical leakage was defined as well localized leak without dissemination into the pleural or abdominal cavity and without systemic clinical manifestations. Type II leakage was defined as leak which disseminates into abdominal or pleural cavity, with consequent severe and systemic clinical manifestations. Based on both clinical and radiological findings, type A leaks are micro-perforations without clinical or radiographic evidence of leak, while type B leaks are leaks

Table 11.1 Classification of LSG leaks

Leak classification		
Time of onset	Early	First 4 postoperative days
	Intermediate	4–9 postoperative days
	Late	≥ 10 postoperative days
Clinical presentation and extent of dissemination	I (subclinical)	Well localized without pleural or abdominal dissemination
	II	Dissemination into pleural or abdominal cavity.
Radiological and clinical findings	A	Micro-perforation. No clinical or radiological evidence of leak.
	B	Detected by radiological studies but without any clinical finding.
	C	Both radiological and clinical evidence.

detected by radiological studies but without any clinical finding, and finally, type C leaks were those which presented both radiological and clinical evidence [2].

11.2.1.2 Pathophysiology and Risk Factors

Gastric leaks are usually due to either ischemic or mechanical causes. Leak features are different depending on the related cause.

Mechanical Aspects

Mechanical aspects refer to stapler misfiring or direct tissue injuries that are related to early leak, which usually appears within 2 days after surgery. These mechanical factors are usually associated with the intrinsic characteristic of the long staple line of LSG but also with an adequate stapling technique. Optimal stapling should allow adequate time for tissue compression and creeping while preventing the production of excessive tensile stress. Waiting at least 15 s before firing is usually recommended to optimize stapling and allow adequate pre-cut compression time. Moreover, optimal stapling is related to proper cartridge choice considering that the thickness of the stomach wall varies, usually decreasing, from the pylorus to the angle of His [2].

Ischemic Aspects

Ischemic leaks typically occur on the fifth or sixth postoperative day. These leaks usually arise from the angle of His after a LSG which is considered as the critical area of this procedure. In that sense, experts recommend to stay away from the gastroesophageal junction on the last firing but at the same time not much away to avoid leaving residual fundus. Certain group recommends 1–2 centimeters as safe distance to avoid stapling too close to the esophagogastric junction in order to avoid ischemic leaks.

Ischemic leaks have also been related to aggressive dissection especially near the posterior aspect of the upper sleeve, leading to devascularization and making that area more susceptible to leakage in addition to thermal injuries to the gastric tube by ultrasonic devices.

11.2.1.3 Clinical Features

Clinical presentation can vary widely between totally asymptomatic patients diagnosed with postoperative routine imaging studies such as upper gastrointestinal series to the signs and symptoms of septic shock.

Simple postoperative tachycardia with or without other signs and symptoms after LSG should be considered as a **warning sign of complication** [3]. Tachycardia may be the earliest sign of staple-line leakage and appear before any other signs of sepsis. In that sense, heart rate above 120 beat/min is a powerful indicator of leak and systemic compromise specially accompanied by other signs of infection.

Fever, usually associated with tachycardia, should raise the index of suspicion of a septic complication and push the surgeon to perform further investigations to dismiss the presence of a leak.

Early leaks may present with sudden abdominal pain while late leaks tend to present with insidious abdominal pain [1]. However, physical examination in obese patients can be a challenge. Peritoneal signs such as rebound tenderness, guarding, or abdominal rigidity may be identified lately in evolved infections.

11.2.1.4 Diagnostic Approach

Staple-line leak diagnosis requires a high index of suspicion specially in subclinical cases and those presenting with unspecific signs or symptoms. Diagnosis is based on clinical features, laboratory findings, and radiological imaging.

Clinical features include signs of sepsis such as tachycardia, fever, and hypotension but also abdominal pain and signs of peritonitis during physical examination. These findings guide the diagnosis but usually further studies are performed to confirm the leak. In a small number of cases that present with septic shock, further investigations can be avoided and surgical treatment must be carried out if leakage is highly suspected.

Laboratory findings include leukocytosis with neutrophilia and high levels of C-reactive protein (CRP) and/or procalcitonin. Elevated levels of creatinine, prolonged clotting times (INR and TTPa), hyperfibrinogenemia, hyperlactatemia, and altered levels of liver enzymes can be altered in cases of organ failure. Some of these parameters can be used as predictors of postoperative leak. Ruiz Tovar et al. found that levels of CRP > 9 mg/L, procalcitonin >0.85 ng/mL, and fibrinogen >600 mg/dL at the first postoperative day should alert the surgeon about the possibility of the occurrence of postoperative septic complications, even before it becomes clinically apparent [4].

Computed tomography (CT) of the abdomen with intravenous and per-oral water-soluble contrast is considered as a part of the diagnostic workup of patients with suspected leak. Findings related to staple-line leak include the presence of abdominal collection or free fluid, extravasation of contrast into the abdominal cavity or the drain tube or persistent pneumoperitoneum (Fig. 11.1). CT is considered the best non-invasive modality for confirmation of a gastric leak as it offers information about leak size and location which is important to decide the best treatment [1].

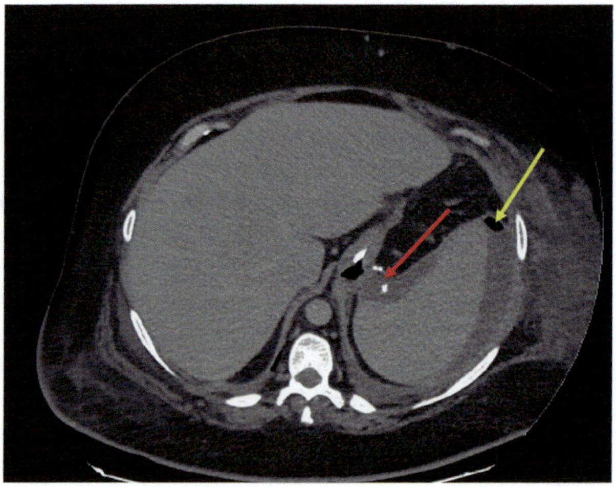

Fig. 11.1 CT scan of a staple-line leak showing the extravasation of oral contrast (red arrow) and pneumoperitoneum (yellow arrow)

Other diagnostic tools are upper gastrointestinal radiography, which may also localize the leak and define its size but is not as useful as CT to define the presence of collections or free pneumoperitoneum. Endoscopy has also been proposed for the diagnosis of gastric leak but is not usually the first step for this aim and often used as a part of leak treatment.

Patient clinical status in combination with laboratory and imaging findings allows surgeons to plan the optimal treatment approach.

11.2.1.5 Strategies for Treatment

Initial management was established based on the time of occurrence and the septic appearance of the patient. Non-septic patients will be managed according to radiological features on UGI series and CT scan. Septic patients will be directly reoperated for abdominal lavage, identification of the site of leak, and primary repair with simple suturing, surgical drainage, and insertion of a feeding jejunostomy. An overview of treatment for patients suffering from staple-line fistula is represented in Fig. 11.2.

General Management

In all cases of leak, the initial approach was insertion of a central line (PICC line), administration of broad-spectrum antibiotics with good anti-fungal coverage. Patients were kept nil per os (NPO) and total parenteral nutrition was started. This conservative management may be sufficient for most patients who presented with a type I fistula.

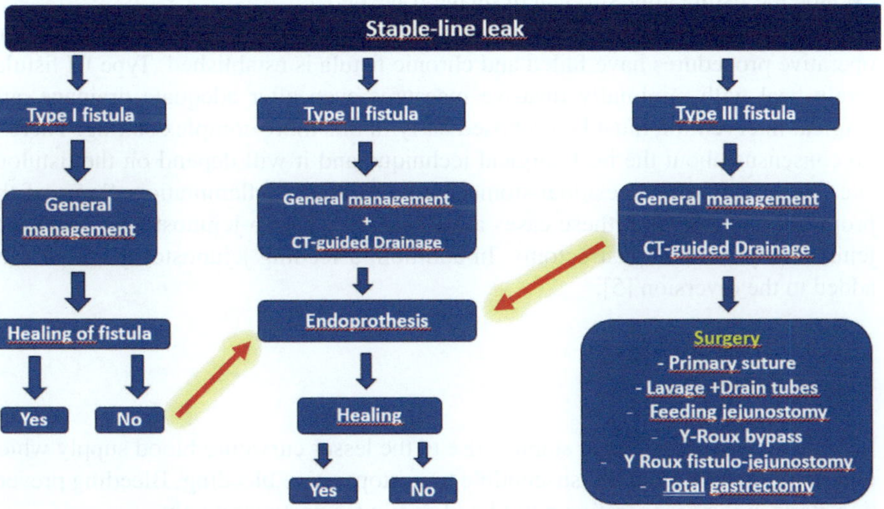

Fig. 11.2 Algorithm for staple-line leak treatment

Stable Patients

Once general measurements have been established, adequate drainage of any intra-abdominal collection visualized on CT scan should be performed either laparoscopically or preferably by CT-guided drainage [5].

In a stable patient with a proximal and mid-aspect gastric sleeve leak (type I fistula non-responding to general management, most type II fistula, and selected type III fistula), the use of an endoscopic stent may be a viable option in an attempt to exclude the defect. An upper endoscopy needs to be performed to assess the size and location of the leak, as well as the viability of the gastric sleeve. As endoscopically covered stents decrease the intraluminal pressure, it allows a conducive environment for the leaking site to heal. Other endoscopic strategies such as clips or fibrin glue have also been tried but stents seem to be more effective for the treatment of sleeve leaks.

The use of an endoscopic covered stent is a safe and effective option in the management of staple-line leaks after sleeve gastrectomy. However, 30 days after the operation, the possibility of the leak site healing by exclusion using a stent is low. Successful placement of a stent allows the patient to be fed orally, and if well, can be monitored as an outpatient. However, the stent migration rate is high (58–59%), and they have to be removed after 6–8 weeks, as the gastric mucosa may be damaged if kept for a more extended period [6].

Unstable Patients and Chronic Fistula

Unstable patient with a contained or uncontained leak warrants an urgent reoperation. The aim of emergency surgical procedure is to control the infection and achieve patient stabilization. Emergency strategies include abdominal lavage, identification of the site of leak, insertion of drain tubes, and the suture of the defect with a feeding jejunostomy if possible [5]. Endoscopic stent insertion can also be useful to exclude the fistula after surgical drainage if needed.

Surgical approach is also the treatment of choice when conservative and non-operative procedures have failed and chronic fistula is established. Type III fistulas rarely heal with minimally invasive measures even after adequate drainage, and surgical intervention must be proposed early in this more complex setting. There is no consensus about the best surgical technique and it will depend on the fistulous site, the quality of the residual stomach, and the local inflammation. Some of the proposed procedures in these cases are Roux-en-Y gastro-jejunostomy, esophago-jejunostomy, or total gastrectomy. In addition, a feeding jejunostomy can also be added to the diversion [5].

11.2.2 Bleeding

LSG involves a long gastric staple close to the lesser curvature blood supply which makes this procedure more susceptible to postoperative bleeding. Bleeding prevention starts in the preoperative period and continues postoperatively.

The preoperative evaluation should include a careful assessment and optimization of risk factors for bleeding including pharmacological treatments (specially anticoagulants) and medical conditions (renal disease, liver failure, or blood diseases). Weight loss prior to surgery is also necessary to reduce hemorrhagic risk because fatty liver is more likely to fracture during retraction and bleed in the perioperative phase. Preoperative weight loss or a lean diet 2–4 weeks before surgery can reduce liver size and consequently the risk of liver injury. Prior abdominal surgery may increase the complexity of the LSG because of the adhesions that must be divided both at the level of the abdominal wall and between the stomach and liver. The more extensive the adhesion, the greater is the chance of bleeding difficulty due to the more extensive dissection [7, 8].

Intraoperatively, an adequate revision of hemostasis emphasizing the most critical bleeding sites such as trocar sites insertion, the omentum, liver, and spleen, as well as the choice of adequate stapler cartridge size, are essential to avoid either intraoperative and postoperative hemorrhage.

11.2.2.1 Staple-Line Bleeding (Intraluminal Bleeding)

Bleeding from the staple line after LSG occurs in 1–2% of patients underwent LSG. Although this complication is less serious than a staple-line leak, some patients may require blood transfusion and/or re-exploration [9].

Staple-line bleeding presents as upper gastrointestinal bleeding (hematemesis and/or melena). This occurs typically in the early postoperative period and remains as self-limited bleeding. However, severe and/or persistent hemorrhages evolve to tachycardia, hypotension, and a drop in hemoglobin and hematocrit levels.

The initial management of upper gastrointestinal bleeding is based on resuscitation measures and discontinuation of subcutaneous heparin, oral anticoagulants, and/or antiplatelet agents. In the immediate postoperative period, it is important to assess the severity of the hemorrhage and rule out a concomitant extraluminal bleeding into the peritoneal cavity. If it is accompanied by hypotension, tachycardia, pallor and vasoconstriction and/or occurs within the first 6 h postoperatively with a decrease in hematocrit levels urgent reoperation will be required. If the bleeding appears more than 48 hours postoperatively without a drop in the hematocrit, a conservative approach is usually the treatment of choice.

Lack of response to medical therapy or persistence of bleeding requires upper endoscopy, although its use in the postoperative period is controversial due to the theoretical risk of staple-line dehiscence. Since most bleeding episodes are self-limited, upper endoscopy should be considered in patients who experience bleeding recurrence after conservative management, those with hemodynamic instability or a hemoglobin drop greater than 2 g/dL. In general, it is recommended to achieve hemostasis with endoscopic clips rather than vasoconstrictive agents to avoid tissue damage or ischemia in the surrounding area. The need for surgical intervention is exceptional [10]. A proposed algorithm for management of upper gastrointestinal bleeding after LSG can be found in Fig. 11.3.

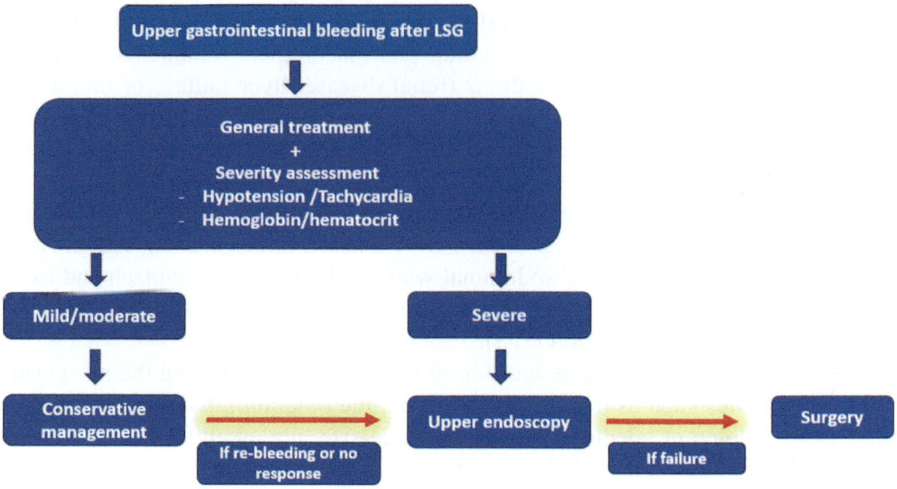

Fig. 11.3 Algorithm for the treatment of upper gastrointestinal bleeding

11.2.2.2 Intraabdominal Bleeding

Intraabdominal bleeding is defined as the hemorrhage that occurs inside the peritoneal cavity. Intraperitoneal bleeding can originate from different anatomical sites during the LGS leading to an intraoperative or postoperative hemorrhage.

Prevention of the intraabdominal bleeding is the best way to avoid this complication. In that sense, adequate revision of hemostasis emphasizing the most critical bleeding is required during the procedure and before abdominal closure. Laparoscopic port placement should be performed carefully and removed under direct view at the end of the procedure to assess adequate hemostasis.

Different critical anatomical sites that should be taken into account, which can lead to intraoperative or postoperative bleeding, are mainly short gastric vessels, major omentum, liver and spleen/splenic hilum.

In all cases of intraabdominal bleeding initial resuscitation with an adequate fluid intake is required. Blood transfusion must be considered in cases of hemoglobin less than 9 mg/dl or if the hemoglobin value drops more than 2 mg/dl [8]. Monitorization of vital signs, drain, urine output, hemoglobin, and hematocrit levels is mandatory.

Hemodynamically stable patients with intraperitoneal bleeding can be treated conservatively or by embolization techniques. CT scan with intravenous contrast should be performed to identify visceral injury and dismiss active bleeding which may require radiological embolization.

Unstable patients will undergo a re-intervention. The main objective should be the identification of the bleeding site, removal of blood clots, peritoneal lavage, and hemostasis with local sealant and mono-polar or bipolar coagulation with drain placement. In case of splenic injury, treatment will vary from splenic preservation with hemostatic procedures or splenectomy in cases of persistent hemorrhage or severe spleen damage.

11.2.3 Splenic Complications

11.2.3.1 Splenic Injuries

Splenic injuries deserve a special mention as a cause of intraabdominal bleeding during or after LSG. The incidence of splenic injury requiring splenectomy during laparoscopic sleeve gastrectomy is as low as 0.1%. Such injuries typically occur due to traction or laceration during the mobilization of the gastric fundus.

The spleen proximity to the surgical field and its extensive vascular supply makes it vulnerable to injury. Even minor trauma can cause significant hemorrhage, requiring immediate intervention. In order to minimize and prevent splenic injury during LSG, it is important to avoid excessive manipulation or unnecessary traction on peri-splenic peritoneal folds and reach the best and most adequate exposure and visualization of all anatomic structures. Another technical aspect for minimizing the risk of splenic injury may include the division of the short gastric vessels as close as possible to the stomach to avoid the risk of a splenic branch damage.

Management depends on patient clinical status and grade of spleen injury ranging from conservative treatment in stable patients with mild to moderate injuries without active bleeding, embolization in stable patients with active bleeding and surgical exploration in unstable patients. Surgical procedures range from conservative measures like direct pressure to splenectomy if bleeding is difficult to control. The American Association for the Surgery of Trauma (AAST) and the World Society of Emergency Surgery (WSES) proposed different classifications for splenic injuries (Tables 11.2 and 11.3) [11].

11.2.3.2 Splenic Infarction

Splenic infarction, although rare during LSG, results from the interruption of the splenic blood vessels. Most splenic infarctions are asymptomatic and incidentally discovered on postoperative period. When symptomatic, patients usually manifest left upper quadrant pain associated or not with fever.

Analgesia is the primary approach for symptomatic cases, typically involving NSAIDs or acetaminophen. Most patients recover fully without surgical intervention. In order to reduce the risk of splenic infarction, it is important to practice preventative measures during surgery, such as avoiding excessive traction and maintaining hydration.

11.2.3.3 Splenic Abscess

Splenic abscess is another rare and potentially life-threatening complication after LSG usually secondary to splenic infarction/ischemia. Patients may present with fever, left upper quadrant abdominal pain, nausea, and vomiting. In most cases, symptoms are non-specific, making the diagnosis challenging. The diagnostic process mainly relies on the combination of clinical presentation, blood tests (namely increased WBC count, CRP, and procalcitonin), and imaging. According to the literature, a contrast-enhanced abdominal CT scan remains the gold standard in the diagnosis since it can provide paramount information regarding the main

Table 11.2 AAST splenic injuries

Grade	Injury description	
I	Hematoma	Subcapsular, < 10% surface area
	Laceration	Capsular tear, < 1 cm parenchymal depth
II	Hematoma	Subcapsular, 10–50% surface area
	Laceration	Intraparenchyma, < 5 cm diameter
III	Hematoma	Subcapsular, > 50% surface area or expanding Ruptured subcapsular or parenchymal hematoma Intraparenchymal hematoma >5 cm
	Laceration	> 3 cm parenchymal depth or involving trabecular vessels.
IV	Laceration	Laceration of segmental or hilar vessels producing major devascularization (> 25% of spleen)
V	Laceration	Completely shatters spleen
	Vascular	Hilar vascular injury which devascularized spleen

characteristics of the splenic abscess (unilocular versus multilocular, presence of inner air component), which may have an impact on treatment choice.

The gold standard treatment for splenic abscess after SG is still under debate. The initial nonoperative approach includes intravenous broad-spectrum antibiotic therapy and percutaneous drainage without splenectomy. Splenectomy should be reserved for patients with complex abscess features, which may include multilocular composition and multiple or recurrent splenic abscesses where percutaneous drainage has failed.

11.2.4 Gastric Pouch Necrosis

Gastric pouch necrosis after LSG is an unusual but severe complication that requires emergency surgery. This complication can arise after endoscopic procedures to control gastric bleeding after LSG specially when adrenaline or etoxisclerol are used to stop the hemorrhage. Gastric vessel injury during the procedure can also lead to postoperative gastric sleeve necrosis. Gastric volvulus is a rare postoperative complication but if occurs may lead to gastric necrosis.

Table 11.3 WSES-AAST equivalence

	WSES CLASS	AAST	Hemodynamic	CT-scan	First-line treatment
Minor	WSES I	AAST I-II	Stable	YES	Conservative + serial clinical laboratory/imaging evaluation. Consider angiography +/– embolization
Moderate	WSES II	AAST III	Stable	YES	
	WSES III	AAST IV-V	Stable	YES	
Severe	WSES IV	AAST I-V unstable	Unstable	NO	Surgical

11.2.5 Esophageal Perforation

Esophageal perforation (EP) is a rare but extremely severe complication after LSG. It is usually related to intraoperative surgical maneuvers as well as orogastric tube insertion to calibrate sleeve size.

The initial clinical and biological presentation of EP has no specific patterns such as isolated tachycardia or fever. Late stages are characterized by signs of inflammation and sepsis. To avoid delay in diagnosis (> 50% of cases) and allow timely management, a high degree of suspicion is required at presentation.

11.2.5.1 Diagnostic and Treatment Strategies

Contrast-enhanced computed tomography (CT) and CT esophagography are the imaging examinations of choice in patients with suspicion of EP. CT is highly sensitive (92–100%) in detecting EP and helps to assess extension to adjacent structures (collection of air or fluid in the mediastinum, pleural, and intra-peritoneal effusions) and to guide initial therapy. CT can also eliminate other conditions that may mimic EP (aortic dissection, esophageal intramural hematoma, etc.). In select cases, contrast-enhanced esophagogram (gastrografin/barium) may provide useful information regarding the location and the contained character of EP. Indirect signs of esophageal injury can also be seen on a plain chest radiograph (pleural effusion, pneumomediastinum, subcutaneous emphysema, hydrothorax, pneumothorax, and collapse of the lung) *(*Fig. 11.4*)*.

Diagnostic endoscopy is useful in patients with suspected EP and doubtful CT findings. Diagnostic endoscopy for EP is reliable and safe in experienced hands; nevertheless, potential risks of enlarging the perforation size and aggravating the contamination of surrounding spaces warrant caution and limit its use as a first-line examination.

Endoscopic treatment is the gold standard for closing EP that occur and are recognized during an endoscopic procedure. New interventional endoscopic techniques, including endoscopic clips, covered metal stents, and endoluminal vacuum

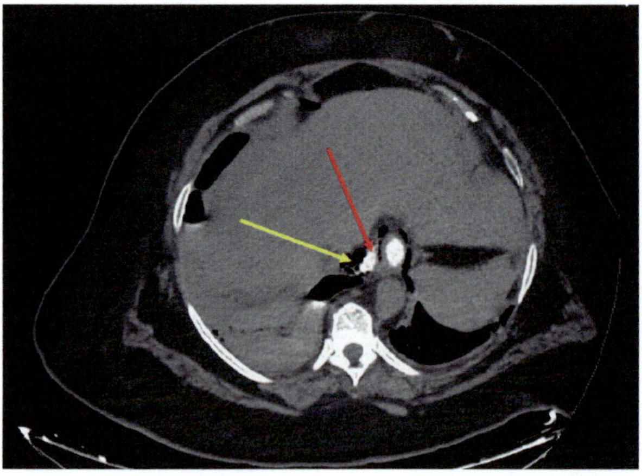

Fig. 11.4 Esophageal perforation during orogastric tube insertion showing contrast leak (red arrow) and extraluminal gas bubbles surrounding the esophagus

therapy, have been developed over the last several years to manage esophageal perforation in an attempt to decrease the related morbidity and mortality. Endoscopic clip placement (through the scope clips, over the scope clips) is currently the standard method for closing small (< 2 cm) luminal perforations. Endoscopic stents (partially or fully covered self-expandable metal stents, self-expandable plastic stents) can be used to cover larger defects or complete unsatisfactory clip closure. Minimal 2–4-week duration of stent placement has been advocated to allow sealing of the perforation. Esophageal stent placement is probably just as effective as surgical repair for the treatment of iatrogenic EP. Endoscopy may be used as definitive treatment either alone or in combination with interventional radiology or surgical procedures (drainage of pleural abscess, or compressive pneumothorax, etc.). Successful closure of esophageal defects by primary or rescue endoluminal vacuum therapy has been recently reported and may represent a promising alternative treatment for EP.

Non-operative Treatment and Minimally Invasive Treatment

Non-operative management (NOM) of EP can be considered in stable patients with early presentation, contained esophageal disruption, and minimal contamination of surrounding spaces if highly specialized surveillance is available. Patients eligible for NOM should be kept on nil per os, administered broad-spectrum antibiotics (aerobic and anaerobic bacteria), and proton pump inhibitor therapy. Early introduction of nutritional support by enteral feeding or total parenteral nutrition is essential for esophageal healing. Endoscopic placement of a nasogastric tube is recommended.

Additional measures should target sepsis control by using percutaneous radiology techniques to drain periesophageal and pleural collections. Drainage of pleural collections and pleural decortication by videothoracoscopy and use of endoscopic techniques (clips, stents, and internal vacuum drainage) are part of an aggressive minimally invasive management of EP.

Surgical Approach

Surgery should be undertaken in all patients who do not meet NOM criteria. General principles of esophageal perforation management include excellent exposure, debridement of non-viable tissue, closure of defect, use of buttress to reinforce esophageal sutures, and adequate tube drainage. The surgical approach should be tailored according to the location of EP [12].

Cervical EP

Cervical EP is unusual during LSG and if occurs is related to orogastric tube insertion. For EP located in the neck, direct repair of the esophageal defect should be attempted whenever feasible. The esophagus is approached through a left neck incision along the anterior border of the sternocleidomastoid muscle or by a collar incision if bilateral cervical exploration is required. Surgical treatment includes circumferential esophageal mobilization to facilitate repair, debridement of the perforation site, single- or double-layer tension-free closure of the perforation, buttressing of the repair with vascularized tissue (sternocleidomastoid muscle, digastric muscle), and adequate drainage. Placement of a feeding tube (nasogastric, jejunostomy) at the time of repair allows early nutritional support and favors healing. If direct repair is not feasible (disruption exceeds 50% of the esophageal circumference, delayed surgical exploration), external drainage is recommended. Construction of a lateral or end esophageal stoma should be considered to decrease contamination of surrounding spaces.

Thoracic EP

Primary repair is the treatment of choice for EP with free perforation of the thoracic esophagus. Management of perforation of the thoracic esophagus relies on immediate interruption of mediastinal and pleural contamination, debridement of the perforation to healthy tissue, tension-free primary repair, and adequate external drainage.

Thoracotomy will usually be required and the degree of pleural effusion or visible wall defect on CT may guide the incision side. A laparotomy or laparoscopy will usually be required in addition to enable construction of a feeding jejunostomy and possibly a decompressive tube gastrostomy. The alternative is a nasogastric tube or a combination of tubes to allow decompression and feeding. In general, a diversionary cervical esophagostoma (for saliva) is not recommended.

The mucosal defect is often longer than the muscular tear; longitudinal myotomy at both ends of the EP is useful to expose mucosal edges for appropriate repair. Two-layer repair, with separate suturing of the mucosa and muscle, has traditionally been recommended. Buttressing the esophageal repair with surrounding viable tissue (intercostal muscle flap, pleural or pericardial patch) has been recommended to decrease the risk of leakage. Drainage of the mediastinum and pleural cavity is required and enteral nutrition remains an essential component of the treatment plan. If direct repair of thoracic EP is not feasible (hemodynamic instability, delayed surgical exploration, extensive esophageal damage), esophageal exclusion, diversion, or resection should be performed. Repair over a large size T-tube can be used to create a controlled esophago-cutaneous fistula and minimize mediastinal and pleural contamination. Complete esophageal diversion or thoracic esophageal resection is required in the presence of large esophageal disruption; creation of a cervical esophagostomy and feeding jejunostomy are mandatory in these patients. If the patient survives, colon interposition or gastric pull-up reconstruction is required 6–12 months after complete diversion or resection of the thoracic esophagus [12].

Abdominal EP

Operative repair is the treatment of choice for patients with free perforation of the abdominal esophagus. Abdominal esophageal perforation should be approached by a midline laparotomy. Following debridement of necrotic tissues, single- or double-layer tension-free closure of the perforation should be performed. It is recommended to buttress the esophageal suture with a gastroplasty using the gastric fundus (i.e., complete or partial fundoplication); however, this maneuver is not possible after LSG as gastric fundus has been excised [13]. Insertion of a nasogastric tube, construction of a feeding jejunostomy, and performance of external drainage of the subphrenic space are also recommended.

11.2.6 Wound Complications

Surgical wound complications after laparoscopic sleeve gastrectomy (LSG) are relatively uncommon compared to open bariatric procedures, primarily due to the minimally invasive nature of the technique. Nevertheless, these complications can have a significant impact on postoperative recovery, patient morbidity, and health-care costs. The main wound-related complications reported in the literature include **surgical site infection (SSI), hematoma, seroma, wound dehiscence, and port-site hernia** [14–16].

Several patient- and procedure-related variables influence wound healing and the likelihood of complications. These include obesity, diabetes, smoking, malnutrition, surgical duration, trocar size and location, and intraoperative technique [14–16]. Optimization of comorbidities, perioperative glucose control, and proper postoperative wound care are essential to minimize risk [15, 17].

11.2.6.1 Surgical Site Infection (SSI)

The incidence of SSI following LSG is generally low, ranging between 1% and 5%, attributed to the use of laparoscopic approaches and perioperative antibiotic prophylaxis [14, 18]. However, the risk remains elevated in patients with obesity-related comorbidities such as diabetes mellitus, poor glycemic control, or immunosuppression [15, 17]. Clinical manifestations include localized erythema, pain, swelling, purulent discharge, and systemic signs such as fever. Management typically involves wound drainage, empirical or culture-guided antibiotic therapy, and, in severe cases, surgical debridement [14, 19].

11.2.6.2 Hematoma and Seroma

Hematomas result from bleeding into the subcutaneous or fascial layers due to inadequate hemostasis, while seromas are sterile accumulations of serous fluid secondary to tissue dissection and lymphatic leakage [16]. Small collections often resolve spontaneously, but larger or symptomatic cases may require percutaneous aspiration or placement of a drain. Preventive strategies include meticulous hemostasis, gentle tissue handling, and the use of closed-suction drainage when appropriate [14, 16].

11.2.6.3 Wound Dehiscence

Wound dehiscence represents partial or complete disruption of the surgical incision and may arise from increased intra-abdominal pressure, infection, or impaired wound healing. Predisposing factors include obesity, malnutrition, and steroid use. Prevention involves adequate fascial closure, minimizing wound tension, and controlling postoperative vomiting or coughing. Management depends on severity, ranging from local wound care to reoperation in cases of evisceration [16, 17].

11.2.6.4 Port-Site Hernia

Although rare (0.5–3%), port-site hernias can develop, particularly at trocar sites ≥10 mm or those inadequately closed [15]. Clinical presentation may include localized swelling, pain, or symptoms of bowel obstruction. Preventive measures include closing the fascial layer of ports larger than 10 mm and avoiding excessive enlargement of the incision. Symptomatic hernias generally require surgical repair [18].

11.3 Early Medical Complications after Sleeve Gastrectomy

Sleeve gastrectomy (SG) has become a cornerstone of bariatric surgery, widely adopted due to its procedural efficiency and favorable metabolic outcomes. While associated with relatively low complication rates, the early postoperative period can be compromised by several medical issues that impede patient recovery. These include dehydration, electrolyte disturbances, acute metabolic and nutritional issues, infectious complications, gastroesophageal reflux, and thrombotic events. Prompt recognition and management by a multidisciplinary team are essential for ensuring optimal patient outcomes [14, 20].

Effective postoperative management requires vigilant in-hospital monitoring of vital signs, urine output, daily weight, and laboratory parameters. Early outpatient follow-up, typically at 2 and 4 weeks post-discharge, is essential to assess oral tolerance, hydration status, and glycemic control. Patients must be educated to recognize and report "red-flag" symptoms, such as persistent vomiting (>48 h), severe dehydration, neurologic symptoms, or a deteriorating mental state, as these may signal a serious complication requiring prompt re-evaluation and potential readmission.

11.3.1 Dehydration and Fluid–Electrolyte Disorders

11.3.1.1 Clinical Features

Dehydration is the most frequent early complication, driven by the significantly reduced gastric capacity, postoperative nausea, vomiting, and potential alterations in thirst sensation [21]. Clinical manifestations range from mild (thirst, dry mucosa, concentrated urine) to severe (tachycardia, orthostatic hypotension, oliguria, confusion, and hypovolemic shock). Concurrently, electrolyte imbalances such as hypokalemia, hypomagnesemia, and metabolic alkalosis are common, particularly when gastrointestinal losses are significant.

11.3.1.2 Diagnosis

Diagnosis relies on a combination of clinical signs (dry mucosa, poor skin turgor, postural hypotension) and laboratory indicators. Key findings include hemoconcentration (BUN/creatinine ratio > 20:1), potential hypernatremia (>145 mEq/L), increased plasma osmolality (>295 mOsm/kg), and concentrated urine (specific gravity >1.025) with reduced sodium excretion [21].

11.3.1.3 Management

Management is stratified by severity. Mild cases typically respond to oral rehydration with small, frequent sips of isotonic, sugar-free fluids. Moderate to severe dehydration requires intravenous (IV) balanced crystalloids, with careful monitoring for fluid overload, particularly in patients with underlying cardiac or renal comorbidities. Close observation of urine output, daily weight, and regular electrolyte checks is required until resolution.

11.3.2 Acute Metabolic Disturbances

11.3.2.1 Clinical Features

Acute metabolic complications, including hyperglycemia and ketosis, can occur early after SG, even in non-diabetic patients, stemming from the surgical stress response and reduced oral intake [22]. Hyperglycemia may develop (often 250–400 mg/dL), presenting asymptomatically or with polydipsia and polyuria. Starvation ketosis can also occur, presenting with nausea, vomiting, abdominal pain, and an acetone odor on the breath.

11.3.2.2 Diagnosis

Diagnosis involves regular (e.g., 4–6 hourly) capillary blood glucose monitoring in the initial 3 days, evaluation for urine or serum ketones in patients with poor oral intake, and a blood gas analysis if an acid-base disorder is suspected. A comprehensive metabolic panel is essential to monitor renal and hepatic function [22].

11.3.2.3 Management

For diabetic patients, pre-existing insulin doses should be titrated downward (often a 50–75% reduction in basal dose) to maintain glycemic targets between 140–180 mg/dL. Oral agents like metformin and sulfonylureas are temporarily held. In the setting of ketosis, IV fluids with dextrose are provided once glucose levels normalize, along with the correction of any concurrent hypokalemia.

11.3.3 Early Nutritional Deficiencies

11.3.3.1 Clinical Features

While most nutritional deficiencies are long-term concerns, acute deficiencies can develop rapidly, especially in the context of prior malnutrition or significant postoperative fasting.

- *Thiamine Deficiency (Wernicke's Encephalopathy):* This is a neurologic emergency characterized by the classic triad of confusion, ataxia, and ophthalmoplegia (e.g., nystagmus). It can progress rapidly to coma and is often precipitated by persistent vomiting [23].

- *Hypoproteinemia:* Early protein malnutrition can also manifest, leading to edema, impaired wound healing, and increased infection risk.

11.3.3.2 Diagnosis

Diagnosis requires a high index of suspicion in at-risk patients (e.g., those with persistent vomiting). This is supported by laboratory assessment of thiamine, albumin, prealbumin, and other micronutrients as indicated.

11.3.3.3 Management

Empiric multivitamin supplementation is standard for all patients from day one. Any clinical suspicion of thiamine deficiency warrants immediate treatment with high-dose IV thiamine (e.g., 500 mg TID for 2–3 days, then 250 mg daily) before administering glucose. Protein supplementation should also be initiated.

11.3.4 Infectious Complications: Pneumonia and Aspiration

11.3.4.1 Clinical Features

Pulmonary infections, including hospital-acquired pneumonia and aspiration pneumonitis, typically occur between postoperative days 2 and 7. Patients with obstructive sleep apnea or prolonged operative times are at higher risk [24]. Pneumonia presents with fever, cough, tachypnea, and purulent sputum. Aspiration may cause sudden-onset hypoxia, respiratory distress, and crackles on auscultation.

11.3.4.2 Diagnosis

Diagnosis is based on clinical assessment and respiratory examination, confirmed by chest X-ray, which may be supplemented by CT imaging. Arterial blood gases and sputum or blood cultures help guide therapeutic choices [24].

11.3.4.3 Management

Management includes prompt empiric antibiotics tailored to patient risk and local flora, early pulmonary physiotherapy with incentive spirometry, and minimizing opioid analgesics to facilitate deep breathing and coughing.

11.3.5 Gastroesophageal Reflux Disease (GERD)

11.3.5.1 Clinical Features

New-onset or de novo GERD develops in 15–30% of SG patients, often within the first postoperative month [25]. Symptoms are primarily postprandial heartburn, acidic regurgitation, and mild dysphagia. Some patients may present with atypical symptoms like chronic cough or laryngitis.

11.3.5.2 Diagnosis

Diagnosis is primarily clinical. Upper endoscopy is reserved for patients with refractory symptoms, alarm signs (e.g., progressive dysphagia, bleeding), or severe discomfort. Esophageal manometry and pH monitoring may be used in cases of diagnostic uncertainty [25].

11.3.5.3 Management

Initial treatment involves an 8-week course of proton-pump inhibitors (e.g., omeprazole 40 mg/day), complemented by lifestyle and dietary modifications (avoiding reclining post-meals, separating solids and liquids, limiting trigger foods). Refractory cases may require surgical conversion to a gastric bypass.

11.3.6 Venous Thromboembolic Events (VTE)

11.3.6.1 Clinical Presentation

VTE occurs early (usually within 2 weeks). Clinical presentation depends on the location: Deep vein thrombosis (DVT) manifests as limb swelling, erythema, pain, and warmth. Pulmonary embolism (PE) presents with acute dyspnea, pleuritic chest pain, tachycardia, and potentially syncope or hypoxemia [26].

11.3.6.2 Diagnosis

Diagnosis is made via duplex ultrasonography for DVT and CT pulmonary angiography (CTPA) for PE. The D-dimer assay is unreliable in the immediate postoperative setting due to inflammatory changes and is not recommended.

11.3.6.3 Management

Effective management hinges on prevention. All patients receive perioperative thromboprophylaxis with weight- and renal-adjusted low-molecular-weight heparin (LMWH), typically continued for 10–14 days post-discharge. A confirmed VTE requires full therapeutic anticoagulation for 3–6 months [26].

11.3.7 Portal–Mesenteric Vein Thrombosis (PMVT)

11.3.7.1 Clinical Features

A rare but critical complication, PMVT typically presents between postoperative days 3 and 7 [27, 28]. The hallmark is severe, diffuse, or periumbilical abdominal pain that is often disproportionate to physical findings and frequently lacks peritonism. Nausea, vomiting, and abdominal distension are common.

11.3.7.2 Diagnosis

The diagnostic modality of choice is a contrast-enhanced abdominal CT, which can visualize the thrombus and identify signs of bowel ischemia. Doppler ultrasound is a useful screening tool.

11.3.7.3 Management

Management requires immediate therapeutic anticoagulation with LMWH. Following stabilization, oral anticoagulants are continued for 3–6 months. Extensive thrombosis or signs of bowel infarction necessitates urgent consultation for endovascular intervention or surgery [27, 28].

References

1. Abou Rached A, Basile M, El Masri H. Gastric leaks post sleeve gastrectomy: review of its prevention and management. World J Gastroenterol. 2014;20(38):13904–10.
2. Iossa A, Abdelgawad M, Watkins BM, Silecchia G. Leaks after laparoscopic sleeve gastrectomy: overview of pathogenesis and risk factors. Langenbeck's Arch Surg [Internet]. 2016;401(6):757–66. https://doi.org/10.1007/s00423-016-1464-6.
3. Kassir R, Debs T, Blanc P, Gugenheim J, Amor IB, Boutet C, Tiffet O. Complications of bariatric surgery: presentation and emergency management. 2016;27:77–81.
4. Alejandro G, Jose JR, Mun L. C-reactive protein , fibrinogen , and procalcitonin levels as early markers of staple line leak after laparoscopic sleeve gastrectomy in morbidly obese patients within an Enhanced Recovery After Surgery (ERAS) program. 2017;
5. Al Hajj G, Chemaly R. Fistula following laparoscopic sleeve gastrectomy: a proposed classification and algorithm for optimal management. Obes Surg. 2018;28(3):656–64.
6. Loo GH, Rajan R, Nik Mahmood NRK. Staple-line leak post primary sleeve gastrectomy. A two patient case series and literature review. Ann Med Surg [Internet]. 2019;44(May):72–6. https://doi.org/10.1016/j.amsu.2019.06.014.
7. Jossart GH. Complications of sleeve gastrectomy: bleeding and prevention. Surg Laparosc Endosc Percutaneous Tech. 2010;20(3):146–7.
8. De Angelis F, Abdelgawad M, Rizzello M. Perioperative hemorrhagic complications after laparoscopic sleeve gastrectomy: four-year experience of a bariatric center of excellence. Surg Endosc. 2016;
9. Khoursheed M, Al-bader I, Mouzannar A, Ashraf A. Postoperative bleeding and leakage after sleeve gastrectomy: a single-center experience. Obes Surg [Internet]. 2016; https://doi.org/10.1007/s11695-016-2215-z.
10. Ruiz de Adana JC, Villalonga Puy R, Del Arco GC. Urgencias del paciente con antecedente de cirugía bariátrica: Referencias-clave para el médico de guardia. In: Sociedad Española de Cirugía de la Obesidad y Enfermedades metabólicas. Madrid; 2019.
11. Coccolini F, Montori G, Catena F, Kluger Y, Biffl W, Moore EE, et al. Splenic trauma: WSES classification and guidelines for adult and pediatric patients. World J Emerg Surg. 2017;12(1):1–26.
12. Chirica M, Kelly MD, Siboni S, Aiolfi A, Riva CG, Asti E, et al. Esophageal emergencies: WSES guidelines. World J Emerg Surg. 2019;14(1):1–15.
13. Bevilacqua E, Aiolfi A, Tornese S, Tringali D, Panizzo V, Micheletto G, et al. Successful laparoscopic treatment of iatrogenic distal esophageal perforation during sleeve gastrectomy. Laparosc Surg. 2018;2:65.
14. Wozniewska P, Diemieszczyk I, Hady HR. Complications associated with laparoscopic sleeve gastrectomy—a review. Prz Gastroenterol. 2021;16(1):5–9.
15. Głuszyńska P, Diemieszczyk I, Szczerbiński Ł, Krętowski A, Major P, Razak Hady H. Risk factors for early and late complications after laparoscopic sleeve gastrectomy in one-year observation. J Clin Med. 2022;11(2):436.
16. Nienhuijs SW, de Zoete JP, Berende CAS, de Hingh IHJT, Smulders JF. Evaluation of laparoscopic sleeve gastrectomy on weight loss and co-morbidity. Int J Surg [Internet]. 2010;8(4):302–4. https://doi.org/10.1016/j.ijsu.2010.03.003.

17. Ullah R, Nazir M, Shahana N, Shuja I, Fazal MA, Nazir K, et al. Frequency of early complications of laparoscopic sleeve gastrectomy using four ports. Cureus. 2024;16(7)
18. Park Y, Park YS, Lee S, Kang SH, Lee E, Ahn SH, et al. Safety and effectiveness of reduced-port laparoscopic sleeve gastrectomy in Asian morbidly obese patients. Sci Rep [Internet]. 2021;11(1):1–11. https://doi.org/10.1038/s41598-021-02999-1.
19. Ruiz-Tovar J, Priego-Jimenez P, Paiva-Coronel GA. Use of Foley's catheter to control port-site bleeding in bariatric surgery. Obes Surg. 2012;22(2):306–8.
20. Glanternik J, Lazzati A, L'Huillier S, Ovize M, Karkas A. Early medical complications after bariatric surgery. J Visc Surg. 2021;158(6):499–509. https://doi.org/10.1016/j.jviscsurg.2021.03.003.
21. Ben-Porat T, El-Shami N, Sherf-Dagan S, Goldenshluger A, Shochat T, Keinan-Boker L. Dehydration and related adverse events after bariatric surgery: incidence, predictors, and management. Obes Surg. 2022 Apr;32(4):1125–35. https://doi.org/10.1007/s11695-022-05915-0.
22. Farrar E, Edwards C. Bariatric surgery complications. In: StatPearls [Internet]. Treasure Island: StatPearls Publishing; 2024. Updated 2024 Jul 1. PMID: 30969715.
23. Bathobakae L, Ozgur SS, Lombardo D, Mekheal N, Michael P. "Bariatric beriberi": a rare case of Wernicke encephalopathy two weeks after laparoscopic sleeve gastrectomy. Cureus. 2023;15(4):e37056. https://doi.org/10.7759/cureus.37056.
24. Grosser R, Romero-Velez G, Pereira X, Moran-Atkin E, Choi J, Camacho DR. Postoperative pneumonia after bariatric surgery during the COVID-19 pandemic: a National Surgical Quality Improvement Program study. Surg Obes Relat Dis. 2022;18(10):1239–45. https://doi.org/10.1016/j.soard.2022.06.015.
25. Fernández-Ananín S, Balagué Ponz C, Sala L, Molera A, Ballester E, Gonzalo B, et al. Gastroesophageal reflux after sleeve gastrectomy: the dimension of the problem. Cir Esp (Engl Ed). 2023;101(Suppl 4):S26–38. https://doi.org/10.1016/j.cireng.2023.05.019.
26. Froehling DA, Daniels PR, Mauck KF, Collazo-Clavell ML, Ashrani AA, Sarr MG, et al. Incidence of venous thromboembolism after bariatric surgery: a population-based cohort study. Obes Surg. 2013;23(11):1874–9. https://doi.org/10.1007/s11695-013-1073-1.
27. Goitein D, Matter I, Raziel A, Hazzan D, Rimon U, Ofer A. Portomesenteric thrombosis following laparoscopic bariatric surgery: incidence, patterns, and risk factors. Surg Endosc. 2013;27(10):3746–52. https://doi.org/10.1007/s00464-013-2949-0.
28. Al Wadaani HA, Al Omar S, AlRaihan J, Alnajjar JS, Elserougi M, Al Jabran H. Post laparoscopic sleeve gastrectomy portal vein thrombosis with venous mesenteric ischemia: a case report with literature review. J Surg Case Rep. 2024;2024(8):rjae462. https://doi.org/10.1093/jscr/rjae462.

12 Critical Care in the Patient Undergoing Sleeve Gastrectomy

Alfredo Serrano-Ruiz

12.1 Introduction

Bariatric surgery, an increasingly prevalent and efficacious intervention for patients exhibiting morbid obesity (BMI $\geq$40 kg/m^2) or complicated obesity (BMI 35–40 kg/m^2 with significant comorbidities), is strategically employed to facilitate sustained weight reduction and reduce the derived metabolic derangements [1]. However, individuals presenting with morbid obesity are burdened by pre-existing comorbidities, making them more susceptible to a greater chance of postoperative morbidity and mortality risks [2]. Therefore, a judicious application of intensive care unit (ICU) resources mandates a rigorous risk stratification schema, grounded in physiological parameters and objective clinical criteria.

Obesity has reached pandemic proportions, with rising prevalence observed across both developed and developing nations. Projections suggest an apex with almost 50% being recorded by 2030, while currently European countries present prevalence rates ranging from 20% to 30%. In light of these alarming trends, a concomitant surge in obese patients admitted to intensive care units (ICUs) is anticipated. Obesity amplifies the propensity for severe disease trajectories necessitating critical care support and mechanical ventilation, as demonstrated in the contexts of trauma, traumatic brain injury, out-of-hospital cardiac arrest, H1N1 pandemic influenza, and, most recently, coronavirus disease 2019 (COVID-19) [3].

Given the altered anatomy and physiology inherent in obese individuals, a high body mass index (BMI) has been reported to correlate with heightened risks. These include intraoperative atelectasis, difficulties in achieving effective face mask ventilation, complexities in airway management, and a reduction in both

A. Serrano-Ruiz (✉)
Nursing and Physiotherapy School, Comillas University, Madrid, Spain
e-mail: aserranor@comillas.edu

J. Ruiz-Tovar (ed.), *Multidisciplinary Management of Sleeve Gastrectomy*,
https://doi.org/10.1007/978-3-032-25644-7_12

cardiorespiratory reserve and overall functional capacity. These factors serve to further complicate surgical interventions in this patient demographic [4].

While obesity is generally acknowledged as a risk factor for various diseases, recent research reveals a more intricate association between body mass index (BMI) and survival, particularly in the setting of critical illness. Large-scale studies involving the general population have established a clear link between increased BMI and elevated mortality risk. However, analyses of hospitalized individuals or those managing chronic conditions present a divergent trend where overweight and moderately obese individuals exhibit lower mortality rates compared to those with normal or severely elevated BMIs [5].

This "obesity paradox," wherein obesity paradoxically confers a survival advantage despite concurrently increasing the risk of obesity-related diseases, has been observed across various medical domains. These span chronic conditions, including heart failure, coronary artery disease, and end-stage renal disease, as well as acute settings such as pneumonia, sepsis, and acute respiratory distress syndrome (ARDS). This highlights the importance of carefully scrutinizing the relationship between obesity and disease outcomes, acknowledging that the impact of adiposity is not invariably detrimental [6].

12.2 ICU Admission Criteria Following Bariatric Surgery

Bariatric surgery is an increasingly employed therapeutic intervention for patients with morbid obesity (BMI ≥40 kg/m^2) or complicated obesity (BMI 35–40 kg/m^2 with comorbidities), aimed at facilitating sustained weight loss and ameliorating associated metabolic dysfunction. However, morbidly obese (MO) patients often present with a high prevalence of pre-existing cardiopulmonary disease and multiple comorbidities, rendering them susceptible to elevated postoperative morbidity and mortality [1, 2].

While the necessity for postoperative ICU admission following bariatric surgery is relatively low, its occurrence is typically linked to patient profiles indicative of elevated risk and the presence of significant comorbidities. Respiratory insufficiency represents the most prevalent complication warranting ICU admission, succeeded by severe surgical emergencies, primarily characterized by hemorrhage and leaks in the surgical sutures or anastomoses. Timely identification of risk factors, including elevated American Society of Anesthesiologists (ASA) physical status classification, surgical reinterventions proximal to the initial procedure, conversions from laparoscopic to open surgical approaches, or the recognition of postoperative complications, is critical for optimizing perioperative management and improving outcomes [7, 8].

Absolute indications for ICU admission following sleeve gastrectomy are predicated upon the presence of hemodynamic instability, respiratory compromise or airway compromise, surgical complications with systemic repercussions, acute organ failure, or neurological compromise precluding airway protection. These categories will now be explicated with specific criteria:

- Hemodynamic Instability: Refractory hypotension, defined as a mean arterial pressure (MAP) less than 65 mmHg or systolic arterial pressure (SAP) less than 90 mmHg, accompanied by clinical signs of tissue hypoperfusion (e.g., altered mental status, cool extremities, elevated serum lactate), necessitating vasopressor administration for its correction. Hemorrhagic shock or active bleeding, evidenced by significant blood loss leading to hemodynamic instability, activation of massive transfusion protocols, or the requirement for more than four units of packed red blood cells within a compressed timeframe, constitutes a critical indication. Hemodynamically destabilizing arrhythmias, such as ventricular tachycardia, fibrillation, complete atrioventricular block with adverse hemodynamic consequences, or acute myocardial ischemia with circulatory compromise, mandate immediate intervention [8, 9].
- Respiratory and Airway Compromise: Situations where patients remain intubated post-intervention or cannot be safely extubated in the immediate recovery period due to depressed level of consciousness, respiratory muscle fatigue, or persistent hypoxemia are deemed relevant. Acute respiratory insufficiency, defined by a PaO2/FiO2 ratio below 200, the sustained requirement for a FiO2 exceeding 0.6 to maintain SpO2 of 92% or greater, or the presence of hypoventilation with elevated PaCO2 and concomitant clinical deterioration, represents another criterion for inclusion. Additionally, pharyngeal edema, cervical hematoma, bleeding in the cervical region, or the identification or suspicion of a difficult airway necessitate specialized care. Finally, severe obstructive sleep apnea requiring assisted ventilation via CPAP/VPAP that cannot be adequately managed on a conventional surgical floor justifies intensive monitoring and treatment [10, 11].
- Surgical Complications: Immediate postoperative care involves close monitoring and early intervention. A leak in the suture line, as indicated by systemic repercussions, calls for evaluation with image testing for support and management [8].
- Infectious Processes: Sepsis or septic shock, defined by an infection complicated by acute organ dysfunction (evidenced by an increase in the Sequential Organ Failure Assessment [SOFA] score ≥ 2) or hypotension requiring vasopressor support after adequate fluid resuscitation, constitutes an indication for ICU transfer [8].
- Neurological Deterioration: Patients exhibiting a Glasgow Coma Scale score ≤ 8 or experiencing neurological deterioration that impairs airway protection necessitate intensive care, potentially entailing endotracheal intubation, mechanical ventilation, hemodynamic stabilization, and continuous neurological monitoring. Recurrent seizures or status epilepticus require urgent management with anticonvulsants and intensive surveillance [12].
- Renal and Metabolic Derangements: Acute renal insufficiency with persistent oliguria or the need for renal replacement therapy stands as a relevant criterion. Similarly, severe metabolic derangements, such as significant lactic acidosis, symptomatic hyperkalemia, or severe sodium abnormalities, necessitate continuous correction and monitoring in an intensive care environment.

- Hematological Abnormalities: Coagulopathy with active bleeding or the need for transfusion protocol activation requires ICU stay [9].
- Finally, transfer to the ICU is prudent for patients who, on account of the preanesthetic evaluation, preexisting comorbidities, or frailty, require preventative intensive monitoring to avert potential complications.

12.3 Airway Management

The escalating prevalence of morbid obesity (MO) introduces unique complexities into perioperative care, particularly concerning airway management. The anatomical and physiological alterations inherent in this population necessitate a strategic, multifaceted approach to minimize respiratory risks and improve patient outcomes. This discourse outlines key considerations for pre-operative evaluation, intraoperative airway management, and postoperative strategies, emphasizing techniques to mitigate potential challenges and optimize patient well-being [12].

A meticulous preoperative assessment forms the bedrock of safe and effective anesthetic management. Beyond standard medical history and physical examination, specific attention must be given to cardiopulmonary conditions common in MO patients, including obstructive sleep apnea (OSA), obesity hypoventilation syndrome (OHS), pulmonary hypertension, and cardiac dysfunction. Polysomnography should be considered for undiagnosed OSA, while arterial blood gas analysis can assess chronic hypoventilation.

Detailed airway assessment involves evaluating neck circumference, thyromental distance, mouth opening, and Mallampati score to identify factors predictive of difficult mask ventilation or laryngoscopy. Radiographic imaging (e.g., lateral neck X-ray) may be warranted in select cases to evaluate the presence of anatomical abnormalities.

Furthermore, healthcare providers have an obligation to provide patients with MO all factors that impact treatment and provide treatment options [12].

Intraoperative and intensive care airway management demands meticulous planning and adherence to evidence-based best practices. The following strategies are critical:

- Positioning: Ramped positioning, achieved by placing blankets or specialized devices beneath the patient's head, neck, and upper torso, optimizes airway alignment and improves visualization during laryngoscopy. This position helps to compensate for the increased neck circumference and adipose tissue deposition in MO patients [13].
- Preoxygenation: Prior to induction, meticulous preoxygenation with 100% oxygen via a tight-fitting face mask or non-invasive ventilation (NIV) is essential to maximize oxygen reserves. A preoxygenation strategy with high-flow nasal cannula (HFNC) can further prolong the safe apnea time during intubation [14].
- Induction Techniques: Rapid sequence induction (RSI) with cricoid pressure is generally indicated to minimize aspiration risk. Careful titration of induction

agents and neuromuscular blockade ensures controlled airway access while minimizing the risk of hemodynamic instability.
- Laryngoscopy Techniques: Direct laryngoscopy may be challenging due to anatomical distortions and limited neck mobility. Video laryngoscopy is strongly recommended as a first-line approach, offering enhanced visualization of the glottic opening and potentially increasing first-pass success rates. Alternative airway adjuncts, such as intubating stylets and laryngeal mask airways (LMAs), should be readily available as rescue devices [15].

Postoperative and postextubation in intensive care airway management in MO patients necessitates close monitoring and vigilance for respiratory complications. Patients should be maintained in a semi-recumbent position to optimize respiratory mechanics and facilitate lung expansion. Prophylactic NIV should be considered, particularly in those with known OSA or OHS, to prevent postextubation respiratory failure and atelectasis. Early mobilization and pulmonary hygiene measures are also essential to promote lung clearance and prevent respiratory infections [12].

12.4 Ventilation

Obesity, particularly abdominal obesity characterized by an android fat distribution, induces marked alterations in respiratory anatomy and physiology, thereby complicating airway management and ventilator settings during mechanical ventilation. The predisposition to respiratory complications is also heightened, with obesity demonstrably associated with an increased risk of developing acute respiratory distress syndrome (ARDS) and infections, particularly pneumonia. Consequently, obese patients requiring mechanical ventilation experience prolonged ICU stays and ventilation durations [12].

This patient group often displays heightened respiratory workload and impaired gas exchange. A critical factor is the reduction in lung volumes, a consequence of cephalic diaphragmatic displacement due to elevated tissue mass within the abdomen and thoracic walls. Functional residual capacity (FRC) diminishes by 5–15% for every 5 kg/m^2 increase in BMI, promoting atelectasis, a process exacerbated by anesthesia and neuromuscular blockade [16].

Obesity is linked with increased abdominal and thoracic tissue mass, which exerts additional hydrostatic pressure on alveoli. When pleural pressure surpasses intra-alveolar pressure, alveolar collapse ensues, predisposing dependent lung regions to compressive atelectasis. It is intuitive that a recruitment maneuver followed by adequate positive end-expiratory pressure (PEEP) would thus prove beneficial. However, the application of higher PEEP levels is often accompanied by hemodynamic compromise and increased requirements for fluids and vasopressors, mandating careful titration. Limiting tidal volumes to 6–8 mL/kg of predicted body weight (PBW) can mitigate ventilator-associated lung injury by normalizing tidal volume for PBW and limiting mechanical pulmonary strain [12, 16].

Obese patients show a higher risk of pulmonary and pulmonary diseases. Therefore, non-invasive ventilation (NIV) is recommended for both prevention and treatment of respiratory failure, specifically by following current physiological data and by recognizing that there is still little support for making statements on this case.

A central observation is a phenomenon termed the "obesity paradox," where, in the general population, obesity is a key risk factor for chronic diseases and mortality, critically ill obese patients may exhibit improved survival, often due to complex interactions between inflammation and protective compensatory mechanisms [6].

12.5 Hemodynamic Monitorization and Support

Managing cardiovascular function in critically ill obese adults requires a comprehensive understanding of their unique pathophysiology. Obesity-related cardiovascular disease results from both fat mass-related and sick fat-related pathologies. Increased blood volume and cardiac output contribute to ventricular hypertrophy, diastolic dysfunction, and, potentially, dilated cardiomyopathy (obesity cardiomyopathy). Additionally, heightened rates of atrial fibrillation and pulmonary hypertension (secondary to increased left atrial pressure, obstructive sleep apnea/hypoventilation syndrome, or thromboembolism) are frequent. Effective management thus necessitates a multifaceted approach [4].

Accurate hemodynamic monitoring becomes critical but can be difficult in obese individuals. Oscillometric measurements tend to be less accurate; therefore, invasive blood pressure monitoring should be considered as standard. Consider transthoracic echocardiography, which helps determine ventricular functions. If transesophageal echocardiography (TEE) is utilized, imaging should be used more precisely when standard transthoracic measures are tough to collect [17].

Furthermore, it is vital to note that hemodynamic parameters in obesity can differ from those in non-obese patients. Indexing these parameters to body surface area might offer some correction for body habitus, though more research is needed to define optimal targets.

Fluid resuscitation calls for precision. The raised blood volume and the potential for heart failure indicate the importance to cautiously track fluid responsiveness. This requires evaluating stroke volume and other hemodynamic characteristics while cautiously administering crystalloid fluid. In individuals who have an existing kidney or cardiovascular condition, a conservative strategy of maintenance of perfusion pressures while closely watching fluid equilibrium is encouraged [17].

Given those difficulties, a precise technique is essential to evaluate the use of vasopressor medications. Some evidence reveals that obese people in septic shock had greater fluid needs, which may show the need to maintain an acceptable blood pressure and flow while minimizing needless fluid overload. Using ideal body weight for vasopressor dosage calculations can guide therapy when taking into account the patient's hemodynamic response, clinical circumstance, and the potential for toxicity [17].

Ultimately, it's important to treat cardiac problems that are occurring. Carefully consider and eliminate any underlying cardiac issues while providing individualized assistance focused on heart problems of the patients.

By combining these methods, physicians must attempt to improve cardiovascular results while restricting potential adverse consequences like fluid overload or underdosing. An awareness of the specific obstacles impacting seriously unwell obese patients enables the use of prompt interventions and specialized therapy to handle hemodynamic problems. These individualized tactics are important to assist people with those problems and enhance outcomes.

12.5.1 Cardiopulmonary Resuscitation on Obese Patients

Managing cardiopulmonary resuscitation (CPR) in obese adults demands a tailored approach, incorporating both fundamental principles and adaptations to anatomical and physiological considerations. The goal is to maximize the effectiveness of interventions and improve the likelihood of positive outcomes.

Obesity is frequently associated with an increased likelihood of difficult mask ventilation and challenges in securing the airway. Regarding airway management, early endotracheal intubation using skilled personnel is of the highest priority, as is using two hands technique for mask seal. These measures can decrease aspirations and support correct oxygenation. Also, the health providers must assess equipment for airway intubation [18].

Ensuring effective chest compressions is essential, but the process may require significantly increased physical force due to the thickness of the chest wall and surrounding adipose tissue. To mitigate rescuer fatigue and maintain the critical compression depth, it is advisable to switch the rescuer performing chest compressions frequently, ideally more often than the standard two-minute cycle. The use of mechanical chest compression devices may be considered when high-quality manual compressions are impractical or compromise provider safety. However, the physical dimensions and contour of the chest wall in patients with extreme obesity may limit the usefulness of many currently available mechanical systems [18, 19].

For managing shockable rhythms (ventricular fibrillation/pulseless ventricular tachycardia), standard energy levels should be utilized. Existing studies generally suggest that the efficacy of defibrillation for a given energy level does not substantially differ in obese patients compared to normal-weight patients.

Although some literature suggests that mortality might be higher in obese patients undergoing ECPR compared to normal-weight patients, this advanced therapy should not be withheld solely on the basis of obesity if it is otherwise clinically indicated according to local protocols [20].

It is important to consider the unique pharmacological considerations present in obese patients, although the precise details are a matter of debate.

Effective teamwork and communication between healthcare professionals ensures that rapid and precise intervention happens, improving treatment efficacy.

By acknowledging particular considerations and employing customized strategies, healthcare practitioners could provide better care in cases of cardiac arrest concerning obese grown-ups. To best support this important aim, continuing educational efforts should concentrate in building capabilities and awareness of customized procedure implementations.

12.6 Pain, Agitation, and Delirium

Pain, agitation, and delirium management in obese critically ill patients presents unique complexities stemming from altered physiology and limited data guiding pharmacotherapy. Optimal strategies prioritize titrating medications to clinical effect, while also considering individual patient characteristics and weight management to minimize complications and mortality [7].

- Opioid analgesics should be carefully titrated, utilizing ideal or adjusted body weight to minimize the risk of oversedation and respiratory depression. For sedatives like propofol and dexmedetomidine, ideal or adjusted body weight is generally preferred to estimate maintenance dose [21].
- Propofol's high lipophilicity might suggest utilizing total body weight. However, the non-linear relationship between total body weight and drug clearance carries a risk of supratherapeutic concentrations. Similarly, dexmedetomidine, despite exhibiting broad distribution, shows decreased clearance in obese patients, reinforcing the importance of basing the dosage on ideal or adjusted body weight. This approach mitigates drug accumulation and reduces the risk of hypotension and other associated adverse effects [22].
- Midazolam, a benzodiazepine, exhibits complex pharmacokinetic behavior in obese patients. While the initial volume of distribution may increase, requiring higher loading doses to attain the desired sedation level, drug clearance is not significantly affected by weight gain. Therefore, the risk of accumulation and overdose with continuous administration is latently elevated, particularly if total body weight is used for maintenance dosing. Consequently, continuous administration should be guided by ideal or adjusted body weight, closely monitoring the clinical response to avert oversedation and its associated adverse effects [22].
- In managing delirium, haloperidol, a typical antipsychotic, and quetiapine, an atypical antipsychotic, are frequently used at standard, non-weight-based doses. While haloperidol's pharmacokinetic properties suggest distribution into adipose tissue, the risk of QTc interval prolongation necessitates rigorous electrocardiographic monitoring. Quetiapine, often preferred by its more favorable adverse effect profile, is similarly utilized at standard doses, although data on its pharmacokinetic behavior in critically ill obese patients remain limited [22].

Individualized care, including consultation with clinical pharmacists, is crucial for safe and efficacious medication management in critically ill obese patients, guiding appropriate drug selection and dose adjustments to optimize therapeutic outcomes while minimizing harm. Intensive care clinical pharmacists play a major part in tracking progress and minimizing the risks to those unique patients.

12.7 Acute Kidney Injury and Renal Support

Acute kidney injury (AKI) represents a frequent and formidable complication within the critical care setting, posing heightened risks for patients with obesity. Obesity, characterized by increased body mass index (BMI), is increasingly prevalent in ICUs and is associated with distinct physiological and metabolic derangements that modify the risk, progression, and outcomes of AKI. This discussion underscores the underlying mechanisms, diagnostic challenges, and management considerations relevant to AKI in obese critically ill patients, synthesizing current evidence and providing guidance for clinical decision-making [23, 24].

Obesity introduces several factors that contribute to increased AKI susceptibility. Alterations in renal hemodynamics, including increased glomerular filtration rate (GFR) and hyperfiltration, coupled with heightened tubular sodium reabsorption, can lead to glomerular injury over time. Adipose tissue stimulates the production of angiotensinogen and aldosterone, thereby activating the renin-angiotensin-aldosterone system, and contributing to glomerular injury. These combined effects increase vulnerability to ischemia-reperfusion injuries and toxicity from nephrotoxic agents [25, 26].

Adiposity promotes a systemic inflammatory state characterized by elevated levels of pro-inflammatory cytokines like TNF-α and IL-6, and increases risk of infection as those same hormonal factors, such as leptin, increase both innate and adaptive immune responses [27].

Alterations to the glomerular structure and other hormonal changes can also affect the kidneys as it struggles to filter blood. Together, these factors exacerbate renal vulnerability.

Identifying AKI in obese patients poses specific challenges. Serum creatinine, a commonly used AKI marker, is influenced by muscle mass, which can vary widely in obesity. This variability complicates interpreting creatinine changes as it may or may not be due to kidney damage as the patients go through treatment.

Consequently, relying solely on serum creatinine may lead to underdiagnosis or delayed recognition of AKI. Additionally, difficulties with bladder catheterization and accurate urine output monitoring may hinder the application of established AKI diagnostic criteria.

Effective management of AKI in obese patients demands a multifaceted approach. Optimizing hemodynamic stability and maintaining adequate renal perfusion pressure are of paramount importance. While high-quality evidence on precise blood pressure targets is lacking, recommendations tend to ensure proper fluid balance. Cautious fluid resuscitation is guided by hemodynamic parameters to prevent both hypovolemia and hypervolemia, and which can increase the risk of further damage or fluid overload and related problems [19, 25, 28].

Due to its potential to both enhance outcomes and increase damage from side effects, the use of pharmaceuticals has to be managed with great care. Consideration should be afforded to the pharmacokinetic changes in obese clients which occur due to modified weight, metabolism, and distribution. The adjustment for the creatinine rates is based on the greatest known creatinine estimate and can be calculated depending on altered creatinine clearance rates depending on body weights. Monitoring by pharmaceuticals is very essential for finding the proper administration and dosage.

When available, renal replacement therapy (RRT) is a critical intervention for managing severe AKI, volume overload, electrolyte imbalances, and metabolic acidosis. Intermittent hemodialysis, prolonged intermittent renal replacement therapy (PIRRT), and continuous renal replacement therapy (CRRT) are treatment modalities that each have unique merits in different scenarios. To establish the treatment program with renal replacement therapies, variables have to be considered, such as hemodynamic balance, resource usage, patient tolerability, and the expertise of available workers.

Future research into the intricacies and nuances of AKI in overweight patients need to enhance the approaches. It's also of significant importance to recognize other considerations about how treatment choices are made. Ultimately, improved methods of identification of the risks to AKI along with targeted therapy and team collaborations will probably enable clinicians to boost results and alleviate problems.

12.8 Nutrition and Elimination

Critically ill surgical patients experience a complex and often maladaptive metabolic response that can significantly impair immune function, delay wound healing, and induce muscle wasting, thereby increasing their risk of morbidity and mortality. Inadequate nutritional intake during this critical period further exacerbates adverse outcomes, emphasizing the importance of targeted nutritional interventions. Over time, the concept of nutritional support has advanced into a broader paradigm of nutrition therapy, aimed at preventing oxidative cellular injury, modulating the immune response, and attenuating the exaggerated metabolic response associated with critical illness [29–31].

In the intensive care setting, early initiation of oral feeding, when feasible, constitutes the preferred approach, as it supports gastrointestinal integrity and enhances recovery. Conversely, neglecting nutritional therapy altogether promotes underfeeding in the postoperative phase, especially after major surgeries, which can hamper convalescence and increase complication rates. Early enteral nutrition (EEN) is strongly recommended for critically ill patients because evidence demonstrates its superiority over delayed enteral feeding and early parenteral nutrition in reducing mortality and improving outcomes. Importantly, EEN can be safely commenced soon after hemodynamic stabilization, even in patients receiving vasopressors, to preserve gut mucosal integrity and mitigate systemic inflammatory responses [29, 30].

Parenteral nutrition, while generally reserved for complex cases involving major surgical complications, is not typically indicated following uncomplicated bariatric procedures. In scenarios where relaparotomy is required, enteral nutrition via nasojejunal tube or needle catheter jejunostomy (NCJ) is preferred over parenteral routes due to its proven benefits in reducing mortality and healthcare costs [32].

Postoperative nutritional management in bariatric patients, particularly those undergoing sleeve gastrectomy, centers on preventing nutritional deficiencies, promoting adequate intake, and providing necessary supplementation to optimize recovery and support long-term weight loss [33, 34].

Malnutrition remains a significant risk in bariatric patients, even in those who are overweight or obese. This risk stems from factors such as severe malabsorption, surgical complications, and altered gastrointestinal physiology, including accelerated gastric emptying characteristic of sleeve gastrectomy. Consequently, artificial nutritional support, including parenteral nutrition, may be warranted in cases of severe malnutrition. A personalized, closely monitored nutritional approach is essential, entailing regular assessment of food intake, supplementation with oral nutritional supplements, and timely initiation of enteral or parenteral nutrition when indicated. Recognizing preoperative nutritional risk allows development of tailored postoperative plans that facilitate optimal recovery and long-term success [33, 34].

12.9 Hematological Monitoring

Following bariatric surgery, several factors contribute to a high incidence of iron deficiency anemia. Reduced dietary intake, impaired intestinal absorption, and menstruation (in women) all play a role. Vitamin B12 absorption is also negatively impacted by procedures like sleeve gastrectomy (SG), Roux-en-Y gastric bypass (RYGB), and biliopancreatic diversion with duodenal switch (BPD/DS), given their disruption of the acidic gastric environment and intrinsic factor production [35].

Though B12 stores can last years, deficiency may emerge postoperatively, impacting both hematopoietic and nervous systems, potentially leading to megaloblastic anemia and irreversible neuropathies. Given the unreliability of serum B12 levels in predicting deficiency, methylmalonic acid (MMA) testing is advised when in doubt. Folic acid absorption, primarily in the small bowel, may be compromised by RYGB or BPD/DS, but low dietary intake or non-adherence to supplements is frequently implicated, especially post-SG. As vitamin B12 deficiency is associated with both folate and iron and it may cause megaloblastic and macrocytic anemia, it is necessary to assess all hematic before folate complements are to be added [35].

Postoperative thromboembolic complications represent a considerable source of morbidity and mortality. Risk factors such as obesity, a history of venous thromboembolism, smoking, and other clinical conditions can increase this risk. There is a wide variation in bariatric surgery. Due to the results of a Cochrane review, the usage of intermittent pneumatic leg compression alongside pharmacological measures can decrease the rate of developing venous thrombosis [36].

Additionally, current suggestions advocate the use of pharmacological prophylaxis, including unfractionated heparin or low-molecular-weight heparin (LMWH), within the first 24 hours postoperatively for all individuals. Twice daily dosing with enoxaparin, dalteparin, or tinzaparin should be considered in patients with a body mass index above 40 kg/m^2. Prophylactic measures may not consistently achieve aXa targets; in high-risk individuals, tracking aXa can enhance individualized dosage [37].

Thromboembolic occurrences after release are a serious risk that is much more elevated in case they had a record. Therefore, for people in danger who go beyond the usual treatments, the postdischarge measures need to be thoroughly looked at. Prophylaxis may not, however, consistently stop thromboembolism, but further evaluation is needed into how they influence prophylaxis methods. Retrievable inferior vena cava filters might help that issue. Portal-mesentric and splenic vein thrombosis can happen [38].

To reduce that unique issue, extra assessment of the current guidelines and strategies may be needed [7].

12.10 Prevention and Treatment of Infection

The increasing global prevalence of obesity necessitates a re-evaluation of antimicrobial dosing strategies, especially within the context of critical illness. While adhering to core pharmacological principles, it is imperative to recognize the distinctive anatomical and physiological alterations in obese patients that significantly impact drug distribution, metabolism, and excretion [28, 39, 40].

A cornerstone of effective antimicrobial treatment in obese adults involves the recognition that standard dosing regimens, commonly based on total body weight (TBW), may yield subtherapeutic drug concentrations at the site of infection, thereby increasing the risk of treatment failure and fostering antimicrobial resistance. It's essential to acknowledge that the volume of distribution, clearance, and elimination half-life can be significantly altered in obese patients due to factors such as increased adipose tissue mass, altered protein binding, and concomitant changes in renal and hepatic function [28, 40].

Central to navigating this complexity is the choice of an appropriate dosing weight descriptor. While TBW might seem intuitive, it can lead to overestimation of drug exposure for hydrophilic agents that preferentially distribute into lean tissues. Alternative weight metrics, including ideal body weight (IBW), adjusted body weight (AdjBW), or lean body weight (LBW), may offer more accurate predictions of drug distribution and target attainment. The selection of the most suitable descriptor must consider the physicochemical properties of the antimicrobial agent, the patient's body composition, and the specific clinical context [28, 39].

Given the intricate interplay of factors influencing antimicrobial pharmacokinetics in obesity, therapeutic drug monitoring (TDM) assumes paramount importance. TDM allows for the individualization of dosing regimens, ensuring that drug concentrations are optimized while minimizing the risk of toxicity. This is particularly critical for antimicrobials with narrow therapeutic windows and high inter-patient variability, such as aminoglycosides and vancomycin. Target-specific AUC/MIC ratios or trough concentrations should be used to guide dose adjustments, guided by established guidelines and institutional protocols [28, 39].

Recognizing that many antimicrobials exhibit time-dependent bactericidal activity, prolonged or continuous infusions of beta-lactam antibiotics may offer advantages over intermittent infusions. Such strategies may enhance target attainment, particularly when treating infections caused by organisms with elevated minimum inhibitory concentrations (MICs) or in patients exhibiting augmented renal clearance [27].

Accurately estimating renal function is also essential for optimizing antimicrobial dosing in obese patients. While the Cockcroft-Gault equation is commonly used, it may overestimate creatinine clearance (CrCl) in obese individuals. Consideration should be given to alternative methods of estimating renal function, including formulas incorporating adjusted body weight or those based on cystatin C, to guide dose adjustments in patients with renal impairment.

While definitive randomized controlled trials specifically addressing antimicrobial dosing in obese individuals remain limited, evolving data and pharmacokinetic modeling analyses support the implementation of the strategies outlined above. The effective pharmacotherapy of infections in obese adults ultimately necessitates integrating a thorough understanding of antimicrobial properties, patient-specific characteristics, meticulous TDM strategies, and emerging data on alternative dosing metrics. As research continues to illuminate the intricacies of antimicrobial pharmacokinetics in obesity, clinicians must adapt their approach to optimize therapeutic outcomes and mitigate adverse effects, thus improving the well-being of this increasingly prevalent patient population [28, 39, 40].

12.11 Disclaimer

The author translated parts of the text/chapters/the work with the help of AI but reviewed, revised, and took accountability for the final submitted version.

References

1. Goubar T, Goubar C, Fenton-Lee D, Stefanidis A, Macdonald PS, Rushworth RL. A population-based study of bariatric surgery trends in Australia: variations reflect continuing inequities in access to surgery. Obes Surg. 2025;35(3):1026–35.
2. World Health Organization. Obesity and Overweight. Available from: https://www.who.int/news-room/fact-sheets/detail/obesity-and-overweight. Accessed on 15 November 2025; 2016
3. Schetz M, De Jong A, Deane AM, Druml W, Hemelaar P, Pelosi P, Pickkers P, Reintam-Blaser A, Roberts J, Sakr Y, Jaber S. Obesity in the critically ill: a narrative review. Intensive Care Med. 2019;45(6):757–69.

4. Kao CL, Sun CK, Lin HJ, Hung KC. Perioperative complications and intensive care unit utilization in super-superobese patients undergoing laparoscopic bariatric surgery. Tzu Chi Med J. 2019;31(4):254–9.
5. Tober C, Quasim T, Kinsella J. Haemodynamics, inflammation and mortality in medical patients with first diagnosis atrial fibrillation within a general intensive care unit. Europe PMC. 2012;
6. Zhou D, Wang C, Lin Q, Li T. The obesity paradox for survivors of critically ill patients. Crit Care. 2022;26(1):198.
7. Stenberg E, dos Reis Falcão LF, O'Kane M, Liem R, Pournaras DJ, Salminen P, et al. Guidelines for perioperative care in bariatric surgery: enhanced recovery after surgery (ERAS) society recommendations: a 2021 update. World J Surg. 2022;46(3):729–51.
8. Morgan DJR, Ho KM, Armstrong J, Baker S. Incidence and risk factors for intensive care unit admission after bariatric surgery: a multicentre population-based cohort study. Br J Anaesth. 2015;115(6):873–82.
9. Holsworth C, Gallagher S. Managing care of critically ill bariatric patients. AACN Adv Crit Care. 2017;28(3):275–83.
10. McKechnie A, Iliff HA, Black R, Ahmad I, Chesworth P, Davis N, et al. Airway management in patients living with obesity: best practice recommendations from the Society for Obesity and Bariatric Anaesthesia. Anaesthesia. 2025;80(11):1103–14.
11. Schetz M, De Jong A, Deane AM, Druml W, Hemelaar P, Pelosi P, et al. Obesity in the critically ill: a narrative review. Intensive Care Med. 2019;45(6):757–69.
12. De Jong A, Wrigge H, Hedenstierna G, Gattinoni L, Chiumello D, Frat JP, et al. How to ventilate obese patients in the ICU. Intensive Care Med. 2020;46(12):2423–35.
13. Singh A, Sharma S, Gupta D. Comparison of ramp and new modified ramp positioning in laryngoscopic view during intubation in patients with morbid obesity: a randomized clinical trial. Anesthesiol Pain Med. 2021;11(3):e114508.
14. Kim M, Lee I, Park S. Preoperative risk evaluation and perioperative management of patients with obstructive sleep apnea: a narrative review. J Dent Anesth Pain Med. 2023;23(4):179–87.
15. Ahn HS, Kim JY, Lee SH. Ultrasound-measured skin-to-epiglottis distance as a predictor of difficult intubation in obese patients: a prospective observational study. J Clin Med. 2025;14(6):2092.
16. Boesing C, Schaefer L, Rocco PRM, Luecke T, Krebs J. Positive end-expiratory pressure optimisation during general anaesthesia in patients with obesity: a narrative review of respiratory and cardiovascular outcomes. Br J Anaesth. 2025;
17. Lagrand WK, van Slobbe-Bijlsma ER, Schultz MJ. Haemodynamic monitoring of morbidly obese intensive care unit patients. Neth J Med. 2013;71(5):234–42.
18. Greif R, Lauridsen KG, Djärv T, Ek JE, Monnelly V, Monsieurs KG, et al. European resuscitation council guidelines 2025 executive summary. Resuscitation. 2025;215(Suppl 1):110770.
19. Lott C, Truhlář A, Alfonzo A, Barelli A, González-Salvado V, Hinkelbein J, et al. European resuscitation council guidelines 2021: cardiac arrest in special circumstances. Resuscitation. 2021;161:38–407.
20. Scquizzato T, Bonaccorso A, Swol J, Gamberini L, Scandroglio AM, Landoni G, et al. Refractory out-of-hospital cardiac arrest and extracorporeal cardiopulmonary resuscitation: a meta-analysis of randomized trials. Artif Organs. 2023;47(5):806–16.
21. Dagher C, Mattar R, Aoun M, Tohme J, Naccache N, Jabbour H. Opioid-free anesthesia in bariatric surgery: a prospective randomized controlled trial. Eur J Med Res. 2025;30(1):320.
22. Erstad BL, Barletta JF. Drug dosing in the critically ill obese patient – a focus on sedation, analgesia, and delirium. Crit Care. 2020;24(1):384.
23. Kounatidis D, Vallianou NG, Stratigou T, Voukali M, Karampela I, Dalamaga M. The kidney in obesity: current evidence, perspectives and controversies. Curr Obes Rep. 2024;13(4):680–702.
24. Schiffl H. Intensive care unit continuous kidney replacement therapy: time to change dosage recommendations? Int Urol Nephrol. 2025;57(2):511–6.
25. Ahn YH, Yoon SM, Lee J, Lee SM, Oh DK, Lee SY, et al. Early sepsis-associated acute kidney injury and obesity. JAMA Netw Open. 2024;7(2):e2354923.

26. Danziger J, Chen KP, Lee J, Feng M, Mark RG, Celi LA, et al. Obesity, acute kidney injury, and mortality in critical illness. Crit Care Med. 2016;44(2):328–34.
27. López-Ortega O, Moreno-Corona NC, Cruz-Holguin VJ, Garcia-Gonzalez LD, Helguera-Repetto AC, Romero-Valdovinos M, et al. The immune response in adipocytes and their susceptibility to infection: a possible relationship with infectobesity. Int J Mol Sci. 2022;23(11):6154.
28. Meng L, Mui E, Ha DR, Stave C, Deresinski SC, Holubar M. Comprehensive guidance for antibiotic dosing in obese adults: 2022 update. Pharmacotherapy. 2023;43(3):226–46.
29. Frías-Toral J, Chapela R, González A, Martinuzzi G, Locatelli I, Llobera J, et al. Managing severe malnutrition post-bariatric surgery using artificial nutrition. Nutrients. 2025;17(6):1234.
30. Chalopin R, Lassen C, Genser B, Aron-Wisnewsky J, Poitou B, Ciangura C, et al. Management of severe malnutrition post-bariatric surgery using artificial nutrition. Obes Surg. 2023;
31. Wobith T, Weimann A. Oral nutritional supplements and enteral nutrition in patients with gastrointestinal surgery. Nutrients. 2021;13(9):3012.
32. Dickerson RN, Andromalos L, Brown JC, Correia MITD, Pritts W, Ridley EJ, et al. Obesity and critical care nutrition: current practice gaps and directions for future research. Crit Care. 2022;26(1):283.
33. Weimann A, Braga M, Carli F, Higashiguchi T, Hübner M, Kłęk S, et al. ESPEN practical guideline: clinical nutrition in surgery. Clin Nutr. 2021;40(5):2443–64.
34. Miedziaszczyk M, Ciabach P, Szałek E. The effects of bariatric surgery and gastrectomy on the absorption of drugs, vitamins, and mineral elements. Pharmaceutics. 2021;13(12):2111.
35. Amaral FCF, Baptista-Silva JCC, Nakano LCU, Flumignan RLG. Pharmacological interventions for preventing venous thromboembolism in patients undergoing bariatric surgery. Cochrane Database Syst Rev. 2020;7
36. Abildgaard A, Madsen SA, Hvas AM. Dosage of anticoagulants in obesity: recommendations based on a systematic review. Semin Thromb Hemost. 2020;46(8):932–69.
37. Benedetti R, Marino S, Tangianu F, Imberti D. Inferior vena cava filters: a clinical review and future perspectives. J Clin Med. 2024;13(6):1761.
38. Märtson AG, Barber KE, Crass RL, Hites M, Kloft C, Kuti JL, et al. The pharmacokinetics of antibiotics in patients with obesity: a systematic review and consensus guidelines for dose adjustments. Lancet Infect Dis. 2025;25(9):e504–15.
39. Castro-Balado A, Varela-Rey I, Mejuto B, Mondelo-García C, Zarra-Ferro I, Rodríguez-Jato T, et al. Updated antimicrobial dosing recommendations for obese patients. Antimicrob Agents Chemother. 2024;68(5):e0171923.
40. Yadav S, Sinha N, Sinha P. Supraglottic jet oxygenation and ventilation assisted fiberoptic intubation in a paralyzed patient with morbid obesity and obstructive sleep apnea: a case report. BMC Anesthesiol. 2019;19:189.

Diet Progression and Lifestyle Modification

13

Ana Martín-Nieto

13.1 Introduction

Obesity is a public health problem that has been increasing in recent years. It represents a major risk factor for the development of numerous diseases such as diabetes, cardiovascular diseases, cancer, metabolic syndrome, and psychological disorders. Although the treatment of choice in these cases is diet, lifestyle modification, or pharmacological therapy, bariatric surgery is considered an option for those patients who do not achieve significant weight reduction or are unable to maintain it in the long term [1].

Sleeve gastrectomy is a surgical procedure that involves reducing the volume of the stomach through the removal of the greater curvature. With this technique, in addition to decreasing stomach size, appetite is also reduced due to the suppression of certain orexigenic hormones [2]. Sleeve gastrectomy is an increasingly popular bariatric surgery option for achieving weight loss; however, its success depends on adequate lifestyle modification. Individuals undergoing this surgical intervention should follow a multidisciplinary weight-control approach that includes dietary changes, increased physical activity, and psychological support [3].

A. Martín-Nieto (✉)
Health Sciences Department, San Juan de Dios School of Nursing and Physical Therapy, Comillas Pontifical University, Madrid, Spain
e-mail: amartinn@comillas.edu

J. Ruiz-Tovar (ed.), *Multidisciplinary Management of Sleeve Gastrectomy*,
https://doi.org/10.1007/978-3-032-25644-7_13

13.2 Physiological and Metabolic Postoperative Fundamentals

Sleeve gastrectomy results in a reduction of gastric volume and a decrease in the number of cells that produce ghrelin. This peptide hormone is responsible for increasing the sensation of hunger by acting directly on the lateral hypothalamus and the arcuate nucleus [2]. Therefore, the immediate consequence is a reduction in appetite, facilitating weight loss through decreased caloric intake [4].

In addition to the reduction in gastric volume and ghrelin levels, there is an increase in glucagon-like peptide-1 (GLP-1). This incretin is secreted by L cells located in the ileum and colon. The increase in GLP-1 leads to early satiety, delayed gastric emptying, enhanced insulin sensitivity, and reduced glucagon secretion, which together contribute to lower blood glucose levels [5].

Finally, the secretion of peptide YY (PYY)—also known as peptide tyrosine-tyrosine—is increased. This peptide regulates appetite by slowing gastric emptying, inhibiting gastric acid secretion, and promoting satiety [6].

The resection of the stomach body reduces mechanical digestion and acid secretion, leading to decreased digestion and absorption of iron, vitamin B12, and other protein-bound nutrients. In addition, because of mid-gastric stenosis, chronic vomiting may occur in the short term. The most common nutritional deficiencies, as will be discussed later, include iron, vitamin B12, calcium, folic acid, copper, and zinc deficiencies [7].

13.3 Diet Progression

Immediately after surgery, the dietary goal should focus on preventing complications, ensuring adequate tolerance to the diet, and avoiding nutritional deficiencies. The volume of food in each intake, and even the type of food best tolerated, will depend on the degree of gastric restriction or malabsorption caused by the intervention [8].

The specific objectives of diet progression following sleeve gastrectomy include [9]:

1. Facilitating the healing of the gastric suture line.
2. Preventing metabolic and mechanical complications.
3. Promoting long-term sustainable dietary re-education and lifestyle modification.

Sleeve gastrectomy is a restrictive procedure, and the reintroduction of diet must be gradual and progressive. The different stages of this process are described in Table 13.1 [9, 10].

In addition, the following general recommendations should be considered [10]:

- It is recommended to eat slowly and chew food thoroughly.

Table 13.1 Diet progression in sleeve gastrectomy

Stage	Dietary period	Dietary form	Recommendations
Stage 0	One week before surgery		Low-calorie diet (approximately 1200 kcal). The recommended protein intake is 60 grams/day
Stage I	The day after surgery	Sips of water	Consume small amounts of water
Stage II	One week after surgery	Full clear liquid diet with protein powder	Try to consume at least 1.5 to 2 liters of fluids, prioritizing those that are high in protein. The intake volume should be progressive, starting with 30 mL every 20–30 min. Avoid liquids containing sugar, carbonation, or caffeine. Liquid vitamin supplementation should be started according to protocol. Protein powder intake is also recommended
Stage III	1–2 weeks after surgery	Liquid diet	Protein-containing liquids (milk, enriched broths, supplements). The protein goal will be 60–80 grams of protein per day
Stage IV	2–4 weeks after surgery	Pureed or mashed diet	It should have a smooth texture, without lumps. Lean protein sources such as chicken, white fish, or eggs are gradually introduced. The goal is to reach 60–80 g of protein per day

(continued)

Table 13.1 (continued)

Stage	Dietary period	Dietary form	Recommendations
Stage V	4–6 weeks after surgery	Soft diet	Increase in texture variety while maintaining a soft diet. Gradual introduction of cooked vegetables, peeled fruit, and soft cereals. The same protein requirements are maintained
Stage VI	From 6–8 weeks after surgery	Regular diet	Maintain a healthy, varied diet adapted to each individual situation. Prioritize natural foods that are high in protein and low in fat and simple sugars. Consume lean proteins. Avoid carbonated beverages, caffeine, alcohol, ultra-processed foods, and sweets

- Drink at least 1.5 to 2 liters of fluids per day.
- Avoid all types of alcohol.
- Avoid carbonated beverages, as they may cause abdominal distension, discomfort, and bloating.
- Monitor for symptoms compatible with dumping syndrome.

Dumping syndrome is a common complication that may occur after surgical intervention. It develops when fatty or sugary foods pass too rapidly from the stomach into the small intestine. Symptoms include nausea, abdominal cramps, palpitations, and diarrhea, among others [10].

13.4 Physical Activity

It has been demonstrated that engaging in physical exercise after surgery can support weight loss and promote its long-term maintenance. In addition, it may increase muscle strength and improve the management of symptoms in patients with obesity who have undergone bariatric surgery. Physical training is an effective strategy to enhance short-term cardiorespiratory fitness following surgery [8].

For physical exercise to provide lasting benefits, aerobic training should be combined with resistance exercises. The duration of exercise programs should be at least 3 months and must be supervised by a qualified professional [11]. Physical activity is therefore considered a fundamental component in the treatment of obesity. It can improve peripheral insulin sensitivity [12] and produce significant improvements in body composition, bone mineral density, muscle strength, and overall physical fitness [13].

There is no clear consensus in the literature regarding the optimal time to initiate physical exercise. Some authors recommend beginning 3 months after surgery, although in certain cases it may be advisable to start earlier, around one-month post-surgery, provided that the patient is in good clinical condition and does not present limiting symptoms [14].

In many cases, to achieve effective lifestyle modification and ensure adherence to regular physical exercise, the implementation of behavioral therapy in postoperative patients is essential.

13.5 Psychological and Behavioral Support

Psychological support for patients undergoing sleeve gastrectomy is essential. It is important to consider that many patients present for surgery with a complex psychological history, which may include anxiety, depression, low self-esteem, negative body image, eating disorders, trauma, or abuse, among others [15, 16]. After surgery, these psychological issues may, in some cases, diminish because of weight loss; however, in some individuals, episodes of binge eating, problematic substance use, suicidal ideation, suboptimal weight loss, or weight regain may reoccur [17]. Consistent with this, several research groups emphasize the importance of psychological support both before and after surgery [18]. Therefore, psychological support is a fundamental component of comprehensive patient care, facilitating adherence to new nutritional and lifestyle habits and preventing long-term weight regain. International guidelines recommend the inclusion of a mental health professional within the multidisciplinary team to ensure the success of the intervention and to prevent potential relapses.

13.6 Nutritional Supplementation

All individuals undergoing bariatric surgery should undergo a preoperative nutritional assessment [7, 19]. Preoperative tests should include screening for nutritional deficiencies, diabetes, renal function, and dyslipidemia. Additionally, specific tests should assess serum levels of vitamin A, zinc, copper, and selenium [20].

Nutritional deficiencies should be corrected prior to surgery. Many professionals recommend a low-carbohydrate diet before surgery to reduce liver size. Since these diets are not nutritionally complete, patients often require targeted supplementation of certain micronutrients [21].

The main recommendations regarding postoperative supplementation following sleeve gastrectomy are summarized below:

- **Iron:**
After surgery, patients should generally be able to maintain adequate iron levels through diet and a comprehensive multivitamin and mineral supplement containing the recommended daily iron intake [22]. However, in some cases following sleeve gastrectomy, a generic multivitamin and mineral supplement may be insufficient to meet requirements, necessitating additional elemental iron. Some authors recommend supplementation with 200 mg of ferrous sulfate, 210 mg of ferrous fumarate, or 300 mg of ferrous gluconate daily. Women of reproductive age and those who are menstruating may require additional supplementation of 50–100 mg of elemental iron per day [23]. For optimal absorption, iron supplements should be taken with citrus-containing foods that provide vitamin C. Moreover, iron and calcium supplements should be spaced 1–2 hours apart to prevent interference with absorption [24].
- **Folic Acid:**
The specific requirements for folic acid following sleeve gastrectomy are not well established. However, these requirements are increased in preconception care, pregnancy, and lactation [25].
- **Vitamin B12:**
There is a high risk of vitamin B12 deficiency following sleeve gastrectomy. Therefore, additional supplementation with high doses of vitamin B12 is required to prevent deficiency. Untreated B12 deficiency can lead to irreversible neuropathy [26].
- **Vitamin D:**
Vitamin D plays a critical role in musculoskeletal health and is essential for calcium absorption and bone mineralization. Following bariatric surgery, optimal serum 25-hydroxyvitamin D (25OHD) levels are not well established but are estimated to be higher than in the general population [27]. Therefore, initiating therapy with 2000–4000 IU of vitamin D3 daily is recommended to maintain serum 25OHD levels. Additionally, once feasible, dietary intake of vitamin D should be encouraged, along with weight-bearing physical activity [28].
- **Calcium:**
Calcium absorption is negatively affected following bariatric surgery. Dietary sources of calcium should be encouraged, as they are better absorbed and have higher bioavailability than supplements. In the case of sleeve gastrectomy, a daily intake of 1200–1500 mg of calcium is recommended [29].
- **Vitamins A, E, and K:**
Patients undergoing sleeve gastrectomy should meet their requirements for vitamins A, E, and K through diet and the use of a comprehensive multivitamin and mineral supplement [30].
- **Zinc and Copper:**
A standard multivitamin and mineral supplement may be insufficient to meet zinc requirements following sleeve gastrectomy. Although the optimal level of zinc supplementation is not well established, some authors recommend starting with 15 mg/day. Specifically for copper, it is recommended that multivitamin and mineral supplements provide at least 2 mg of copper [31].

- **Selenium:**
  There is no consensus in the scientific literature regarding selenium supplementation after sleeve gastrectomy. However, some authors recommend the use of a multivitamin and mineral supplement containing selenium or the consumption of Brazil nuts [32, 33].
- **Thiamine (Vitamin B1):**
  Many patients present with thiamine deficiency following bariatric surgery [34]. In some cases, multivitamin supplements do not provide sufficient thiamine to meet the needs of all patients. Some authors recommend that all patients take 12 mg of thiamine daily, and preferably a dose of 50 mg one or two times daily from a B-complex vitamin [35]. If patients experience dysphagia, prolonged vomiting, poor nutritional intake, intolerance to vitamin supplements, or high alcohol consumption, additional thiamine supplementation should be administered immediately to prevent Wernicke's encephalopathy [36].

In conclusion, following sleeve gastrectomy and due to rapid weight loss, long-term follow-up is essential. The nutritional goal is to prevent malnutrition, ensure adequate caloric and protein intake, and provide personalized nutritional education tailored to each patient's digestive symptoms. Finally, to reduce complications caused by micronutrient deficiencies, periodic blood tests and the use of a comprehensive multivitamin and mineral supplement are recommended.

References

1. Özdoğan Y, Elibol E, Avlanmış Ö, Çelebi-Acungan A, Özdoğan Y, Elibol E, et al. Evaluation of the nutritional status of morbid obesity patients in the first six months after sleeve gastrectomy. Nutr Hos. 2024;41(5):976–83.
2. Roa PE, Kaidar-Person O, Pinto D, Cho M, Szomstein S, Rosenthal RJ. Laparoscopic sleeve gastrectomy as treatment for morbid obesity: technique and short-term outcome. Obes Surg. 2006;16(10):1323–6.
3. Enríquez-Schmidt J, Mautner Molina C, Kalazich Rosales M, Muñoz M, Ruiz-Uribe M, Fuentes Leal F, et al. Moderate-intensity constant or high-intensity interval training? Metabolic effects on candidates to undergo bariatric surgery. Nutr Metab Cardiovasc Dis. 2024;34(7):1681–91.
4. Givon-Madhala O, Spector R, Wasserberg N, Beglaibter N, Lustigman H, Stein M, et al. Technical aspects of laparoscopic sleeve gastrectomy in 25 morbidly obese patients. Obes Surg. 2007;17(6):722–7.
5. McCarty TR, Jirapinyo P, Thompson CC. Effect of sleeve gastrectomy on ghrelin, GLP-1, PYY, and GIP gut hormones: a systematic review and meta-analysis. Ann Surg. 2020;272(1):72.
6. Batterham RL, Cowley MA, Small CJ, Herzog H, Cohen MA, Dakin CL, et al. Gut hormone PYY(3-36) physiologically inhibits food intake. Nature. 2002;418(6898):650–4.
7. Mechanick JI, Youdim A, Jones DB, Timothy Garvey W, Hurley DL, Molly McMahon M, et al. Clinical practice guidelines for the perioperative nutritional, metabolic, and nonsurgical support of the bariatric surgery patient – 2013 update: cosponsored by American Association of Clinical Endocrinologists, the Obesity Society, and American Society for Metabolic & bariatric surgery. Surg Obes Relat Dis. 2013;9(2):159–91.
8. Bellicha A, van Baak MA, Battista F, Beaulieu K, Blundell JE, Busetto L, et al. Effect of exercise training before and after bariatric surgery: a systematic review and meta-analysis. Obes Rev. 2021;22(Suppl 4):e13296.

9. Park S, Kim S, Kim S, Shin AR, Park Y. Nutritional intervention for a patient with sleeve gastrectomy. Clin Nutr Res. 2023;12(3):177–83.
10. Bertoni L, Valentini R, Zattarin A, Belligoli A, Bettini S, Vettor R, et al. Assessment of protein intake in the first three months after sleeve gastrectomy in patients with severe obesity. Nutrients. 2021;13(3):771.
11. Coen PM, Tanner CJ, Helbling NL, Dubis GS, Hames KC, Xie H, et al. Clinical trial demonstrates exercise following bariatric surgery improves insulin sensitivity. J Clin Invest. 2015;125(1):248–57.
12. Sigal RJ, Kenny GP, Boulé NG, Wells GA, et al. Effects of aerobic training, resistance training, or both on glycemic control in type 2 diabetes: a randomized trial. Ann Intern Med de. 2007;147(6):357–69.
13. Hansen D, Decroix L, Devos Y, Nocca D, Cornelissen V, Dillemans B, et al. Towards optimized care after bariatric surgery by physical activity and exercise intervention: a review. Obes Surg. 2020;30(3):1118–25.
14. Alyafei AA, AlMukhaini SK. The impact of sleeve gastrectomy combined with lifestyle interventions on anthropometric and health outcomes in adults: a systematic review and meta-analysis. Cureus. 2025;17(6):e85587.
15. Burgmer R, Legenbauer T, Müller A, de Zwaan M, Fischer C, Herpertz S. Psychological outcome 4 years after restrictive bariatric surgery. Obes Surg. 2014;24(10):1670–8.
16. Strain GW, Kolotkin RL, Dakin GF, Gagner M, Inabnet WB, Christos P, et al. The effects of weight loss after bariatric surgery on health-related quality of life and depression. Nutr Diabetes de. 2014;4(9):e132.
17. King WC, Chen JY, Courcoulas AP, Dakin GF, Engel SG, Flum DR, et al. Alcohol and other substance use after bariatric surgery: prospective evidence from a U.S. multicenter cohort study. Surg Obes Relat Dis. 2017;13(8):1392–402.
18. Sogg S, Lauretti J, West-Smith L. Recommendations for the presurgical psychosocial evaluation of bariatric surgery patients. Surg Obes Relat Dis. 2016;12(4):731–49.
19. Parrott J, Frank L, Rabena R, Craggs-Dino L, Isom KA, Greiman L. American Society for Metabolic and Bariatric Surgery Integrated Health Nutritional Guidelines for the surgical weight loss patient 2016 update: micronutrients. Surg Obes Relat Dis. 2017;13(5):727–41.
20. Remedios C, Bhasker AG, Dhulla N, Dhar S, Lakdawala M. Bariatric nutrition guidelines for the Indian population. Obes Surg. 2016;26(5):1057–68.
21. O'Kane M, Parretti HM, Pinkney J, Welbourn R, Hughes CA, Mok J, et al. British obesity and metabolic surgery society guidelines on perioperative and postoperative biochemical monitoring and micronutrient replacement for patients undergoing bariatric surgery – 2020 update. Obes Rev. 2020;21(11):e13087.
22. McGrice MA, Porter JA. The micronutrient intake profile of a multicentre cohort of Australian LAGB patients. Obes Surg. 2014;24(3):400–4.
23. Salgado W, Modotti C, Nonino CB, Ceneviva R. Anemia and iron deficiency before and after bariatric surgery. Surg Obes Relat Dis. 2014;10(1):49–54.
24. Bays H, Kothari SN, Azagury DE, Morton JM, Nguyen NT, Jones PH, et al. Lipids and bariatric procedures part 2 of 2: scientific statement from the American Society for Metabolic and Bariatric Surgery (ASMBS), the National Lipid Association (NLA), and obesity medicine association (OMA). Surg Obes Relat Dis. 2016;12(3):468–95.
25. Shawe J, Ceulemans D, Akhter Z, Neff K, Hart K, Heslehurst N, et al. Pregnancy after bariatric surgery: consensus recommendations for periconception, antenatal and postnatal care. Obes Rev. 2019;20(11):1507–22.
26. Vitamins and minerals: A model for safe addition to foods | European Journal of Nutrition [Internet]. [citado 29 de octubre de 2025]. Disponible en: https://link.springer.com/article/10.1007/s00394-003-0391-9
27. Busetto L, Dicker D, Azran C, Batterham RL, Farpour-Lambert N, Fried M, et al. Practical recommendations of the obesity management task force of the European Association for the Study of obesity for the post-bariatric surgery medical management. Obes Facts. 2017;10(6):597–632.

28. Aills L, Blankenship J, Buffington C, Furtado M, Parrott J. ASMBS allied health nutritional guidelines for the surgical weight loss patient. Surg Obes Relat Dis. 2008;4(5 Suppl):S73–108.
29. Curhan GC, Willett WC, Rimm EB, Stampfer MJ. A prospective study of dietary calcium and other nutrients and the risk of symptomatic kidney stones. N Engl J Med. 1993;328(12):833–8.
30. James H, Lorentz P, Collazo-Clavell ML. Patient-reported adherence to empiric vitamin/mineral supplementation and related nutrient deficiencies after Roux-en-Y gastric bypass. Obes Surg. 2016;26(11):2661–6.
31. Papamargaritis D, Aasheim ET, Sampson B, le Roux CW. Copper, selenium and zinc levels after bariatric surgery in patients recommended to take multivitamin-mineral supplementation. J Trace Elem Med Biol. 2015;31:167–72.
32. Nett P, Borbély Y, Kröll D. Micronutrient supplementation after biliopancreatic diversion with duodenal switch in the long term. Obes Surg octubre de. 2016;26(10):2469–74.
33. Dolan K, Hatzifotis M, Newbury L, Lowe N, Fielding G. A clinical and nutritional comparison of biliopancreatic diversion with and without duodenal switch. Ann Surg. 2004;240(1):51–6.
34. Garg T, Birge K, et al. A postoperative nutritional consult improves bariatric surgery outcomes. Surg Obes Relat Dis. 2016;12(5):1052–6.
35. Parrott J, Frank L, Rabena R, Craggs-Dino L, Isom KA, Greiman L. American Society for metabolic and bariatric surgery integrated health nutritional guidelines for the surgical weight loss patient 2016 update: micronutrients. Surg Obes Relat Dis. 2017;13(5):727–41.
36. Aasheim ET. Wernicke encephalopathy after bariatric surgery: a systematic review. Ann Surg. 2008;248(5):714–20.

14 Weight Loss and Remission of Comorbidities After Sleeve Gastrectomy

Carlos Guijarro-Moreno and Ana Sanchez-Gollarte

14.1 Introduction

Bariatric surgery (BS) is the most effective long-term therapy for severe obesity. Contemporary guidelines from ASMBS/IFSO recommend BS for individuals with BMI $\geq$35 kg/m^2 regardless of comorbidities and consider surgery for BMI 30–34.9 kg/m^2 with metabolic disease or inadequate response to nonsurgical therapy [1]. SG and RYGB account for the large majority of procedures performed globally. Beyond weight reduction, the primary clinical aim is to reverse obesity-related organ dysfunction and reduce long-term cardiometabolic risk. The impact on diabetes, blood pressure, lipids, OSA, and steatotic liver disease has reoriented surgery from purely restrictive/absorptive models to 'metabolic' interventions affecting endocrine signaling, bile acids, and the microbiome. This chapter synthesizes foundational evidence and pragmatic takeaways for clinicians selecting and following patients after SG.

14.2 Definitions and Reporting Standards

1. Weight-loss metrics—Changes should be reported as percent total weight loss (%TWL) and, where useful, percent excess weight loss (%EWL). Baseline definitions (e.g., ideal body weight for EWL) must be explicit to enable cross-study comparisons. Mean, median, and interquartile ranges are preferred for skewed distributions.

C. Guijarro-Moreno (✉) · A. Sanchez-Gollarte
Servicio de Cirugía General y del Aparato Digestivo, Hospital Universitario del Henares, Madrid, Spain
e-mail: asgollarte@gmail.com

J. Ruiz-Tovar (ed.), *Multidisciplinary Management of Sleeve Gastrectomy*,
https://doi.org/10.1007/978-3-032-25644-7_14

2. Diabetes remission—An international consensus defines T2D remission as HbA1c <6.5% for ≥3 months in the absence of glucose-lowering therapy [2]. Historic categories of 'partial' and 'complete' remission used stricter glycemic thresholds; authors should state criteria clearly. Medication reduction and improved glycemic control, while valuable, should not be conflated with remission.
3. Remission of other comorbidities—Typical definitions include: Hypertension (normotension without antihypertensives); Dyslipidemia (normal lipid profile without lipid-lowering therapy); OSA (resolution on polysomnography or discontinuation of PAP therapy with normalized symptoms); MASLD/NASH (histologic or noninvasive resolution of steatohepatitis and/or improvement in fibrosis stage).
4. Methodologic considerations—Intention-to-treat analyses, clear handling of loss to follow-up, and standardized timepoints (e.g., 12, 24, 60 months) improve interpretability. Composite endpoints (e.g., 'metabolic success') should be deconstructed into components.

14.3 Mechanisms of Weight Loss and Metabolic Improvement After SG

SG removes ~75–80% of the stomach along the greater curvature, producing gastric restriction and accelerated gastric emptying. Metabolically, SG reduces ghrelin (orexigenic), enhances distal nutrient delivery, and increases postprandial GLP-1 and PYY, improving insulin secretion and satiety [3–5]. Bile acid signaling (FXR/TGR5 pathways), changes in vagal tone, and gut microbiome shifts likely contribute to enterohepatic and central effects on appetite and insulin sensitivity. In T2D, early glycemic improvements often precede maximal weight loss, underscoring weight-independent mechanisms and improved β-cell function [4, 5]. These physiologic changes explain why comorbidity improvement can occur even when weight-loss magnitude is modest, and why durability hinges on both anatomy and behavior.

14.4 Weight-Loss Outcomes After SG

1. Short- to mid-term (1–3 years)—Most series report ~25–30% TWL at 1–2 years after SG, with considerable interindividual variability [6–9]. Compared with RYGB, SG tends to yield slightly less weight loss on average, though between-group differences are often modest in the short term [8, 9].
2. Long-term (5–10+ years) and durability—Randomized and prospective cohort data show durable weight loss following SG, with meaningful maintenance at 5–10 years, though average long-term weight loss tends to be greater after RYGB [8–11]. The SLEEVEPASS and SM-BOSS randomized trials demonstrated that both SG and RYGB maintain substantial weight reduction at extended follow-up, with RYGB generally achieving higher %EWL [8, 9]. Weight regain occurs

in a subset; contributors include sleeve dilation, behavioral factors, and hormonal adaptations [10, 11].

3. Predictors of weight-loss response—Higher baseline BMI, younger age, fewer eating disinhibition traits, and stronger program adherence correlate with greater %TWL. Technical factors (bougie size, antral preservation, hiatal repair when indicated) may influence outcomes and reflux risk [10–12]. Multidisciplinary follow-up with nutrition, psychological support, physical activity, and, when appropriate, adjunct pharmacotherapy can sustain results.

14.5 Remission of Obesity-Related Comorbidities After SG

1. Type 2 diabetes—Short term: SG produces high rates of glycemic improvement and remission within the first 1–2 years, aided by weight loss and enhanced incretin signaling [2, 4, 5, 13]. In randomized comparisons to medical therapy, metabolic surgery (including SG) consistently outperforms intensive medical/lifestyle interventions for glycemic control and medication reduction [13–15]. Durability and relapse: Remission rates decline over time due to weight regain and progressive β-cell dysfunction. Across long-term cohorts, durable remission persists in a substantial minority; RYGB tends to show higher long-term remission probability than SG, though between-procedure differences vary by study and patient profile [8, 9, 14]. Predictors: Shorter diabetes duration, lower preoperative HbA1c, absence of insulin therapy, preserved C-peptide, and greater postoperative weight loss predict remission and durability [2, 13–16].
2. Hypertension—Many SG recipients achieve remission or reduced medication burden. Randomized and observational data suggest RYGB may be superior for long-term hypertension remission, but SG still confers clinically meaningful improvements in blood pressure control [8, 9, 17]. Trials comparing surgery vs medical therapy (e.g., in resistant hypertension) demonstrate large treatment effects favoring surgery overall [18].
3. Dyslipidemia—SG improves triglycerides and HDL-C; LDL-C responses are variable and often medication-dependent. Comparative studies frequently show greater lipid normalization after RYGB, but SG nevertheless reduces atherogenic profiles and medication needs in many patients [8, 9, 19].
4. Obstructive sleep apnea—Weight loss after SG yields substantial reductions in apnea–hypopnea index and symptomatic improvement. Remission—stringently defined—ranges widely across studies, often in the 50–70% range at 1–3 years, with continued improvements tied to weight maintenance [20, 21]. Formal reassessment with sleep testing is recommended before withdrawing PAP therapy.
5. MASLD/NASH—Bariatric surgery improves steatosis, ballooning, and inflammation, with many patients achieving NASH resolution and some experiencing fibrosis regression. SG cohorts mirror these benefits, though procedure-specific histologic differences remain debated [22–24]. Use of noninvasive tools (e.g., FIB-4, elastography) can guide surveillance.

6. Other conditions—SG reduces symptoms and medication burden in osteoarthritis and GERD-associated respiratory complaints; fertility and PCOS-related features often improve. Micronutrient issues are less pronounced than after malabsorptive procedures but require lifelong monitoring [12, 25].

14.6 GERD and Barrett's Esophagus After SG

SG is associated with de novo GERD and may increase the risk of erosive esophagitis and Barrett's esophagus relative to RYGB [26–28]. Mechanisms include decreased compliance, increased intragastric pressure, and potential hiatal hernia underrecognition. Patient selection is critical: preoperative reflux or large hiatal hernia may favor RYGB; hiatal repair during SG can mitigate symptoms in selected patients [12, 26]. Endoscopic surveillance should be individualized, particularly for persistent reflux. Algorithms typically begin with PPI optimization, assessment of sleeve anatomy, and consideration of conversion to RYGB when symptoms remain refractory.

14.7 Comparative Effectiveness: SG Versus RYGB

Head-to-head trials (SLEEVEPASS, SM-BOSS) and meta-analyses indicate: Weight loss—RYGB > SG at longer follow-up on average, though both are effective [8–11]. T2D remission—RYGB frequently shows higher remission rates and durability; SG remains effective, especially in early T2D [8, 9, 14–16]. Hypertension/dyslipidemia—RYGB advantage is commonly observed; SG still yields significant improvements [8, 9, 17, 19]. GERD—SG carries higher GERD risk; RYGB often improves reflux [26–28]. Nutritional impact—Both require supplementation; RYGB entails greater malabsorptive risk [12]. Procedure choice should integrate metabolic targets, reflux status, nutritional considerations, and patient preference.

14.8 Safety, Complications, and Nutritional Follow-Up

Perioperative mortality after SG is very low in contemporary series. Major early complications include staple-line leak and bleeding; late complications include stricture, GERD, and weight regain. Standardized perioperative care pathways reduce length of stay and complications [10–12]. Nutritional management—Lifelong supplementation (multivitamin with minerals, vitamin D, iron as indicated, and periodic B12/folate monitoring) is recommended for SG. Regular biochemical surveillance (e.g., every 6–12 months) detects deficiencies early. Protein intake targets (~60–80 g/day or individualized by lean mass), resistance exercise, and behavioral support are central to weight maintenance [12, 25]. Adjunct anti-obesity pharmacotherapy (e.g., GLP-1 receptor agonists) can be considered for inadequate weight loss or regain, tailored to glycemic and reflux status.

14.9 Practical Management and Follow-Up

Preoperative: Standardized evaluation (metabolic profiling, OSA screening, reflux assessment, psychosocial readiness). Define remission criteria prospectively for each condition and set shared goals. Postoperative: Early follow-up (1–3–6–12 months) focusing on hydration, protein targets, micronutrients. Comorbidity tracking with protocolized medication de-escalation (e.g., antihypertensives, hypoglycemics) to avoid hypotension/hypoglycemia as weight and insulin sensitivity improve. Reflux management pathway (PPI trial, imaging/endoscopy, consider hiatal revision or conversion to RYGB for refractory GERD). Lifestyle: Encourage progressive physical activity, structured meal patterns, and avoidance of grazing. Team-based care and long-term engagement improve durability as much as initial operative choice.

14.10 Conclusions

SG delivers substantial, durable weight loss with clinically important remission of T2D, hypertension, dyslipidemia, OSA, and MASLD in many patients. Compared with RYGB, SG generally yields slightly less weight loss and lower long-term remission rates for some comorbidities, while posing a higher risk of GERD. Careful selection, meticulous technique, and longitudinal multidisciplinary follow-up maximize remission and durability and mitigate adverse effects (Figs. 14.1 and 14.2, Tables 14.1 and 14.2).

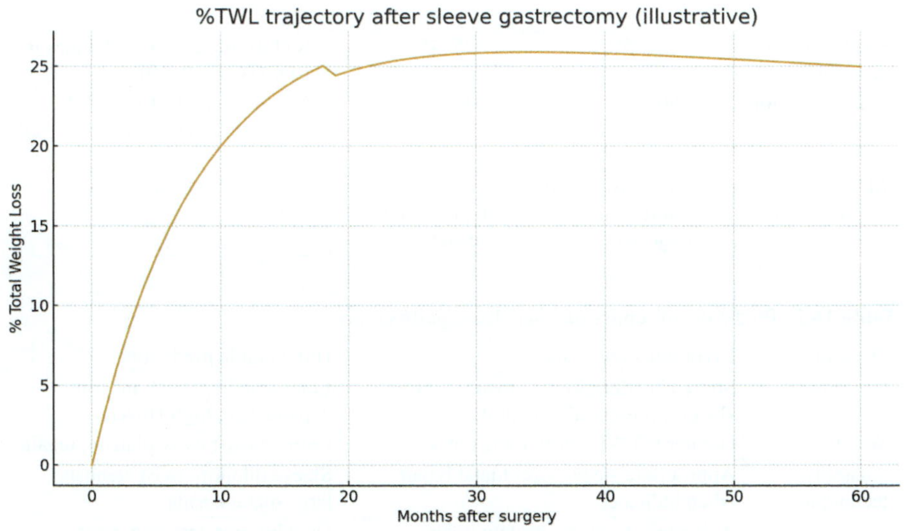

Fig. 14.1 Typical %TWL trajectory after sleeve gastrectomy (illustrative)

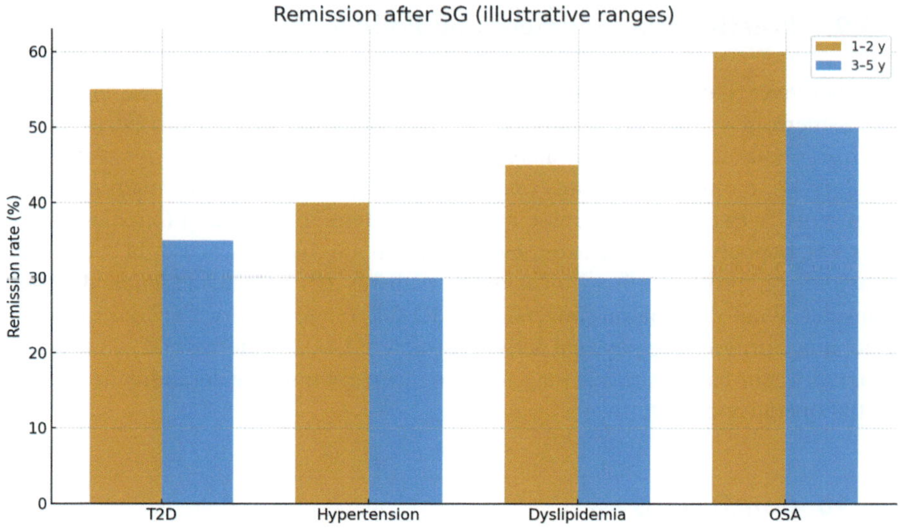

Fig. 14.2 Remission after SG at 1–2 years vs 3–5 years (illustrative ranges)

Table 14.1 Typical remission/improvement after sleeve gastrectomy (illustrative ranges)

Comorbidity	Early (1–2 year)	Mid-term (3–5 year)	Notes
T2D remission (consensus)	~40–60%	~25–45%	Higher with shorter T2D duration, no insulin [2, 13–16]
Hypertension remission	~30–50%	~20–40%	Medication burden falls even without full remission [8, 9, 17, 18]
Dyslipidemia remission	~35–55%	~25–45%	RYGB often greater changes in LDL/TG [8, 9, 19]
OSA remission	~50–70%	~40–60%	Confirm with testing; PAP de-escalation recommended [20, 21]
MASLD/NASH improvement	Steatosis/NASH improve in majority	Fibrosis regression in subset	Weight maintenance key [22–24]

Table 14.2 Predictors of remission after sleeve gastrectomy

Domain	Favorable predictors	Unfavorable predictors
Glycemic	Short T2D duration; no insulin; lower HbA1c; preserved C-peptide	Long-standing T2D; insulin dependence; high HbA1c
Weight	Greater %TWL; early robust loss	Limited loss; early plateau; regain
Anatomy/technique	Appropriate sleeve size; hiatal repair when indicated	Sleeve dilation; twist/stenosis; large hiatal hernia
Behavior	Adherence to visits, protein goals, activity	Disinhibition, grazing, poor follow-up

References

1. Eisenberg D, Shikora SA, Aarts E, Aminian A, Angrisani L, Cohen RV, et al. 2022 American Society for Metabolic and Bariatric Surgery (ASMBS) and International Federation for the Surgery of Obesity and Metabolic Disorders (IFSO): indications for metabolic and bariatric surgery. Surg Obes Relat Dis. 2022;18(12):1345–1356.
2. Riddle MC, Cefalu WT, Evans PH, Gerstein HC, Nauck MA, Ohkuma T, et al. Consensus report: definition and interpretation of remission in type 2 diabetes. Diabetes Care. 2021;44(10):2438–2444.
3. Karamanakos SN, Vagenas K, Kalfarentzos F, Alexandrides TK. Weight loss, appetite suppression, and changes in fasting and postprandial ghrelin and peptide-YY levels after Roux-en-Y gastric bypass and sleeve gastrectomy: a prospective, double blind study. Ann Surg. 2008;247(3):401–407.
4. Peterli R, Wölnerhanssen BK, Peters T, Devaux N, Kern B, Christoffel-Courtin C, et al. Improvement in glucose metabolism after bariatric surgery: comparison of laparoscopic Roux-en-Y gastric bypass and laparoscopic sleeve gastrectomy: a prospective randomized trial. Ann Surg. 2009;250(2):234–241.
5. le Roux CW, Welbourn R, Werling M, Osborne A, Kokkinos A, Laurenius A, et al. Gut hormones as mediators of appetite and weight loss after Roux-en-Y gastric bypass. Ann Surg. 2007;246(5):780–785.
6. Himpens J, Dapri G, Cadière GB. Long-term results of laparoscopic sleeve gastrectomy for obesity. Ann Surg. 2010;252(2):319–324.
7. Kehagias I, Karamanakos SN, Argentou M, Kalfarentzos F. Randomized clinical trial of laparoscopic Roux-en-Y gastric bypass versus laparoscopic sleeve gastrectomy for the management of patients with BMI
8. Salminen P, Helmiö M, Ovaska J, Juuti A, Leivonen M, Peromaa-Haavisto P, et al. Effect of laparoscopic sleeve gastrectomy vs laparoscopic Roux-en-Y gastric bypass on weight loss at 5 years among patients with morbid obesity: the SLEEVEPASS randomized clinical trial. JAMA. 2018;319(3):241–254.
9. Peterli R, Wölnerhanssen BK, Peters T, Vetter D, Kröll D, Borbély Y, et al. Effect of laparoscopic sleeve gastrectomy vs laparoscopic Roux-en-Y gastric bypass on weight loss in patients with morbid obesity: the SM-BOSS randomized clinical trial. JAMA. 2018;319(3):255–265.
10. Courcoulas AP, Christian NJ, Belle SH, Berk PD, Flum DR, Garcia L, et al. Weight change and health outcomes at 3 years after bariatric surgery among individuals with severe obesity. JAMA. 2013;310(22):2416–2425.
11. Sjöström L, Narbro K, Sjöström CD, Karason K, Larsson B, Wedel H, et al. Effects of bariatric surgery on mortality in Swedish obese subjects. N Engl J Med. 2007;357(8):741–752.
12. Mechanick JI, Youdim A, Jones DB, Garvey WT, Hurley DL, McMahon MM, et al. Clinical practice guidelines for the perioperative nutritional, metabolic, and nonsurgical support of the bariatric surgery patient—2013 update. Endocr Pract. 2013;19(2):337–372.
13. Schauer PR, Kashyap SR, Wolski K, Brethauer SA, Kirwan JP, Pothier CE, et al. Bariatric surgery versus intensive medical therapy in obese patients with diabetes. N Engl J Med. 2012;366(17):1567–1576.
14. Mingrone G, Panunzi S, De Gaetano A, Guidone C, Iaconelli A, Leccesi L, et al. Bariatric surgery versus conventional medical therapy for type 2 diabetes. N Engl J Med. 2012;366(17):1577–1585.
15. Ikramuddin S, Korner J, Lee WJ, Connett JE, Inabnet WB, Billington CJ, et al. Roux-en-Y gastric bypass vs intensive medical management for the control of type 2 diabetes, hypertension, and hyperlipidemia: the Diabetes Surgery Study randomized clinical trial. JAMA. 2013;309(21):2240–2249.
16. Arterburn DE, Bogart A, Sherwood NE, Sidney S, Coleman KJ, Haneuse S, et al. A multisite study of long-term remission and relapse of type 2 diabetes mellitus following gastric bypass. Obes Surg. 2013;23(1):93–102.

17. Jakobsen GS, Småstuen MC, Sandbu R, Nordstrand N, Hofsø D, Lindberg M, et al. Association of bariatric surgery vs medical obesity treatment with long-term medical complications and obesity-related comorbidities. JAMA. 2018;319(3):291-301. 18. Schiavon CA, Bersch-Ferreira ÂC, Santucci EV, Oliveira JD, Torreglosa CR, Bueno PT, et al. Effects of bariatric surgery in obese patients with hypertension: the GATEWAY randomized trial (Gastric Bypass to Treat Obese Patients With Steady Hypertension). Circulation. 2018;137(11):1132–1142.
18. Schiavon CA, Bersch-Ferreira ÂC, Santucci EV, Oliveira JD, Torreglosa CR, Bueno PT, et al. Effects of bariatric surgery in obese patients with hypertension: the GATEWAY randomized trial (Gastric Bypass to Treat Obese Patients With Steady Hypertension). Circulation. 2018;137(11):1132–1142.
19. Nguyen NT, Varela JE, Sabio A, Tran CL, Stamos M, Wilson SE. Resolution of hyperlipidemia after laparoscopic Roux-en-Y gastric bypass. J Am Coll Surg. 2006;203(1):24–29.
20. Greenburg DL, Lettieri CJ, Eliasson AH. Effects of surgical weight loss on measures of obstructive sleep apnea: a meta-analysis. Am J Med. 2009;122(6):535–542.
21. Ashrafian H, Toma T, Rowland SP, Harling L, Tan A, Efthimiou E, et al. Bariatric surgery or non-surgical weight loss for obstructive sleep apnoea? A systematic review and comparison of meta-analyses. Obes Surg. 2015;25(7):1239–1250.
22. Lassailly G, Caiazzo R, Buob D, Pigeyre M, Verkindt H, Labreuche J, et al. Bariatric surgery reduces features of nonalcoholic steatohepatitis in morbidly obese patients. Gastroenterology. 2015;149(2):379–388.
23. Mummadi RR, Kasturi KS, Chennareddygari S, Sood GK. Effect of bariatric surgery on non-alcoholic fatty liver disease: systematic review and meta-analysis. Clin Gastroenterol Hepatol. 2008;6(12):1396–1402.
24. Lee Y, Doumouras AG, Yu J, Brar K, Banfield L, Gmora S, et al. Complete resolution of non-alcoholic fatty liver disease after bariatric surgery: a systematic review and meta-analysis. Clin Gastroenterol Hepatol. 2019;17(6):1040–1060.e11.
25. Parrott J, Frank L, Rabena R, Craggs-Dino L, Isom KA, Greiman L. American Society for Metabolic and Bariatric Surgery integrated health nutritional guidelines for the surgical weight loss patient 2016 update: micronutrients. Surg Obes Relat Dis. 2017;13(5):727–741.
26. Oor JE, Roks DJ, Ünlü Ç, Hazebroek EJ. Laparoscopic sleeve gastrectomy and gastroesophageal reflux disease: a systematic review and meta-analysis. Am J Surg. 2016;211(1):250–267.
27. Soricelli E, Casella G, Rizzello M, Calì B, Alessandri G, Basso N. Sleeve gastrectomy and crural repair in obese patients with gastroesophageal reflux disease and/or hiatal hernia. Surg Obes Relat Dis. 2013;9(3):356–361.
28. Qumseya BJ, Qumsiyeh Y, Ponniah SA, Estores D, Yang D, Johnson-Mann CN, et al. Barrett's esophagus after sleeve gastrectomy: a systematic review and meta-analysis. Gastrointest Endosc. 2021;93(2):343–352.e2.

Challenges and Long-Term Complications of Sleeve Gastrectomy

15

Sara Morejon Ruiz

15.1 Introduction: Criteria for Bariatric Surgery and Sleeve Gastrectomy According to Current Guidelines

Obesity has emerged as one of the leading global public health concerns, with significant implications for morbidity, mortality, and quality of life among affected individuals. According to the World Health Organization (WHO), in 2022 more than 1 billion people were living with obesity—approximately one in eight individuals worldwide. This figure has more than doubled since 1990, and projections indicate that without effective interventions, over half of all adults and one-third of children and adolescents will be obese by 2050 (The Guardian).

In both Europe and the Americas, the prevalence of obesity has reached alarmingly high levels. In the Region of the Americas, the combined prevalence of overweight and obesity among adults exceeds 67%, the highest rate globally (World Health Organization). In the United States, for instance, obesity rates have surpassed 40% in several states, with a continuing upward trend in recent years (Pan American Health Organization).

In response to this crisis, bariatric surgery has become a highly effective therapeutic tool for the management of morbid obesity and its associated comorbidities, including type 2 diabetes, arterial hypertension, and obstructive sleep apnea. Among the most commonly performed procedures is the sleeve gastrectomy, which involves the resection of a substantial portion of the stomach, thereby reducing its capacity and altering hormonal secretion patterns. These changes promote weight loss and metabolic improvement.

However, despite its effectiveness, sleeve gastrectomy is not exempt from long-term complications. These may include gastroesophageal reflux disease (GERD),

S. Morejon Ruiz (✉)
Department of General Surgery and Digestive Surgery, Hospital Universitario del Henares, Coslada, Madrid, Spain

J. Ruiz-Tovar (ed.), *Multidisciplinary Management of Sleeve Gastrectomy*,
https://doi.org/10.1007/978-3-032-25644-7_15

nutritional deficiencies, weight regain, and progressive dilation of the gastric sleeve, among others. Understanding the underlying pathophysiological mechanisms of these complications is essential to optimize long-term outcomes and enhance the quality of life of patients undergoing this procedure.

Within this context, it is crucial to conduct a detailed analysis of the surgical technique, its pathophysiological implications, and the strategies for prevention and management of related complications. Such an analysis provides a comprehensive and updated perspective on the current state of bariatric surgery in the treatment of obesity and the long-term challenges that accompany it.

15.2 Criteria for Bariatric Surgery Indication: American and European Guidelines

Bariatric surgery has become the most effective intervention for the treatment of morbid obesity and its associated comorbidities, particularly type 2 diabetes, arterial hypertension, and metabolic disorders. Major international scientific societies have established precise criteria for selecting candidates for bariatric surgery, based on accumulated clinical evidence, with the objective of maximizing benefits and minimizing risks.

15.3 Criteria According to American Guidelines

The American Society for Metabolic and Bariatric Surgery (ASMBS) and the American Diabetes Association (ADA), leading authorities in metabolic and bariatric surgery, have issued recommendations based on body mass index (BMI) and the presence of obesity-related comorbidities:

- **BMI ≥ 40 kg/m^2:**
  A clear indication for bariatric surgery in patients with morbid obesity, given the high associated morbidity and mortality, and the low probability of long-term success with non-surgical treatments.
- **BMI ≥ 35 kg/m^2 with obesity-related comorbidities:**
  The presence of conditions such as type 2 diabetes, arterial hypertension, obstructive sleep apnea, dyslipidemia, or cardiovascular disease represents a strong indication for surgical intervention.
- **BMI 30–34.9 kg/m^2 with poorly controlled type 2 diabetes:**
  Bariatric/metabolic surgery should be considered in selected patients, particularly when metabolic disease does not respond adequately to optimal medical therapy. This expanded criterion has transformed the surgical approach to obesity as a **metabolic therapy**.

Additionally, it is essential to demonstrate failure of conventional medical treatments (diet, exercise, pharmacotherapy) and ensure that the patient is willing and able to adhere to a multidisciplinary postoperative follow-up program.

15.4 Criteria According to European Guidelines

European guidelines, such as those developed by the European Association for the Study of Obesity (EASO) and the European Society for Bariatric Surgery (ESBS), share similar principles, though they place greater emphasis on multidisciplinary evaluation and individualized therapy.

- **BMI ≥ 40 kg/m²**, or.
- **BMI ≥ 35 kg/m² with severe obesity-related comorbidities**, including sleep apnea, resistant hypertension, type 2 diabetes, or coronary artery disease.

In patients with BMI between 30 and 35 kg/m² and severe refractory metabolic disease, bariatric surgery may be considered in specialized centers after comprehensive evaluation.

European guidelines also stress the importance of thorough psychological, nutritional, and medical assessment to ensure patient suitability, as well as long-term follow-up to prevent complications and nutritional deficiencies.

15.5 Selection of Surgical Procedure: Sleeve Gastrectomy Versus Other Techniques

The selection of the most appropriate bariatric procedure should be based on an individualized analysis that considers the patient's clinical characteristics, associated comorbidities, personal preferences, and the pathophysiological implications of each technique.

15.5.1 Indications for Sleeve Gastrectomy

Sleeve gastrectomy (SG) has become a widely used and recommended technique for patients with moderate to severe obesity (BMI between 35 and 50 kg/m²) who do not present with significant gastroesophageal reflux disease (GERD) or large untreated hiatal hernias.

This restrictive procedure involves the longitudinal resection of the stomach, creating a narrow gastric tube that limits food intake and reduces ghrelin production, thereby promoting satiety.

The advantages of sleeve gastrectomy include lower technical complexity compared with Roux-en-Y gastric bypass (RYGB), shorter operative time, and a more favorable short-term complication profile. Moreover, since it is not a primarily malabsorptive procedure, it carries a lower risk of severe nutritional deficiencies.

However, careful patient selection is critical, as sleeve gastrectomy may exacerbate or induce GERD symptoms, contraindicating its use in patients with severe reflux or large hiatal hernias not surgically corrected.

15.6 Comparison with Other Techniques

Roux-en-Y gastric bypass (RYGB) remains the gold standard for patients with severe obesity (BMI > 40 kg/m^2), particularly when accompanied by severe GERD or poorly controlled type 2 diabetes. Its combined restrictive and malabsorptive mechanisms promote greater weight loss and metabolic improvement, though at the cost of higher surgical complexity and an increased risk of long-term nutritional deficiencies [13, 15, 16].

For patients with super-obesity (BMI > 50 kg/m^2), biliopancreatic diversion or duodenal switch procedures offer more substantial weight loss and metabolic control, albeit with higher nutritional and technical risks.

15.7 Conclusion

The decision regarding the indication and choice of bariatric surgical procedure must be grounded in evidence-based criteria and international recommendations. Sleeve gastrectomy represents a safe and effective option for selected patients with BMI between 35 and 50 kg/m^2, without significant GERD, who prefer a restrictive technique with a lower risk of malabsorption.

In all cases, multidisciplinary evaluation and long-term follow-up remain essential pillars for achieving successful outcomes and preventing postoperative complications.

Table 15.1 Comparison of the main bariatric surgery techniques, including their primary indications, advantages, and limitations or contraindications.

Table 15.1 Comparison of bariatric surgery techniques

Procedure	Main indications	Advantages	Limitations/ contraindications
Sleeve gastrectomy	BMI 35–50 kg/ m^2, no significant GERD, preference for restrictive approach	Technically simple, minimal malabsorption, effective weight control	May worsen GERD, risk of stenosis, moderate nutritional deficiencies
Roux-en-Y gastric bypass (RYGB)	BMI > 40 kg/ m^2, severe GERD, or poorly controlled type 2 diabetes	Effective reflux control, superior metabolic improvement	Higher complexity, increased nutritional risk, longer operative time
Biliopancreatic diversion/ duodenal switch	BMI > 50 kg/ m^2, severe obesity, advanced diabetes	Greater weight loss and metabolic control	Highly complex, severe nutritional risks, requires strict lifelong follow-up
Adjustable gastric banding	Less common, used in carefully selected patients	Reversible and minimally invasive	Lower efficacy, high rate of band-related complications

This table evaluates the different surgical options based on their indications, benefits, and drawbacks as defined in the current guidelines

15.8 Pathophysiology and Surgical Technique of Sleeve Gastrectomy

15.8.1 Anatomy and Pathophysiological Principles

Sleeve gastrectomy (vertical gastrectomy) consists of the longitudinal resection of the stomach, leaving behind a narrow, tubular gastric sleeve with a residual volume of approximately 80–150 mL. This reduction limits oral intake and modifies gastric hormonal secretion. The procedure is primarily restrictive, but also induces secondary metabolic effects through the reduction of ghrelin production—the orexigenic hormone mainly secreted in the gastric fundus along the greater curvature [17].

The resection extends from 4 to 6 cm proximal to the pylorus up to the angle of His, preserving both the pylorus and the lesser curvature. This anatomical modification leads to several key physiological effects:

- **Reduced gastric volume and compliance**, increasing intraluminal pressure and promoting early satiety.
- **Decreased ghrelin secretion**, resulting in appetite suppression and metabolic improvement.
- **Altered gastric emptying**, which is initially accelerated but may become abnormal in the presence of complications or suboptimal surgical technique.
- **Changes in motility and gastric compliance**, which may cause postoperative symptoms in some patients.

These mechanisms explain the sustained weight loss and improvement of metabolic comorbidities, but they also underlie potential complications such as stenosis or gastroesophageal reflux [18].

15.8.2 Surgical Technique: Technical Aspects

15.8.2.1 Calibration and Gastric Tube Sizing

The caliber of the gastric sleeve is a critical determinant of outcomes. A bougie (calibration tube) ranging from 32 to 40 French (Fr) is typically used to guide resection, with 36 Fr being the most common standard. A smaller diameter (<32 Fr) increases the risk of stenosis, while larger calibers (>40 Fr) may lead to sleeve dilation and reduced restriction [19].

The bougie is introduced orally to the antrum and positioned along the lesser curvature to ensure a uniform sleeve and prevent narrowing.

15.8.2.2 Staple Line and Number of Cartridges

The resection is performed using endoscopic linear staplers, typically with 60 mm cartridges, requiring 5–8 firings depending on gastric length.

Staple selection is crucial: thicker loads (green or black) are used for the antrum due to greater wall thickness, while thinner loads (blue or purple) are reserved for the fundus.

The staple line must be executed precisely to prevent leaks, stenosis, or bleeding. The use of reinforcement or oversewing remains controversial, though some studies suggest it may reduce leak rates [20].

15.8.2.3 Critical Anatomical Landmarks

- **Pylorus preservation**: Essential to prevent early gastric emptying and dumping syndrome.
- **Complete fundus resection**: Required to reduce ghrelin production and prevent residual gastric distension.
- **Division of gastroepiploic and short gastric vessels**: Necessary to mobilize the greater curvature and minimize bleeding.
- **Angle of His management**: A common site for stenosis or twisting; proper visualization and orientation are crucial to prevent complications.

15.8.2.4 Operative Duration and Laparoscopic Approach

Average operative time ranges from 60 to 120 min, depending on the surgeon's experience and the patient's anatomy.

The standard laparoscopic approach offers reduced postoperative morbidity and faster recovery.

In selected cases, robot-assisted surgery is used to enhance precision during stapling.

15.8.3 Pathophysiological Implications of Technique

- **Tube size and complications**: An overly narrow sleeve increases the risk of stenosis and vomiting; an excessively wide one reduces weight-loss efficacy and predisposes to dilation.
- **Residual stomach length**: Retained fundus or excessive curvature may contribute to GERD and sleeve dilation.
- **Torsion or "kinking"**: Improper orientation can cause functional obstruction, elevate intraluminal pressure, and lead to obstructive symptoms.
- **Pyloric preservation and gastric emptying**: While pyloric integrity prevents dumping, altered motility can cause delayed gastric emptying.

15.9 Contraindications to Sleeve Gastrectomy

Although sleeve gastrectomy is a widely adopted and effective bariatric procedure, not all patients are suitable candidates. Contraindications must be carefully assessed.

15.9.1 Absolute Contraindications

- **Severe gastroesophageal reflux disease (GERD):**
  Sleeve gastrectomy may exacerbate reflux due to increased intragastric pressure and reduced gastric volume, facilitating acid reflux into the esophagus. In these cases, Roux-en-Y gastric bypass is preferred, as it both reduces gastric volume and diverts the alimentary flow, minimizing acid exposure.
- **Severe gastrointestinal anatomical abnormalities:**
  Patients with major structural anomalies (e.g., congenital malformations, extensive prior gastric or intestinal surgery) may not be suitable for sleeve formation.
- **Active or recent gastric cancer:**
  Sleeve gastrectomy should not be performed in patients with current or recent gastric malignancy due to risks of tumor dissemination and postoperative complications.

15.9.2 Relative Contraindications

- **Active psychiatric disorders:**
  Patients with severe psychiatric illness (e.g., psychosis or active eating disorders) require careful evaluation, as they may struggle to adhere to postoperative behavioral and dietary changes essential for long-term success.
- **Severe intra-abdominal adhesions:**
  Adhesions from prior surgeries may complicate laparoscopic access and increase the risk of intraoperative injury.
- **Uncontrolled severe comorbidities:**
  Bariatric surgery, including sleeve gastrectomy, is contraindicated in patients with uncontrolled conditions such as advanced heart failure, renal failure, or other major systemic diseases that increase surgical risk.

15.10 Pathophysiological Importance of the Surgical Technique

Sleeve gastrectomy profoundly affects the **digestive physiology** and **hormonal regulation of appetite**. Key pathophysiological implications include:

- **Altered ghrelin production:**
  Resection of the gastric fundus—the main site of ghrelin secretion—leads to a significant decrease in circulating ghrelin levels, reducing appetite and contributing to sustained weight loss.
- **Reduced gastric volume and modified gastric emptying:**
  The creation of a narrow gastric tube limits food intake and alters gastric emptying dynamics, influencing satiety and nutrient absorption.

- **Modified nutrient transit:**
  Although intestinal continuity remains intact (unlike gastric bypass), the reduced gastric volume may affect nutrient absorption and predispose to micronutrient **deficiencies** (vitamin B12, iron, calcium) over time.
- **Risk of gastroesophageal reflux:**
  Increased intragastric pressure following sleeve formation can predispose to GERD, particularly in patients with pre-existing reflux or Barrett's esophagus.

15.11 Long-Term Complications After Sleeve Gastrectomy

15.11.1 Stenosis (Excessive Restriction or Narrowing of the Gastric Sleeve)

15.11.1.1 Pathophysiology

After sleeve gastrectomy, a narrow tubular stomach is created. If the caliber is excessively tight, torsion or "kinking" of the gastric tube occurs, or if there is residual curvature with excessive scarring, a true or functional stenosis may develop. Scar formation secondary to hematoma or staple-line leakage may also lead to fibrosis, wall retraction, and luminal narrowing. This results in increased intraluminal pressure, proximal dilation of the tube, altered gastric emptying, and symptoms of partial obstruction such as food intolerance, vomiting, early satiety, and undesired additional weight loss.

Mechanically, a sharply angulated tube can promote turbulent flow, stasis, and secondary mural hypertrophy or fibrotic adaptation.

15.11.1.2 Incidence

The reported incidence of clinically significant stenosis after sleeve gastrectomy ranges between 0.5% and 3.5% across different series, as documented in the systematic review and meta-analysis by Eguchi et al. [1]

15.11.1.3 Treatment

First-line therapy is endoscopic balloon dilation, with an overall success rate of approximately 77.8%, according to the same meta-analysis [2].

In more complex or refractory cases, self-expandable metal stents or surgical revision (conversion to gastric bypass or stricturoplasty) may be required.

15.11.1.4 Prognosis

Early diagnosis and endoscopic management generally result in excellent outcomes, avoiding the need for major surgery. Delayed recognition, however, may lead to malnutrition, oral intolerance, and the eventual need for revisional surgery.

15.11.2 Persistent Vomiting and Chronic Nausea

15.11.2.1 Pathophysiology

Postoperative vomiting after sleeve gastrectomy may have multiple etiologies:

- Gastric sleeve stenosis or narrowing (see section A).
- Delayed or impaired gastric emptying due to altered motility and reduced gastric compliance.
- Gastroesophageal reflux disease (GERD), with mucosal irritation leading to nausea.
- Dietary intolerance secondary to rapid ingestion, dense solids, or excessive meal volumes.
- Poor adherence to nutritional recommendations, causing inadequate intake and reflex or rejection vomiting.

15.11.2.2 Incidence

In the retrospective study by AlShahrani et al. (2022) involving 117 patients, persistent vomiting occurred in 23.1% of cases [3].

15.11.2.3 Treatment

- Endoscopic or radiologic evaluation when mechanical obstruction is suspected.
- Dietary modifications: small, frequent meals; fluids between meals; avoidance of dense solids; slow eating.
- Prokinetic or antiemetic agents when motility disorders are present.
- In reflux-induced cases, appropriate anti-reflux therapy.

15.11.2.4 Prognosis

With early intervention and nutritional counseling, most cases resolve or significantly improve. Persistent vomiting leading to **malnutrition** may require further investigation or surgical revision.

15.11.3 Neurological Disorders and Nutritional Deficiencies with Neurological Manifestations

15.11.3.1 Pathophysiology

Although sleeve gastrectomy is primarily a restrictive procedure without a strong malabsorptive component, the reduced gastric volume, decreased gastric acid secretion, and lower intrinsic factor production can impair the absorption of key micronutrients (notably vitamin B12). Combined with reduced intake, vomiting, or intolerance, this may cause neurological complications such as peripheral neuropathy, plexopathy, ataxia, myelopathy, or Wernicke's encephalopathy from thiamine (B1) deficiency.

In a retrospective study of 592 patients, 7 (1.18%) developed postoperative neurological complications [4].

15.11.3.2 Incidence
Approximately 1.18% according to the aforementioned series.

15.11.3.3 Treatment
- Periodic monitoring of CBC, iron, ferritin, vitamin B12, thiamine (B1), folate, calcium, vitamin D, and copper.
- Targeted supplementation as indicated by laboratory findings.
- In established neuropathy: physiotherapy, neurological management, and intensive nutritional support.

15.11.3.4 Prognosis
Prognosis depends on timely detection. Early treatment allows complete recovery in most cases, while delayed recognition may result in irreversible neurological sequelae.

15.11.4 Dietary Adaptation Problems and Psychological Effects

15.11.4.1 Pathophysiology
After sleeve gastrectomy, the patient must adapt to: reduced gastric capacity, new eating patterns (small frequent meals, proper chewing, separating liquids from meals), decreased tolerance to certain foods, and changes in satiety and appetite.

If this adaptation is inadequate, "grazing" (frequent snacking), caloric compensation, vomiting, intolerances, and weight regain may occur. Psychologically, rapid body change can trigger body image dysphoria, anxiety, depression, persistent or new eating disorders, and "addiction transfer" (ceasing overeating but developing other addictions such as alcohol use).

In a study of 32 patients, the prevalence of anxiety and depression at 1 year was 65.6% and 46.9%, respectively [5].

15.11.4.2 Incidence
High: in some studies, over 30% reported anxiety symptoms and approximately 11% reported depression [5].

15.11.4.3 Treatment
- Preoperative psychiatric evaluation and postoperative follow-up.
- Nutritional education program (small frequent meals, avoid liquids during meals, chew thoroughly, stop eating with early satiety).
- Support groups, cognitive-behavioral therapy for eating disorders, and monitoring of alcohol or substance use.

15.11.4.4 Prognosis
Quality of life usually improves after surgery, but without psychological and nutritional support, outcomes may worsen, leading to weight regain or psychological distress.

15.11.5 Gastroesophageal Reflux Disease (GERD)/ Esophageal Deterioration

15.11.5.1 Pathophysiology

Creating a narrow gastric sleeve reduces gastric accommodation capacity and increases intraluminal pressure, favoring reflux. If this is combined with an untreated hiatal hernia or lower esophageal sphincter dysfunction, the risk of esophagitis, Barrett's esophagus, and strictures rises.

This was reported in the *Meta-analysis of Long-term* De Novo *Acid Reflux-Related Outcomes Following Sleeve Gastrectomy: Evidence Against the Need for Routine Postoperative Endoscopic Surveillance* (2023), which included 32 studies with ≥4 years of follow-up after sleeve gastrectomy and evaluated the risk of new GERD, esophagitis, and Barrett's esophagus [6].

15.11.5.2 Incidence

According to that study, the proportion of patients developing new GERD symptoms was significant, though exact numbers varied between studies [6].

15.11.5.3 Treatment

Diagnosis via endoscopy and pH-impedance/manometry when indicated.

Treatment includes proton pump inhibitors, H2 blockers, and lifestyle/dietary modifications (avoid large meals, don't lie down after eating, elevate the head of the bed).

If reflux is severe or complications occur (Barrett's, severe esophagitis), conversion to Roux-en-Y gastric bypass should be considered.

This procedure shows a lower incidence of reflux compared to sleeve gastrectomy, according to the meta-analysis *Long-Term Outcomes in Sleeve Gastrectomy* versus *Roux-en-Y Gastric Bypass: A Systematic Review and Meta-Analysis of Randomized Trials* published in 2025 [7].

15.11.5.4 Prognosis

Reflux can be medically controlled in many patients, but untreated chronic reflux may lead to serious complications. The choice of surgical technique preoperatively is crucial.

15.11.6 Nutritional Deficiencies, Malnutrition, Muscle Loss/ Sarcopenia

15.11.6.1 Pathophysiology

Sleeve gastrectomy reduces gastric volume and absolute caloric intake, and partially alters acid secretion, which may decrease micronutrient absorption. Although not a purely malabsorptive procedure, severe restriction and suboptimal intake combined with vomiting or intolerances can lead to malnutrition.

Rapid weight loss can induce protein catabolism, muscle mass loss, and sarcopenia if protein intake and physical activity are not adequately maintained.

A study conducted in Taiwan by Lin et al. (2023) reported that the proportion of patients with moderate to severe nutritional risk increased from 3.3% before surgery to 20% at 12 months [8].

15.11.6.2 Incidence

In a study of 209 patients followed for 6 years, hemoglobin, ferritin, and vitamin B12 deficiencies increased to 36.7%, 43.3%, and 11.7%, respectively, according to Huang et al. [9].

Furthermore, a meta-analysis by Martínez et al. (2024), which included 54 articles with ≥5 years of follow-up, found that the most prevalent deficiency was vitamin D (~35.8%), followed by vitamins E, A, K, and B12 (~8.5%) [10].

15.11.6.3 Treatment

- Routine and personalized supplementation: lifelong daily multivitamin, with annual monitoring of vitamins A, D, E, K, B12, folate, iron, ferritin, magnesium, phosphorus, and calcium.

  A study showed that use of a "specialized" multivitamin (WLS Optimum) improved hemoglobin, folate, and vitamin D levels compared to standard supplementation or no use [11].
- Adequate protein intake (>1 g/kg ideal body weight) and resistance exercise to preserve muscle mass.
- Balanced diet, regular nutritional follow-up, and management of vomiting or food intolerances.

15.11.6.4 Prognosis

With appropriate follow-up and supplementation, most deficiencies can be prevented or controlled. However, non-adherence to supplementation or follow-up may result in chronic anemia, osteoporosis, fractures, fatigue, and decreased quality of life.

15.11.7 Weight Regain, Sleeve Dilation, and Need for Revisional Surgery

15.11.7.1 Pathophysiology

The restrictive effect of the gastric sleeve may diminish over time if the sleeve dilates, the patient resumes larger meal volumes, increases grazing frequency, or fails to maintain proper nutritional and exercise follow-up.

This leads to increased functional gastric volume, reduced satiety, higher caloric intake, and consequently, weight regain.

A meta-analysis including studies with ≥7 years of follow-up reported an estimated late weight regain rate of 27.8% and a revisional surgery rate of 19.9%, according to García-Pérez et al. [12].

15.11.7.2 Incidence

The overall revisional surgery rate at ≥3 years is approximately 10.4%, increasing to 22.6% in patients with ≥10 years of follow-up, according to the meta-analysis by López-Martínez et al. [13, 15, 16].

15.11.7.3 Treatment

- Continuous education on lifestyle habits, regular consultations for nutrition and physical activity.
- Anatomical evaluation by imaging or endoscopy if sleeve dilation is suspected.
- In cases of significant dilation and recurrence, consider conversion to gastric bypass or band addition, based on individual assessment [13, 15, 16].

15.11.7.4 Prognosis

With timely intervention and lifestyle modification, failure can be effectively managed. Without it, additional surgery may be required.

15.12 Nutritional Approach: Definition, Monitoring, Supplementation, and Follow-Up

15.12.1 Definitions and Key Concepts

After sleeve gastrectomy, the reduced stomach limits the amount of food that can be ingested per meal, leading to a lower intake of calories, protein, and micronutrients.

Although intestinal absorption is not directly bypassed, the reduction in gastric volume, gastric acid, and intrinsic factor—combined with lower tolerance and possible vomiting—predisposes patients to nutritional deficiencies.

15.13 Micronutrients at Highest Risk

- **Vitamin D**: Several studies show that deficiency in 25-OH vitamin D is the most prevalent long-term deficiency. For example, Baldini et al. found that after 2 years, more than 30% of patients still had low vitamin D levels [14].
- **Vitamin B12**: Though less frequent than after gastric bypass, it remains relevant. In a 6-year study, B12 deficiency was observed in approximately 11.7% of patients [9].
- **Iron/Ferritin/Hemoglobin**: Iron-deficiency anemia is common, particularly in women of reproductive age and in patients with reduced intake or frequent vomiting [9].

- **Calcium, Magnesium, Phosphorus**: Reduced intake of these minerals has been documented [5].
- **Fat-Soluble Vitamins (A, E, K)**: According to meta-analyses, deficiencies occur in approximately 13.4% (vitamin A), 16.5% (E), and 9.6% (K) of patients after ≥5 years [10].

15.14 Monitoring and Frequency

Laboratory evaluations should be performed preoperatively (baseline) and then every 6–12 months during the first 2–3 years, followed by at least annually for life.

Recommended laboratory panel: complete blood count, serum iron, ferritin, transferrin, vitamins B12, folate, thiamine (B1) if persistent vomiting, 25-OH vitamin D, calcium, phosphorus, magnesium, and parathyroid hormone if vitamin D deficiency is present; assess serum multivitamin levels as indicated.

15.15 Supplementation

- **Daily multivitamin for life**
  For example, a study comparing a specialized supplement (WLS Optimum 1.0/2.0) versus a standard supplement and non-users found better hemoglobin, folate, and vitamin D levels among users of the specialized formula [11].
- **Iron supplementation** for women and patients with anemia or significant weight loss.
- **Calcium + Vitamin D:** at least **1200–1500** mg of **elemental calcium per day** plus **2000 IU of vitamin D** (or more according to serum levels).
- **Vitamin B12**: if low levels or neurological symptoms are present, consider intramuscular or sublingual supplementation.
- **Protein**: target intake >1 g/kg of ideal body weight per day, with nutritional counseling and protein supplementation if oral intake is insufficient.
- **Patient education**: ensure understanding that surgery does not eliminate the need for proper nutrition and supplementation.

15.16 Pathophysiological Importance

Chronic deficiency can lead to anemia, fatigue, bone deterioration (osteopenia/osteoporosis), fractures, sarcopenia, higher surgical risk in future interventions, and severe neurological manifestations such as neuropathy or encephalopathy.

Therefore, continuous follow-up is essential.

15.17 Other Relevant Complications

- **Cholelithiasis**: rapid weight loss promotes gallstone formation.
- **Incisional or internal hernias, adhesions, late intestinal obstruction**: laparoscopic surgery reduces but does not eliminate this risk.
- **Venous thrombosis (portal/mesenteric vein)**: very rare, but reported after sleeve gastrectomy.
- **Decreased bone density/Osteoporosis**: due to vitamin D and calcium deficiency, low protein intake, and reduced body mass.
- **Gynecological or endocrine problems**: hormonal changes after rapid weight loss may alter menstrual cycles and fertility, although specific data for sleeve gastrectomy remain limited.
- Table 15.2 footnote: Summary of main complications after sleeve gastrectomy: clinical features, pathophysiology, treatment, and prognosis.

Table 15.2 Summary of complications after sleeve gastrectomy

Complication	Main clinical feature	Pathophysiology	Treatment	Prognosis
Stenosis	Food intolerance, vomiting, early satiety	Anatomical/functional narrowing due to fibrosis, scarring, or tube torsion	Endoscopic balloon dilation (77.8% success); stent or surgery if refractory	Good if diagnosed early; surgery for complex cases
Persistent vomiting	Nausea, recurrent vomiting, food intolerance	Stenosis, delayed emptying, reflux, or poor nutritional adherence	Address underlying cause (dilation, reflux control, education)	Improves with management; chronic cases lead to malnutrition
GERD	Heartburn, regurgitation, esophagitis, possible Barrett's	Increased pressure, reduced capacity, hiatal hernia, or sphincter dysfunction	PPIs, H2 blockers, lifestyle changes; conversion to bypass if severe	Generally controllable; risk of esophageal complications if untreated
Nutritional deficiencies	Excessive weight loss, fatigue, muscle weakness	Reduced intake, partial malabsorption, vomiting, and protein catabolism	Vitamin/protein supplements, strict follow-up, and exercise	Significant risk if uncontrolled; improves with intervention
Weight regain	Late weight gain, increased hunger	Progressive sleeve dilation, loss of restriction, and increased grazing	Nutritional counseling, exercise, possible revisional surgery	Revisional surgery in 10–22.6%; prevention requires strict follow-up

This table details the clinical features, underlying causes, and management strategies for the most common long-term complications

15.18 Concluding Considerations

- Sleeve gastrectomy is an effective technique but carries long-term risks that must be anticipated and managed.
- The clinical team should establish a multidisciplinary follow-up protocol (surgery, nutrition, psychology, endocrinology) starting preoperatively.
- The surgical technique must ensure an appropriate sleeve caliber, avoiding excessive narrowing or torsion, and address any hiatal hernia to minimize GERD risk.
- Implement a strict lifelong supplementation program and systematic analytical follow-up.
- Educate patients about nutritional requirements, the importance of follow-up, adherence to supplements, exercise, and healthy eating habits.
- Detect early symptoms such as persistent vomiting, food intolerance, reflux, or neurological or psychological alterations to intervene before sequelae develop.
- Document complications in clinical practice to contribute to improved long-term data and outcomes.

References

1. Park JY. Diagnosis and management of postoperative complications after sleeve gastrectomy. J Metab Bariatr Surg. 2022;11(1):1–12.
2. Eguchi M, Nogueira R, Balthazar da Silveira CA, Vidotto L, Kasakewitch JP, Eckerdt Lech G, et al. Endoscopic management of gastric stenosis after sleeve gastrectomy: a systematic review and single-arm meta-analysis. Obes Surg. 2025;
3. AlShahrani A, et al. Early and late complication of sleeve gastrectomy. Int J Community Med Public Health. 2022;9(7)
4. Tabbara M, Carandina S, Bossi M, Polliand C, Genser L, Barrat C. Rare neurological complications after sleeve gastrectomy. Obes Surg. 2016;26(12):2843–8.
5. Al Khalifa K, Al Ansari A. Quality of life, food tolerance, and eating disorder behavior after laparoscopic gastric banding and sleeve gastrectomy-results from a middle eastern center of excellence. BMC Obesity. 2018;5(1):44.
6. Hajibandeh S, Hajibandeh S, Ghassemi N, Evans D, Cheruvu CV. Meta-analysis of long-term de novo acid reflux–related outcomes following sleeve gastrectomy: evidence against the need for routine postoperative endoscopic surveillance. Curr Obes Rep. 2023;12(3):395–405.
7. Monteiro Delgado L, Fabretina de Souza V, Fontel Pompeu B, de Moraes Ogawa T, Pereira Oliveira H, Sacksida Valladão VDC, et al. Long-term outcomes in sleeve gastrectomy versus roux-en-Y gastric bypass: a systematic review and meta-analysis of randomized trials. Obes Surg. 2025;35(8):3246–57.
8. Liao WC, Wang TJ, Liu CY, Liu TP, Liang SY, Chang KS. Risk of malnutrition in adults who have undergone sleeve gastrectomy: a retrospective study. Nutrients. 2023;15(17):3858.
9. Mulita F, et al. Long-term nutritional deficiencies following sleeve gastrectomy: a 6-year single-centre retrospective study. Menopause Rev. 2021;20(4):170–6.
10. Chen L, Chen Y, Yu X, Liang S, Guan Y, Yang J, Guan B. Long-term prevalence of vitamin deficiencies after bariatric surgery: a meta-analysis. Langenbeck's Arch Surg. 2024;409(1):226.
11. Heusschen L, Berendsen AA, Deden LN, Hazebroek EJ, Aarts EO. Nutritional deficiencies 3 years after sleeve gastrectomy can be limited by a specialized multivitamin supplement. Obes Surg. 2022;32(11):3561–70.

12. Clapp B, Wynn M, Martyn C, Foster C, O'Dell M, Tyroch A. Long term (7 or more years) outcomes of the sleeve gastrectomy: a meta-analysis. Surg Obes Relat Dis. 2018;14(6):741–7.
13. Mechanick JI, et al. Clinical practice guidelines for the perioperative nutrition, metabolic, and nonsurgical support of the bariatric surgery patient – 2019 update. Endocr Pract. 2019;25(12):1346–59.
14. Busetto L, et al. Practical recommendations of the obesity management task force of the European Association for the Study of obesity for the post-bariatric surgery medical management. Obes Facts. 2017;10(6):597–632.
15. Angrisani L, et al. Bariatric surgery worldwide 2013. Obes Surg. 2015;25(10):1822–32.
16. Peterli R, et al. Sleeve gastrectomy vs. roux-en-Y gastric bypass in morbid obesity: 5-year outcomes of a randomized controlled trial. Ann Surg. 2018;268(3):446–53.
17. Peterli R, Wölnerhanssen BK, Peters T, et al. Sleeve gastrectomy vs. roux-en-Y gastric bypass in morbid obesity: 5-year outcomes of a randomized controlled trial. Ann Surg. 2018;268(3):446–53.
18. Gagner M, Buchwald JN. Minimally invasive bariatric surgery: an overview. Obes Surg. 2013;23(9):1584–94.
19. Rosenthal RJ, Diaz AA, Arvidsson D, et al. International sleeve gastrectomy expert panel consensus statement: best practice guidelines based on experience of >12,000 cases. Surg Obes Relat Dis. 2013;9(1):8–19.
20. Parikh M, Issa R, McCrillis A, et al. Surgical strategies that may decrease leak after laparoscopic sleeve gastrectomy: a systematic review and meta-analysis. Surg Obes Relat Dis. 2013;9(6):748–55.

Nutritional Sequelae and Specific Supplementation Requirements

16

Maria Jose Castro-Alija, Ghazal Zolfaghari,
Irene Albertos-Muñoz, and Jose María Jimenez-Perez

16.1 Introduction

Sleeve gastrectomy (SG) has emerged as the predominant bariatric surgical procedure worldwide, accounting for more than 60% of all metabolic and bariatric operations, which collectively surpass 500,000 annual interventions globally. This surgical modality is celebrated for its efficacy in inducing sustained weight loss and ameliorating obesity-related comorbidities, while maintaining anatomical continuity without intestinal bypass [1–3]. Yet, sleeve gastrectomy (SG) is associated with a progressive increase in the prevalence of anemia and micronutrient deficiencies, particularly iron, ferritin, and vitamin B12, despite its restrictive mechanism without intestinal bypass [4, 5].

The pathophysiological underpinnings of nutritional depletion post-SG are multifactorial, stemming primarily from the resection of approximately 75–80% of the gastric volume, including the acid-producing fundus and parietal cell mass. This results in diminished gastric acid secretion and intrinsic factor production, integral to protein digestion and vitamin B12 absorption, respectively. Concurrently, reduced gastric reservoir capacity prompts substantial caloric and nutrient intake restriction, while also perturbing hormonal regulators of appetite and nutrient handling. These factors collectively precipitate a milieu of potential macronutrient insufficiency—most notably protein malnutrition—and micronutrient deficits across diverse vitamin and mineral classes [4, 6–8].

Empirical evidence from seminal randomized controlled trials with decade-long follow-up (e.g., the SLEEVEPASS trial) elucidates the prevalence and temporal

M. J. Castro-Alija (✉) · G. Zolfaghari · I. Albertos-Muñoz · J. M. Jimenez-Perez
Research Group on Multidisciplinary Assessment and Intervention in Healthcare and Sustainable Lifestyles (VIMAS+), University of Valladolid, Valladolid, Spain
e-mail: mariajose.castro@uva.es; gzolfaghari@uva.es; irene.albertos@uva.es; jose.maria.jimenez@uva.es

J. Ruiz-Tovar (ed.), *Multidisciplinary Management of Sleeve Gastrectomy*,
https://doi.org/10.1007/978-3-032-25644-7_16

dynamics of these deficiencies. Data indicate persistent vitamin D insufficiency affecting approximately 11% of patients, calcium and vitamin B12 deficits persisting in 3–5%, and iron deficiency manifesting in 14–41% depending on surgical procedure (SG versus Roux-en-Y gastric bypass).

Moreover, long-term follow-up reveals anemia rates rising from 7% preoperatively to 18% at 60 months, alongside ferritin deficiency escalating to 27% and vitamin B12 deficiency to 11.7% at 6 years, necessitating routine supplementation and monitoring to mitigate risks [4, 5]. Ferritin-defined iron deficiency, despite greater incidence in bypass surgeries, remains clinically significant after SG, especially in vulnerable cohorts such as menstruating women. Crucially, adherence to supplementation regimens significantly influences these outcomes, with SG patients demonstrating notably lower long-term compliance (71%) relative to bypass counterparts (89%), thereby amplifying deficiency risks [7, 9].

The clinical sequelae of these deficiencies are not trivial. Vitamin B12 and folate scarcity may provoke megaloblastic anemia, neuropathy, and cognitive disturbances, whereas iron depletion's hematologic consequences exacerbate fatigue and impair physical and occupational functioning. Hypovitaminosis D and resultant calcium malabsorption threaten skeletal integrity, predisposing to osteopenia, osteoporosis, and fracture risk. These nutrient insufficiencies, compounded by often inadequate and non-standardized supplementation, underscore the necessity for rigorous, lifelong nutritional surveillance and evidence-informed, tailored supplementation protocols [4, 7, 10, 11].

Contemporary recommendations stress routine uses of specialized bariatric multivitamins with high-dose vitamin D, calcium citrate, and individualized iron/vitamin B12 therapy, utilizing oral or parenteral routes based on tolerance and absorption capability. Multidisciplinary management leveraging dietitians, endocrinologists, surgeons, and primary care providers is paramount to maintain adherence and optimize nutritional status [12–15].

In conclusion, sleeve gastrectomy epitomizes advancement in obesity therapeutics yet imposes complex, multifactorial nutritional challenges that demand precision, personalization, and lifelong vigilance to forestall insidious deficiencies undermining the surgery's profound health benefits. This chapter synthesizes the most recent high-quality evidence to elucidate the optimized management strategies for nutritional sequelae and supplementation after SG, guiding clinicians toward improving patient-centered outcomes and quality of life.

16.2 Pathophysiology of Nutritional Sequelae After Sleeve Gastrectomy

16.2.1 Anatomical and Physiological Alterations

Sleeve gastrectomy (SG) involves a longitudinal resection of approximately 75–80% of the stomach, encompassing the gastric fundus and greater curvature, producing a narrow, tubular gastric remnant. This markedly reduces gastric capacity while preserving pyloric continuity, resulting in a restrictive, non-malabsorptive surgical modification. Unlike Roux-en-Y gastric bypass (RYGB), which diverts nutrient flow and reduces surface area for absorption, SG primarily alters gastric structure and physiology without bypassing the small intestine. Consequently, SG engenders nutrient-processing limitations rooted in gastric, rather than intestinal, dysfunction [16–19].

The elimination of parietal cell–rich regions—especially the fundus and corpus—leads to hypochlorhydria and decreased intrinsic factor synthesis. The resultant hypoacidic environment compromises multiple nutrient-processing steps:

- **Protein digestion:**
  Reduced gastric acid hampers protein denaturation and pepsin activation, leading to incomplete proteolysis.
- **Mineral solubilization:**
  Acidic conditions are required for ionizing minerals such as calcium, magnesium, and iron; reduced acidity impairs their bioaccessibility.
- **Vitamin B12 absorption:**
  Liberation of cobalamin from dietary proteins requires both hydrochloric acid and intrinsic factor. Their combined reduction predisposes to long-term B12 deficiency.

This multifactorial disruption underlies the progressive development of macro- and micronutrient deficiencies that often manifest months to years postoperatively [4, 7, 20, 21].

16.2.2 Hormonal Alterations and Metabolic Impact

A defining endocrine change post-SG is the pronounced reduction in circulating ghrelin levels, attributable to the removal of ghrelin-secreting X/A-like cells in the gastric fundus. Plasma ghrelin declines by up to 68%, curbing hunger signals and contributing to early satiety and reduced caloric intake. Concurrently, levels of incretin hormones such as glucagon-like peptide-1 (GLP-1) and peptide YY (PYY) rise significantly postprandially, enhancing insulin sensitivity and post-meal glucose control. However, these hormonal modulations also influence gastrointestinal motility, nutrient transit, and potentially micronutrient transport mechanisms, whose long-term consequences remain under investigation.

The mechanical properties of the sleeve remnant further affect physiology. Elevated postprandial intragastric pressures may exacerbate gastroesophageal reflux symptoms, indirectly influencing nutrient adequacy by deterring food intake and promoting selective dietary restriction [22–27].

16.2.3 Gut Microbiome Shifts

Emergent metagenomic data indicate that SG precipitates substantial remodeling of the gut microbiota, albeit with individual variability. Postoperative microbial profiles show increased diversity and an enrichment of taxa associated with improved metabolic profiles, including reduced systemic inflammation and enhanced insulin sensitivity. However, these microbiome alterations can also perturb processes involved in bile acid metabolism, short-chain fatty acid synthesis, and vitamin biosynthesis (notably B vitamins and vitamin K). Such shifts may variably affect fat-soluble vitamin absorption and mineral bioavailability, suggesting the microbiome as a novel axis in post-SG nutritional pathophysiology [28–31].

16.3 Major Nutritional Sequelae

Sleeve gastrectomy (SG) effectively promotes weight loss but increases the risk of nutrient deficiencies due to reduced stomach capacity and altered absorption. Micronutrient and mineral deficiencies, particularly iron, ferritin, vitamin B12, folate, vitamin D, calcium, and zinc, are prevalent and often worsen over time without supplementation. Macronutrient deficiencies are less emphasized in post-SG outcomes, though inadequate protein intake can lead to muscle loss if caloric consumption remains low long-term [32–34].

16.3.1 Macronutrient Considerations Post-SG

Macronutrient deficiencies are not as extensively documented as micronutrient issues after SG, as the procedure primarily affects absorption rather than overall caloric intake. However, reduced stomach volume limits total food consumption, potentially leading to inadequate protein, carbohydrate, or fat intake if patients do not adhere to balanced diets [35–37].

- **Protein and Overall Caloric Intake**
  Average daily intake post-SG is around 1256 kcal at 26 months, with 21% from protein, 54% from carbohydrates, and 26% from fat [38]. Protein malnutrition can occur if intake falls below 60–80 g/day, contributing to muscle mass loss and sarcopenia, especially in the first year when weight loss is rapid [39].
  Food **frequency** questionnaires show no significant differences in estimated nutrient intake between supplemented and unsupplemented groups, but overall caloric restriction heightens deficiency risks [40]. Long-term studies indicate sustained weight loss (64.9% excess weight loss at 6 years) correlates with controlled macronutrient balance, but excessive restriction may exacerbate micronutrient issues indirectly [4].

- **Carbohydrates, Fats, and General Risks**
  Carbohydrate and fat deficiencies are rare as primary concerns, but low-fat diets post-SG can worsen fat-soluble vitamin absorption [41]. In super-obese cohorts, SG maintains comparable short-term weight loss to other procedures without notable macronutrient shortfalls, though nutritional monitoring is crucial to prevent imbalances [42]. Further research is needed on macronutrient-specific outcomes, as current evidence focuses more on micronutrients; guidelines recommend 1.2–1.5 g/kg ideal body weight of protein daily to mitigate muscle loss [39].

16.3.2 Micronutrient and Mineral Deficiencies Post-SG

SG restricts food intake and removes part of the stomach that produces intrinsic factor, contributing to malabsorption of key micronutrients and minerals. These deficiencies can manifest as anemia, fatigue, neurological issues, and bone health problems if not monitored and managed.

- **Vitamin B12 and Folate Deficiencies**
  Impaired gastric acid and intrinsic factor synthesis reduce cobalamin cleavage and binding affecting up to 11.7% of patients at 6 years post-SG [4]. Neurological and hematologic sequelae (e.g., paresthesia, megaloblastic anemia) may emerge years after surgery, necessitating parenteral or high-dose oral supplementation [7, 43, 44].
  Folate absorption occurs in the proximal small intestine but is heavily dependent on dietary intake from fortified foods and leafy vegetables, which decline postoperatively. Dual deficiencies with B12 exacerbate megaloblastic anemia, posing particular risks to women of reproductive age [44, 45].
  In comparative studies, B12 deficiency rates are low overall (3.8% preoperatively, 6.6% at 24 months in SG groups) but higher in procedures like Roux-en-Y gastric bypass (RYGB) compared to SG (relative risk 1.86, 95% CI 1.15–3.02, $p = 0.012$) [33, 34]. Folate deficiency remains low postoperatively, at 1.4% preoperatively and 1.7% at 6 years [4]. with no significant changes over time [5]. Preoperative correction of these deficiencies prevents early postoperative recurrence, as seen in groups receiving pre-SG supplementation where no new B12 or folate deficits developed at 3 or 12 months. In unsupplemented groups, deficiencies persisted despite postoperative multivitamins [40].
- **Vitamin D and Calcium Deficiencies**
  Vitamin D deficiency is prevalent both pre- and post-SG, with 43% of patients having levels below 20 ng/mL at 26 months postoperatively (mean 20.9 ± 10.5 ng/mL) [38]. Preoperative rates reach 39.5% [40], and deficiencies can contribute to secondary hyperparathyroidism, though elevated parathyroid hormone (PTH) levels show no significant change (2.9% preoperatively to 1.7% at 6 years,

$p = 0.606$) [4]. Calcium deficiency affects 68% of patients at 26 months (levels <1.1 mmol/L) without hyperparathyroidism [38]. Bone mineral density monitoring is advised, as these deficiencies heighten osteoporosis risk [41]. Preoperative optimization reduces postoperative risks [40].

- **Iron and Related Deficiencies**
  Iron deficiency is one of the most common issues after SG, often leading to anemia due to decreased acid production in the stomach, which impairs iron absorption. Preoperative anemia affects about 7% of patients, rising to 25% at 36 months and 18% at 60 months postoperatively. Ferritin levels, indicating iron stores, start at 6% deficiency preoperatively and increase steadily to 27% at 60 months [5]. Serum iron deficiency decreases initially from 13% at baseline to 6% at 24 months but rebounds to 20% by 60 months. In a cohort of 40 patients evaluated 26 months post-SG, anemia was present in 28%, and iron deficiency in 38% [38].
  Long-term data from 60 patients at 6 years showed hemoglobin deficiency worsening to 36.7% and ferritin to 43.3% [4].
  Anemia and ferritin deficiency are strongly correlated (Pearson $r = 0.774$, $p = 0.041$), with risk factors including age ≥ 40 years, preoperative anemia, and insufficient iron supplementation. Routine iron supplementation is recommended, but current guidelines may underestimate required dosages [5].
- **Zinc and Other Minerals**
  Zinc deficiency occurs in 6.6–7.9% of patients preoperatively and persists or worsens in some cohorts, with 20% deficiency at 6 years (no significant change, $p = 0.139$) [4]. Comparative data show superior zinc levels in SG versus RYGB patients at 24 months (6.6% vs. 30% deficiency, $p = 0.002$) [33]. Magnesium and phosphorus deficiencies are noted at 29.7% and 5.3% preoperatively, respectively, remaining stable at 20% and 3% at 6 years ($p = 0.139$ and $p = 0.539$) [4]. Fat-soluble vitamins (A, E, K) and thiamine (B1) deficiencies are also reported, particularly in long-term follow-up, with rates up to 78.3% in similar gastric procedures [46]. These are linked to reduced intake and absorption, emphasizing the need for lifelong supplementation [39, 41].

16.4 Prevalence and Risk Factors Across Time Points

- **Short-term (3–12 months):** Anemia prevalence is 6–10%, with low B12 and folate rates but rising ferritin issues [5]. Preoperative deficiencies in 25-hydroxyvitamin D (39.5%), iron (26.3%), and zinc (7.9%) persist without correction [40].
- **Long-term (24–60 months):** Deficiencies accumulate, e.g., anemia at 18–25%, ferritin at 27%, and iron at 20% by 60 months [4, 5]. Hypoabsorptive procedures like RYGB pose higher risks than restrictive SG, but SG still requires vigilant monitoring [34, 41, 42]. High-risk groups include super-obese patients (BMI ≥50 kg/m^2), those with comorbidities, and poor adherence to supplements [42].

Preoperative screening and correction prevent up to 100% of early deficiencies in optimized groups [40]. Adherence decreases over time due to behavioral factors, necessitating multidisciplinary strategies like telemedicine [41].

16.5 Monitoring after Sleeve Gastrectomy

Nutritional complications can develop insidiously and progress to severe clinical sequelae; thus, rigorous, lifelong nutritional surveillance is mandatory after SG.

Nutritional screening is recommended at 3, 6, 12, and 24 months post-SG, followed by annual assessments for life. High-risk patients (rapid weight loss, pregnancy, persistent symptoms) require more frequent follow-up [13, 15].

1. **Regular Laboratory Surveillance**

   Scheduled, proactive biochemical evaluations enable early detection of subclinical deficiencies. This is vital since many deficiencies (e.g., iron, B12) accumulate slowly and may remain asymptomatic until advanced.
2. **Addressing High-Risk Situations**

   Pregnancy requires trimester-specific lab assessments and supplementation adjustments to prevent maternal and fetal complications [13, 15].

   Persistent vomiting and rapid weight loss necessitate urgent assessment for thiamine deficiency to prevent Wernicke's encephalopathy and other severe complications.
3. **Laboratory Panel Includes**

   - Complete blood count with indices to evaluate for anemia type and severity.
   - Iron studies: serum iron, ferritin, transferrin saturation.
   - Serum vitamin B12, methylmalonic acid may be used for confirmation.
   - Serum folate.
   - Calcium, albumin-adjusted calcium, and parathyroid hormone (PTH) to assess calcium homeostasis.
   - 25-hydroxy vitamin D (25[OH]D) concentration.
   - Additional assessments of zinc, copper, selenium, thiamine (vitamin B1), vitamins A, E, and K guided by symptoms and risk profile.

   SG preserves intestinal continuity but alters gastric physiology, impairing digestion and absorption of critical micronutrients, especially those requiring gastric acid and intrinsic factor for uptake (e.g., vitamin B12, iron). Early detection by biochemical markers allows timely intervention, preventing irreversible complications like neurological damage from B12 deficiency or bone demineralization due to calcium/vitamin D deficiency [13, 15, 47].
4. **Behavioral and Educational Interventions**

   Continuous follow-up with a multidisciplinary team (surgeon, dietitian, psychologist) promotes adherence to supplements and dietary recommendations. Education tools such as written guidelines, digital reminders, and support groups improve long-term outcomes [13].

5. **Physical Activity**

   It is recommended to start walking slowly from the very first day, depending on the patient's condition, to prevent any possible embolism. Exercise regimens, especially weight-bearing and resistance training, are recommended to preserve bone density and muscle mass, helping mitigate SG-related risks of sarcopenia and osteoporosis [13].

16.6 Nutritional and Supplementation Strategies for Optimal Recovery and Long-Term Health After Sleeve Gastrectomy

The European Society for Clinical Nutrition and Metabolism (ESPEN) has published comprehensive guidelines on clinical nutrition in surgery, including specific recommendations applicable to sleeve gastrectomy (SG) patients [12, 48].

16.7 Nutritional Strategies (Table 16.1)

1. **Early Oral Feeding (Day 1)**

   Initiating oral intake, clear liquids only, within hours after surgery in most patients, adapting the amount and type of food according to individual tolerance and gastrointestinal function. However, it is strongly recommended that patients start eating even if they do not feel hungry. 64 ounces of fluids a day. One ounce every 10 min. It is better to maintain this minimum fluid intake for the first month and not reduce it. Protein intake should also be started and continued along with slow walking. This early feeding approach reduces the risk of undernutrition and supports recovery, avoids dehydration, maintains hydration, minimizes gastric load and irritation to promote healing.
2. **Gradual Diet Progression**

   The diet is progressively advanced from clear fluids to full liquids, then pureed and soft foods, and finally to a regular textured diet, typically completed by 6–8 weeks postoperatively. This progression minimizes gastrointestinal intolerance and ensures adequate nutrient intake as gastric capacity improves.

   - **Early Postoperative Period (1 Week Post-Surgery)**

     Full liquid diet augmented with protein powder supplements should be in small frequent meals (6–9 times/day). This prevents catabolism by meeting protein targets, supports wound healing, and maintains lean body mass.

     Protein target: 60–80 g/day or 1.2 g/kg ideal body weight (IBW)

     The important part can be teaching the patient how to chew carefully and slowly.
   - **Transition Phase (1–2 Weeks Post-Surgery)**

     In this stage, patients consume full liquids alongside the gradual introduction of protein-rich soft foods such as eggs, tofu, yogurt, and soy milk. This phase

Table 16.1 Nutritional management for sleeve gastrectomy at one glance

Phase	Timing	Nutritional strategy	Protein target	Supplementation
Early Oral feeding	Day 1 (hours after surgery)	Clear liquids only; start early oral intake even if no hunger; maintain hydration (64 oz./day)	Start protein intake with slow walking	None specified here; support hydration
Early postoperative period	1 week post-surgery	Full liquid diet + protein powder; small frequent meals (6–9/day); teach careful chewing	60–80 g/day or 1.2 g/kg ideal body weight (IBW)	Protein supplements
Transition phase	1–2 weeks post-surgery	Full liquids + gradual introduction of protein-rich soft foods (e.g., eggs, tofu, yogurt, soy milk); 4–6 small meals/day	Maintain protein and caloric adequacy	Protein-rich soft foods
Soft/puree diet	2–6 weeks post-surgery	Pureed/soft foods (porridge, mashed veggies, soft fish, tender meats); avoid irritants (carbonated, caffeine, alcohol)	60–80 g/day or 1.2 g/kg IBW	Protein supplements + lean protein foods
Normal diet	From 6 weeks onward	Nutrient-dense regular textured diet; emphasize lean protein, veggies, whole grains; avoid sugar, excess fats, caffeine	60–80 g/day or ~ 1.2 g/kg IBW	Lifelong multivitamins, calcium citrate, vitamin D, iron, vitamin B12

aims to progressively reintroduce textured foods while ensuring that protein and caloric intake remain adequate to support healing and weight management. Patients are encouraged to eat 4 to 6 small, balanced meals daily, allowing close monitoring for any signs of food intolerance or gastrointestinal discomfort. This approach promotes adaptation to new dietary demands while minimizing post-surgical complications such as nausea or vomiting.

- **Soft/Puree Diet (2–6 Weeks Post-Surgery)**

  This stage of the postoperative dietary progression involves transitioning the patient to a soft/puree diet lasting from approximately 2–6 weeks after surgery. During this stage, patients consume pureed and soft foods such as porridge, mashed vegetables, soft fish, and tender meats, focusing on textures that are easier to digest and gentle on the newly formed gastric sleeve. The initial caloric goal is around 500–700 kcal per day, with progressive advancement toward 1000 or more kilocalories by the end of this period to support healing and maintenance of energy balance. Adequate protein intake is emphasized, maintained between 60 and 80 grams per day through the inclusion of lean protein sources and protein supplements. Patients are encouraged to chew thoroughly and avoid consumables that could irritate the gastric mucosa or delay gastric emptying, such as carbonated beverages, caffeine, alcohol, and highly fibrous foods. The overarching objective during this phase is to facilitate the gradual adaptation of the gastrointestinal tract to more solid foods while preventing postoperative complications such as dumping syndrome and gastroesophageal reflux.

- **Normal Diet (From 6 Weeks Post-Surgery Onward)**

  This stage marks the transition to a normal diet beginning around 6 weeks' post-surgery, during which patients progressively adopt a nutrient-dense diet with regular texture, emphasizing lean protein sources, vegetables, and whole grains to support sustained weight loss and nutritional adequacy. The recommended caloric intake ranges from 1000 to 1400 kcal per day depending on individual energy needs and weight loss goals, while protein intake should be maintained at 60–80 grams daily or approximately 1.2 grams per kilogram of ideal body weight, focusing on high biological value sources such as lean meats, dairy, and plant-based proteins. Lifestyle recommendations include avoiding sugary foods, excess fats, carbonated beverages, alcohol, and caffeine, alongside promoting adequate hydration and continued use of lifelong supplementation, including multivitamins, calcium citrate, vitamin D, iron, and vitamin B12. Regular clinical follow-ups and nutritional assessments remain critical to monitor for and correct potential nutrient deficiencies, gastrointestinal symptoms, or dumping syndrome, ensuring optimal long-term outcomes in surgical patients.

3. **Protein Intake**

   Adequate protein provision is crucial and generally range from 60 to 80 grams daily or approximately 1 to 1.2–1.5 grams per kilogram of ideal body weight to preserve lean body mass and promote healing.

16.8 Key Supplementation Recommendations Post-Sleeve Gastrectomy (Table 16.2)

After sleeve gastrectomy (SG), routine supplementation with iron, vitamin B12, and multivitamins is essential to prevent deficiencies that can lead to anemia and impaired long-term health. Iron supplementation should be prioritized due to rising ferritin deficiency rates, starting at 200–300 mg elemental iron daily, potentially higher for high-risk patients. Vitamin B12 injections or sublingual forms (1000 mcg weekly) are recommended lifelong, alongside calcium (1200–1500 mg/day) and vitamin D (2000–3000 IU/day) to support bone health. Monitoring via blood tests every 3–6 months initially, then annually, ensures optimal recovery and sustained metabolic benefits.

Table 16.2 Supplementation for sleeve gastrectomy at one glance

Phase	Nutrient/intervention	Recommended dose
Immediate post-Op (0–6 months)	**Multivitamin**	≥200% DV of key micronutrients; folate 400–800 mcg/day
	Vitamin B12	1000 mcg IM monthly or sublingual daily
	Iron	45–60 mg elemental iron twice daily (with vitamin C)
	Calcium + magnesium (via fluids)	Ca 500 mg + Mg 200–400 mg as part of hydration
	Hydration / electrolytes	1.5–2 L/day as tolerated
Protein (early)	**Protein intake**	60–80 g/day or 1.0–1.5 g/kg ideal body weight
Long-term (≥6 months to lifelong)	**Vitamin B12**	1000 mcg weekly sublingual or monthly IM
	Folate	400–800 mcg/day (via multivitamin)
	Iron	200–300 mg elemental iron daily; IV if ferritin <30 ng/mL or poor oral response
	Calcium (citrate)	1200–1500 mg/day, split doses
	Vitamin D3	2000–3000 IU/day
	Zinc	8–11 mg/day
	Other vitamins (A, E, K)	Provided in multivitamin
	Omega-3 / probiotics	Optional; evidence emerging
Special cases	**High-risk patients (≤40 years, preoperative anemia)**	Increase iron to 300 mg/day; correct B12/iron 3 months pre-op
	Weight regain / poor EWL (<60% at 5 years)	Reassess nutrient absorption and adherence
Monitoring schedule	**Blood tests**	3, 6, 12 months; then annually

16.9 Immediate Postoperative Supplementation for Recovery

In the first 3–6 months post-SG, the focus is on mitigating acute nutritional gaps to support wound healing, reduce inflammation, and prevent complications like post-operative nausea or readmissions. Patients often experience rapid weight loss (up to 44.3% excess weight loss at 3 months), which can exacerbate deficiencies if dietary intake is limited [49].

1. **Multivitamin Therapy**

   A high-potency bariatric-specific multivitamin containing at least 200% of the daily value for key micronutrients is advised daily. This covers broad needs, including folate (400–800 mcg) to maintain low deficiency rates postoperatively [5, 50].

2. **Vitamin B12**
   Administer 1000 mcg intramuscularly monthly or sublingually daily from week 1, as deficiency risks climb to 48% by 5 years due to reduced intrinsic factor [49]. Over 46% of patients need this in follow-up [50].
3. **Iron Supplementation**
   Start with 45–60 mg elemental iron twice daily, taken on an empty stomach with vitamin C to enhance absorption. This counters the initial drop in serum iron (from 13% to 6% deficiency at 24 months) and prevents early anemia [5]. About 51% of patients require iron supplements in the first 2 years [50].
4. **Hydration and Anti-Nausea Support**
   While not a supplement, electrolyte solutions with added calcium (500 mg) and magnesium (200–400 mg) help during the enhanced recovery phase, reducing hospital stays from 52 to 30 h when paired with protocols [51].
5. These measures align with evidence showing no increase in readmissions ($P = 0.498$) when supplementation is integrated into recovery plans [51].

16.10 Long-Term Strategies for Sustained Health

Beyond the initial recovery, deficiencies evolve, with ferritin levels dropping to 27% at 60 months and anemia stabilizing at 18–25% from 36 months onward. Long-term supplementation must be personalized, with annual blood work to track hemoglobin, ferritin (>50 ng/mL target), B12 (>300 pg/mL), and folate levels [5].

1. **Vitamin B12 and Folate Management**
   Vitamin B12 deficiency remains low initially but requires proactive dosing due to gastric fundus removal [5]. Sublingual or nasal forms bypass absorption issues, with 46.3% of patients supplemented in observational data [50]. Folate deficiency stays minimal (under 5%), but 41.5% receive it routinely to support red blood cell production. Routine B12 therapy is non-negotiable post-SG for neurological and hematologic health [5, 49, 50].
2. **Vitamin D, Calcium, and Bone Health**
   Calcium malabsorption risks osteopenia; aim for 1200–1500 mg/day from citrate forms (better absorbed without acid), split doses to avoid GI upset. Pair with 2000–3000 IU vitamin D3 daily, as 26.8% of patients need it. This duo supports the 61% excess weight loss at 5 years while preventing secondary hyperparathyroidism [49, 50].
3. **Iron and Anemia Prevention**
   Iron storage declines steadily post-SG, correlating strongly with anemia (Pearson $r = 0.774$, $p = 0.041$). Routine oral iron (200–300 mg elemental daily) is recommended lifelong, but guidelines may underestimate needs—consider intravenous iron for ferritin <30 ng/mL or non-responders. High-risk groups (age ≤ 40 years, preoperative anemia, or inadequate prior supplementation) face 2–3 times higher anemia odds, necessitating stricter dosing. Zinc (8–11 mg/day)

co-supplementation (36.6% usage rate) prevents interference with iron absorption [5, 50].

4. **Additional Micronutrients**

    - **Other Vitamins**: Water-soluble vitamins (A, E, K) via multivitamins suffice, but monitor if weight regain occurs (up to 39% at 5 years) [49, 52].
    - **Probiotics and Omega-3 s**: Emerging evidence suggests fish oils and microbiome support (e.g., prebiotics) to enhance protein uptake and reduce inflammation, fitting into postoperative metabolic modulation. However, data specific to SG is limited, warranting further trials [53].

5. **Protein**

    Target intakes ranging from 60 to 80 grams daily (or 1.0–1.5 g/kg ideal body weight), with early use of protein supplements recommended due to reduced appetite, altered gastric capacity, and intolerance to large food volumes [12, 54, 55].

16.11 Risk Factors and Personalized Approaches

16.11.1 Certain Profiles Demand Intensified Strategies

- **Younger Patients (≤40 years)**
  Higher anemia risk; escalate iron to 300 mg/day and monitor quarterly.
- **Preoperative Deficiencies**
  Baseline anemia triples postoperative odds—prehab with 3 months of iron/B12 corrects this [5].
- **Weight Regain or Reoperations**
  If excess weight loss dips below 60% at 5 years, reassess absorption; conversions to bypass may arise in 10–20% [52].

Subgroup analyses highlight insufficient supplementation as a key modifiable factor. Integrate with lifestyle: high-protein diets (>60 g/day) and exercise boost outcomes, but supplements bridge gaps [5].

16.12 Monitoring and Future Considerations

Blood tests at 3, 6, 12 months, then yearly, guide adjustments—e.g., if ferritin plateaus below 100 ng/mL, increase iron. While SG yields metabolic wins like improved lipids (triglycerides down, $p < 0.05$) and cardiac function. Unaddressed deficiencies could undermine these. Current protocols reduce complications, but partial data on optimal dosing (e.g., for zinc or emerging agents like poloxamer for lipid control) suggests need for longitudinal studies. Adhering to these strategies ensures SG's benefits endure, promoting recovery and vitality [5, 49, 53].

16.13 Supplementation in Special Patient Populations After Sleeve Gastrectomy (Table 16.3)

Effective nutritional management after sleeve gastrectomy requires tailored strategies for distinct high-risk groups to mitigate complications and optimize recovery. For example, those with preoperative anemia, younger age (≤40 years), gastroesophageal reflux disease (GERD), high body mass index (BMI >45 kg/m^2), mild obesity (BMI 30–34.9 kg/m^2), or candidates for combined procedures like liver transplantation face heightened risks of nutritional deficiencies, particularly in iron, vitamin B12, ferritin, and vitamin D. Routine multivitamin supplementation is essential, but tailored strategies, including higher-dose iron and lifelong B12 monitoring, are recommended to mitigate long-term complications like anemia and suboptimal micronutrient levels, with close follow-up every 3–6 months.

16.14 Nutritional Risks in High-Risk Groups

Patients undergoing SG often experience altered absorption and intake due to reduced stomach volume, leading to deficiencies that can worsen over time. In populations with preoperative anemia or age ≤ 40 years, the risk of postoperative anemia rises significantly, with pooled prevalence increasing from 7% at baseline to 18% at 60 months. Ferritin deficiency, a marker of iron stores, steadily climbs from 6% preoperatively to 27% at 60 months, correlating strongly with anemia (Pearson $r = 0.774$, $p = 0.041$). Insufficient iron supplementation exacerbates this, highlighting the need for proactive management in these groups [5].

For patients with GERD, SG can induce or worsen symptoms in up to 84.1% of cases, potentially complicating oral supplementation adherence due to gastrointestinal adverse events (6.9% vs. 3.6% without GERD, $p < 0.05$). This population also shows decreased weight loss and higher revisional surgery needs (0.6% vs. 0.3%, $p < 0.05$), indirectly increasing nutritional vulnerability [56].

Table 16.3 Supplementation recommendations in special populations after sleeve gastrectomy

Nutrient	Special population risk	Recommended supplementation	Monitoring frequency
Iron/ferritin	Preoperative anemia, age ≤ 40, high-BMI	45–200 mg elemental iron daily; pair with vitamin C for absorption	Every 3 months (hemoglobin, ferritin)
Vitamin B12	Gastric atrophy, females, long-term (>36 months)	1000 μg sublingual weekly or IM monthly	Every 3–6 months (serum levels)
Vitamin D/ calcium	All, especially mild obesity, transplant candidates	2000–4000 IU D + 1200–1500 mg calcium citrate daily	Every 3 months (25-OH D, PTH)
Folic acid	Routine for all	400–800 μg daily (in multivitamin)	Annually if stable

High-BMI, high-risk patients (e.g., mean BMI 66 kg/m^2, multiple comorbidities averaging 9.6 per patient) demonstrate durable excess weight loss (48% at 73 months) but require vigilant monitoring for micronutrient shortfalls, as long-term data show persistent risks despite no perioperative mortality [57].

In mildly obese individuals (BMI 30–34.9 kg/m^2), short-term outcomes are favorable with 76.5% excess weight loss at 12 months and low complication rates (1.6% hemorrhage), yet vitamin D levels remain suboptimal even with multivitamins [58, 59].

Combined SG with liver transplantation in morbidly obese patients (median BMI 42 kg/m^2) poses unique challenges, including 45.5% 90-day survival and risks from factors like age > 60 years, BMI >45, or high-risk donors (ET-DRI >1.6), where metabolic syndrome amplifies deficiency potential [60]. Preoperative deficiencies in iron (22%), vitamin B12 (3.8%), and others are common across cohorts, worsening to 36.7% anemia and 43.3% low ferritin at 6 years without targeted intervention [4].

16.15 Tailored Supplementation Strategies

Supplementation should begin preoperatively to correct deficits and continue lifelong, adjusted for individual risks. For anemia-prone groups (younger patients or those with baseline low hemoglobin), routine iron supplementation reduces incidence, though current guideline doses (e.g., 45–60 mg elemental iron daily) may prove inadequate, necessitating doses up to 100–200 mg with monitoring for ferritin every 3 months [5, 50]. In one cohort, 51.2% required iron, underscoring its prevalence [50].

Vitamin B12 deficiency affects up to 46.3% postoperatively, particularly in patients with gastric atrophy (61.7% prevalence), where levels drop significantly despite support ($p = 0.024$ overall, $p = 0.023$ in females) [50, 61]. Routine sublingual or intramuscular B12 (1000 μg weekly or monthly) is advised for all SG patients, with more frequent dosing in atrophy-confirmed cases [50, 61]. Folic acid supplementation (41.5% usage) maintains low deficiency rates (1.7% at 6 years) when paired with B12 [4, 50].

Calcium and vitamin D needs are elevated due to reduced acid secretion; 37.8% and 26.8% of patients require these, respectively, with vitamin D often remaining suboptimal (<30 ng/mL) despite daily multivitamins (400–800 IU) [50, 58]. High-risk groups, including transplant candidates, benefit from 1200 to 1500 mg calcium citrate and 2000–4000 IU vitamin D daily, monitored quarterly to prevent secondary hyperparathyroidism (elevated PTH in 1.7–2.9%) [4, 62].

In GERD patients, liquid or chewable formulations improve tolerance, as solid pills may worsen reflux [56]. For high-BMI or mildly obese subgroups, standard multivitamins suffice initially, but escalation to zinc (36.6% usage) and magnesium (20% deficiency) is needed if symptoms like fatigue emerge [50, 59]. Phosphorus (3–5.3% low) rarely requires separate attention [4].

16.16 Long-Term Management and Follow-Up

Deficiencies evolve dynamically: serum iron dips to 6% at 24 months but rebounds to 20% at 60 months, while B12 and folate stay low with supplementation [5, 58]. In special populations, annual endoscopy for atrophy in B12 non-responders and DEXA scans for bone health in vitamin D-deficient cases are prudent [61, 62]. For transplant patients, prioritizing standard donors and listing severely obese individuals higher reduces procedural risks, allowing better supplementation adherence [60].

Overall, 70.5% comorbidity resolution in mild obesity and 77% diabetes improvement in high-risk groups affirm SG's benefits, but unsupplemented patients risk 15.1% major complications [56, 57, 59]. Patient satisfaction scores (4.4–4.6/5 for body image and tolerance) improve with consistent regimens. While data support these approaches, further research on optimal dosing in transplant or GERD cohorts could refine protocols, emphasizing personalized, multidisciplinary care to sustain outcomes beyond 6 years.

Integrating these targeted strategies within multidisciplinary care frameworks aligns with the latest global clinical practice guidelines, underscoring personalized and vigilant nutritional care as critical for sustainable postoperative success following sleeve gastrectomy [12, 63–65].

References

1. Mejaddam A, Carlsen HK, Larsson I, Eeg-Olofsson K, Lugner M, Ottosson J, et al. Long–term effects of gastric bypass and sleeve gastrectomy in type 2 diabetes: a matched retrospective cohort study from Sweden. Lancet Reg Health Eur. 2025;58:101430.
2. Nocca D, Gagner M, Biertho L, Cuenca-Abente F, Nedelcu M. Sixth international consensus conference on sleeve gastrectomy. Surg Endosc. 2025; https://doi.org/10.1007/S00464-025-11974-0.
3. Loss SW. FACT SHEET – metabolic and bariatric. Surgery. 2025;2025:1–2.
4. Mulita F, Lampropoulos C, Kehagias D, Verras GI, Tchabashvili L, Kaplanis C, et al. Long-term nutritional deficiencies following sleeve gastrectomy: a 6-year single-centre retrospective study. Przegl Menopauzalny. 2021;20:170.
5. Nie Y, Tian Z, Wang P, Liu B, Zhang N, Zhou B, et al. Prevalence of anemia and related nutrient deficiencies after sleeve gastrectomy: a systematic review and meta-analysis. Obes Rev. 2023;24:e13516.
6. Alexandrou A, Armeni E, Kouskouni E, Tsoka E, Diamantis T, Lambrinoudaki I. Cross-sectional long-term micronutrient deficiencies after sleeve gastrectomy versus roux-en-Y gastric bypass: a pilot study. Surg Obes Relat Dis. 2014;10:262–8.
7. Saarinen I, Strandberg M, Hurme S, Helmiö M, Grönroos S, Juuti A, et al. Nutritional deficiencies after sleeve gastrectomy and roux-en-Y gastric bypass at 10 years: secondary analysis of the SLEEVEPASS randomized clinical trial. Br J Surg. 2025;112:132.
8. Hany Emile S, Elfeki H. Nutritional deficiency after sleeve gastrectomy: a comprehensive literature review. EMJ Gastroenterol. 2017:99–105.
9. Soewarno. Nutritional deficiencies after sleeve gastrectomy and roux-en-Y gastric bypass at 10 years: secondary analysis of the SLEEVEPASS randomized clinical trial. BJS Acad. 2025;11:296–300.
10. Ganipisetti VM, Naha S. Bariatric surgery malnutrition complications. StatPearls; 2023

11. Haughton S, Gentry S, Parretti HM. Nutritional deficiencies following bariatric surgery: a rapid systematic review of case reports of vitamin and micronutrient deficiencies presenting more than two years post-surgery. Clin Obes. 2025;15:e70035.
12. Weimann A, Bezmarevic M, Braga M, et al. ESPEN guideline on clinical nutrition in surgery – update 2025. Clin Nutr. 2025;53:222–61.
13. Steenackers N, de Boer L, Dekempeneer C, Deleus E, Lannoo M, Mertens A, et al. Current clinical practice guidelines for nutritional screening before and after sleeve gastrectomy and roux-En-Y gastric bypass: a scoping review. Curr Obes Rep. 2025; https://doi.org/10.1007/S13679-025-00606-2.
14. Chelsea and Westminster Hospital NHS Foundation Trust. Dietary guidance after gastric bypass or sleeve gastrectomy surgery. Available from: https://www.chelwest.nhs.uk/your-visit/patient-leaflets/bariatric-dietetics/dietary-guidance-after-gastric-bypass-or-sleeve-gastrectomy-surgery; 2025
15. Shiau J, Biertho L. Bariatric surgery: postoperative management. Can Adult Obes Clin Pract Guidel. 2020:1–15.
16. Brethauer SA, Schauer PR. Sleeve gastrectomy. In: Bariatr Surg what every Provid needs to know; 2023. p. 89–100.
17. Katayama RC, Herbella FAM. Surgical technical key points of laparoscopic sleeve gastrectomy: how I do it. J Vis Surg. 2025; https://doi.org/10.21037/JOVS-25-7/COIF.
18. Spiegel HU, Skawran S. From longitudinal gastric resection to sleeve gastrectomy – revival of a previously established surgical procedure. J Gastrointest Surg. 2010;15:219.
19. Rodriguez M. Vertical sleeve gastrectomy. 2013.
20. Caron M, Hould FS, Lescelleur O, Marceau S, Lebel S, Julien F, et al. Long-term nutritional impact of sleeve gastrectomy. Surg Obes Relat Dis. 2017;13:1664–73.
21. Lupoli R, Lembo E, Saldalamacchia G, Avola CK, Angrisani L, Capaldo B. Bariatric surgery and long-term nutritional issues. World J Diabetes. 2017;8:464.
22. Mans E, Serra-Prat M, Palomera E, Suñol X, Clavé P. Sleeve gastrectomy effects on hunger, satiation, and gastrointestinal hormone and motility responses after a liquid meal test. Am J Clin Nutr. 2015;102:540–7.
23. Al Hussaini SK, Al Wazee SGS. Ghrelin and leptin changes post-sleeve gastrectomy. Acad Int J Med Updat. 2024;2:21–32.
24. Advanced Obesity Surgery. How gastric sleeve surgery decreases the "hunger hormone" in Sydney. Available from: https://www.advancedobesitysurgery.com.au/how-gastric-sleeve-surgery-decreases-the-hunger-hormone-for-major-weight-loss/; 2025
25. Sharma G, Nain P, Sethi P, Ahuja A, Sharma S. Plasma ghrelin levels after laparoscopic sleeve gastrectomy in obese individuals. Indian J Med Res. 2019;149:544.
26. Sethi P, Thillai M, Nain PS, Ahuja A, Aulakh N, Khurana P. Role of hunger hormone "ghrelin" in long-term weight loss following laparoscopic sleeve gastrectomy. Niger J Surg. 2018;24:121.
27. Basso N, Soricelli E, Casella G, Di Rocco G, Redler A. Longitudinal sleeve gastrectomy: current perspectives. Open Access Surg. 2014:35.
28. Welsch EC, Barron MR, Storage KM, Kazen AB, Aboulalazm FA, Kirby JR, et al. Gut microbiome and bile acid changes after male rodent sleeve gastrectomy: what comes first? Am J Physiol Regul Integr Comp Physiol. 2025;329:R410–21.
29. Voermans B, Gerdes V, Nieuwdorp M. Gut microbiota alterations and their role in the pathophysiology of obesity following bariatric surgery. Expert Rev Endocrinol Metab. 2025;20:291–305.
30. Komori E, Kato-Kogoe N, Imai Y, et al. Gastrectomy-induced alterations in gut microbiota linked to changes in oral and gastric microbiota. Front Microbiol. 2025;16:1599503.
31. Gong S, Zhang X, Chen X, Wan P, Zhou L, Zhang J. The impact of bariatric surgery on gut microbiota: a bibliometric analysis of research trends and scientific contributions. Front Microbiol. 2025;16:1523809.
32. Silva M, Lau E, Varela A, Freitas P, Carvalho D. Micronutrient deficiencies in post-bariatric patients – an undervalued consequence. Rev Port Endocrinol Diabetes Metab. 2024;18

33. Ferraz ÁAB, Carvalho MRC, Siqueira LT, Santa-Cruz F, Campos JM. Micronutrient deficiencies following bariatric surgery: a comparative analysis between sleeve gastrectomy and roux-en-Y gastric bypass. Rev Col Bras Cir. 2018;45:1–9.
34. Kwon Y, Ha J, Lee YH, Kim D, Lee CM, Kim JH, et al. Comparative risk of anemia and related micronutrient deficiencies after roux-en-Y gastric bypass and sleeve gastrectomy in patients with obesity: an updated meta-analysis of randomized controlled trials. Obes Rev. 2022; https://doi.org/10.1111/OBR.13419.
35. Derbyshire Joint Area Prescribing Committee. Protein intake after bariatric surgery: information for patients; 2017–2020
36. Bertoni L, Valentini R, Zattarin A, Belligoli A, Bettini S, Vettor R, et al. Assessment of protein intake in the first three months after sleeve gastrectomy in patients with severe obesity. Nutrients. 2021;13:771.
37. Carey S, Rd MS. Sleeve gastrectomy nutritional guidelines. Nutrit Staff. 2012:1–19.
38. Alvarez V, Cuevas A, Olivos C, Berry M, Farías MM. Déficit de micronutrientes a más de un año de postoperatorio en gastrectomía en manga. Nutr Hosp. 2014;29:73–9.
39. Patel JJ, Mundi MS, Hurt RT, Wolfe B, Martindale RG. Micronutrient deficiencies after bariatric surgery: an emphasis on vitamins and trace minerals. Nutr Clin Pract. 2017;32:471–80.
40. Schiavo L, Pilone V, Rossetti G, Romano M, Pieretti G, Schneck AS, et al. Correcting micronutrient deficiencies before sleeve gastrectomy may be useful in preventing early postoperative micronutrient deficiencies. Int J Vitam Nutr Res. 2019;89(1–2):22–8.
41. Reytor-González C, Frias-Toral E, Nuñez-Vásquez C, Parise-Vasco JM, Zambrano-Villacres R, Simancas-Racines D, et al. Preventing and managing pre- and postoperative micronutrient deficiencies: a vital component of long-term success in bariatric surgery. Nutrients. 2025;17:741.
42. ElSafty M, Khaled Sabra H, Ahmed Orebi H, Futooh Z, Shinkar A, et al. Comparative outcomes of one anastomosis gastric bypass and sleeve gastrectomy: a retrospective analysis of weight loss and micronutrient deficiencies in superobese patients at 12 months. Br J Surg. 2025; https://doi.org/10.1093/BJS/ZNAF128.318.
43. Côté M, Pelletier L, Nadeau M, Bouvet-Bouchard L, Julien F, Michaud A, et al. Micronutrient status 2 years after bariatric surgery: a prospective nutritional assessment. Front Nutr. 2024;11:1385510.
44. Humięcka M, Sawicka A, Kędzierska K, Binda A, Jaworski P, Tarnowski W, et al. Prevalence of nutrient deficiencies following bariatric surgery – long-term, prospective observation. Nutrients. 2025;17:2599.
45. Haughton S, Gentry S, Parretti HM. Nutritional deficiencies following bariatric surgery: a rapid systematic review of case reports of vitamin and micronutrient deficiencies presenting more than two years post-surgery. Clin Obes. 2025; https://doi.org/10.1111/COB.70035.
46. Teixeira Farinha H, Bouriez D, Grimaud T, Rotariu AM, Collet D, Mantziari S, et al. Gastrointestinal disorders and micronutrient deficiencies following oncologic esophagectomy and gastrectomy. Cancer. 2023;15:3554.
47. Derbyshire Joint Area Prescribing Committee. Monitoring and medication after bariatric surgery; 2017–2020
48. Ryu S-W. Nutritional support after gastrectomy. Foregut Surg. 2022;2:47.
49. Kikkas EM, Sillakivi T, Suumann J, Kirsimägi T, Tikk T, Värk PR. Five-year outcome of laparoscopic sleeve gastrectomy, resolution of comorbidities, and risk for cumulative nutritional deficiencies. Scand J Surg. 2019;108:10–6.
50. Pech N, Meyer F, Lippert H, Manger T, Stroh C. Complications, reoperations, and nutrient deficiencies two years after sleeve gastrectomy. J Obes. 2012;2012:828737.
51. Demirpolat MT, Şişik A, Yildirak MK, Basak F. Enhanced recovery after surgery promotes recovery in sleeve gastrectomy: a randomized controlled trial. J Laparoendosc Adv Surg Tech. 2023;33:452–8.
52. Langer FB, Shakeri-Leidenmühler S, Bohdjalian A, Schoppmann S, Zacherl J, Felberbauer FX, et al. Strategies for weight regain after sleeve gastrectomy. Surg Laparosc Endosc Percutan Tech. 2010;20:159–61.

53. Martindale RG. Novel nutrition strategies to enhance recovery after surgery. JPEN J Parenter Enteral Nutr. 2023;47:476–81.
54. Rhode B Vitamin and mineral supplementation after gastric bypass. Pamtremble.com; 2000
55. Lopez RC, Gallanis AF, Davis JL. The essentials of vitamin and mineral supplementation after total gastrectomy. J Gastrointest Cancer. 2025;56:130.
56. DuPree CE, Blair K, Steele SR, Martin MJ. Laparoscopic sleeve gastrectomy in patients with preexisting gastroesophageal reflux disease: a national analysis. JAMA Surg. 2014;149:328–34.
57. Eid GM, Brethauer S, Mattar SG, Titchner RL, Gourash W, Schauer PR. Laparoscopic sleeve gastrectomy for super obese patients: forty-eight percent excess weight loss after 6 to 8 years with 93% follow-up. Ann Surg. 2012;256:262–5.
58. Capoccia D, Coccia F, Paradiso F, Abbatini F, Casella G, Basso N, et al. Laparoscopic gastric sleeve and micronutrients supplementation: our experience. J Obes. 2012;2012:672162.
59. Noun R, Chakhtoura G, Nasr M, Skaff J, Choucair N, Rkaybi N, et al. Laparoscopic sleeve gastrectomy for mildly obese patients (BMI 30–35 kg/m^2): operative outcome and short-term results. J Obes. 2012; https://doi.org/10.1155/2012/813650.
60. Manzia TM, Sensi B, Gentileschi P, Quaranta C, Toti L, Baiocchi L, et al. Safety and efficacy of simultaneous liver transplantation and sleeve gastrectomy in morbid obese patients with end-stage liver disease: the LT-SG study. Liver Transpl. 2025;31:770–80.
61. Adalı Y, Binnetoğlu K. Evaluación de la respuesta a suplementación de vitamina B12 en pacientes con atrofia en materiales de gastrectomía de manga. Cir Cir. 2022;90:17–23.
62. Al-Mulhim AS. Laparoscopic sleeve gastrectomy and nutrient deficiencies: a prospective study. Surg Laparosc Endosc Percutan Tech. 2016;26:208–11.
63. Li Y, Zhang T. Advances in perioperative nutritional management in metabolic and bariatric surgery. Diabetes Metab Syndr Obes. 2025;18:2191.
64. Farias DA, Ward MA, Buckmaster BA, Shabbir R, Jefferies RS, Ogola GO, et al. Achieving optimal nutritional goals in management of patients with sleeve gastrectomy leaks with endoluminal vacuum therapy. Surg Obes Relat Dis. 2025; https://doi.org/10.1016/J.SOARD.2025.08.022.
65. Tewksbury C, Mahoney L, Shover R, Schiavone PA. Considerations in nutrition support for long-term bariatric surgery care. Nutr Clin Pract. 2025;40:1065–72.

17 Impact of Physical Activity on Postoperative Outcomes

Artur Marc-Hernández and Adrián García-Valverde

17.1 Introduction

Currently, there is consistent evidence on the benefits of bariatric surgery, especially sleeve gastrectomy (SG), which is a cost-effective procedure and provides substantial advantages for patients with morbid obesity [1]. All of these benefits have a positive impact on both physiological and psychological dimensions.

Regarding physiological advantages, weight loss is highlighted as one of the main effects and objectives. This outcome is considered one of the indicators of success when at least 50% of excess weight loss (EWL) is achieved. Fortunately, a wide evidence base is available, including systematic reviews and meta-analyses, that have examined the mentioned effect of SG. These studies revealed that the patients undergoing SG could achieve between 39.9% and 49.3% of EWL in only 6 months [2], whereas a higher loss between 57.5% and 81.8% of EWL may be achieved after 12 months of surgery [3, 4]. As would be expected this reduction is accompanied by other physiological advantages, such as a resolution rate in diabetes levels up to 82.8% [5], a decrease of hypertension on 73.3% of cases [4], a referral of hypercholesterolemia on 21.4% of cases [4], and high resolution of sleep apnoea [4–6].

In addition to these benefits, improvements in psychological outcomes have been reported in the literature. For example, in the short time, SG induces patients to reduce anxiety and depression [7, 8], as well as to increase their self-esteem and perception of body image [9, 10].

Similarly, further studies have shown a significant improvement in physical health after SG, increasing physical functioning and mobility of patients [11]. In addition, this surgery has the ability to increase the patient's mental health despite

A. Marc-Hernández (✉) · A. García-Valverde
Department of Education and Humanities, European University of Madrid, Madrid, Spain
e-mail: adrian.garcia@universidadeuropea.es

J. Ruiz-Tovar (ed.), *Multidisciplinary Management of Sleeve Gastrectomy*,
https://doi.org/10.1007/978-3-032-25644-7_17

the fact that the improvement is usually lower than any other parameter, as these patients generally report poor mental health than the general population [12]. Finally, social functioning has also been reported to improve following SG, with patients demonstrating greater social engagement and work performance [13].

All of these issues have an influence on the lifespan of patients with SG. In fact, it has been reported that patients may increase their life expectancy by approximately 6.1 years following surgery [14]. This gain may be even greater in patients with diabetes, whose life expectancy could increase by up to 9.3 years [14]. However, this finding is not isolated, since this trend has been reproduced in several research. For example, a retrospective cohort study of bariatric patients, most of whom underwent SG, reported that the 10-year mortality risk among patients with morbid obesity treated with SG was 48% lower than that of patients who did not undergo surgery [15]. In addition, a sub-analysis examining surgical procedure type indicated that patients with diabetes undergoing SG experienced an almost 50% reduction in mortality risk [16].

As evidenced by previous studies, SG offers significant clinical advantages for patients, establishing it as a cost-effective surgical intervention that improves both quality of life and life expectancy. However, this surgical procedure also has specific drawbacks which should be minimised, although they are not worrying, to optimise the results of the surgery. The following sections focus exclusively on surgery-related limitations that can be addressed through physical exercise. These issues may arise in both the short and long-term following the surgical intervention.

17.2 Adverse Effects Following Sleeve Gastrectomy

17.2.1 Fat-Free Mass

The primary drawback of surgery is related to muscle or fat-free mass (FFM) loss after treatment. It is generally assumed that when weight loss occurs, at least 25% of this loss is attributable to reductions in FFM [17], although some studies indicate that FFM losses may account for up to 39% of total weight loss [18].

Given the above, it is pertinent to consider that the loss of FFM may be exacerbated by the confluence of several factors, such as protein intake and the speed at which the loss of body weight occurs [19, 20]. These factors are particularly relevant following SG. Firstly, patients experience restricted caloric intake after surgery, leading to reduced protein consumption. Secondly, concomitant substantial weight loss facilitates a decrease in FFM. In fact, 55% of FFM loss observed at 12 months post-surgery occurs within the first 3 months [21]. As a result, a marked reduction in FFM is typically observed during the early postoperative period.

In recent years, several meta-analyses have studied the effects of SG on FFM showing that, continuing the third months of surgery, the loss of FFM achieves 5.99 kg, increasing to 7.49 kg and 9.64 kg in the sixth and twelfth months [22]. Similarly, focusing on skeletal muscle mass, a loss of approximately 7.3 kg has been reported in patients 12 months after surgery [21].

The loss of skeletal muscle mass is associated with poorer surgical outcomes due to its essential physiological role. Firstly, skeletal muscle allows storage and use of glucose [23–25], which several authors have discussed about the potential of muscle as an endocrine organ [26, 27]. In addition, they are a key component in the functional capacity of the subject, especially in patients with bariatric surgery, since loss of FFM is associated with lower basal metabolic rate and weight regain after surgery [28–31].

17.2.2 Bone Mineral Density

Another significant risk following SG is a decrease in bone mineral density (BMD), a trend that parallels the loss of FFM. Several studies have shown a decrease in BMD of approximately 2.62% to 4.04% between the sixth and twelfth postoperative month [32]. In this sense, specific anatomical areas appear particularly vulnerable to these changes, with the femoral neck (−5.4%) and total hip (−6.6%) [32, 33]. This decline in BMD introduces a significant long-term risk, particularly for elderly patients in whom this loss may become chronic [33]. Within this framework, some studies have reported not only an increase in the incidence of osteopenia after 2 years of SG [33] but also a corresponding rise in fracture risk of up to 38% [34].

17.2.3 Suboptimal Weight Loss, Weight Regain, and Comorbidities Relapses

In terms of weight loss, there are two main drawbacks that may appear after SG: sub-optimal weight loss and weight regain.

Sub-optimal weight loss is a concept that refers to patients who do not achieve satisfactory weight loss, defined as a loss of 50% of EWL within 12–18 months after surgery [35]. Other authors focus on capability of response of the patients after surgery, categorising as 'non-responder' those subjects who show a loss body weight lower than 20% [36–38]. Ultimately, both definitions converge on the same core phenomenon: patients whose post-surgical weight loss is clinically insufficient. Although this represents a less frequent outcome, its prevalence is not negligible, with reported rates ranging from 7.5% to 11.3% of patients within 12 months of SG [36, 38, 39].

The concept of weight regain has been described in multiple ways in the literature, including as an increase of ≥10 kg from the *nadir* weight, a regain of ≥25% of EWL, or ≥ 15% from the total weight at *nadir* [40]. This is a more common and concerning issue in the medium and long-term following SG. For instance, weight regain is reported to show up in approximately 5.7% of patients after 2 years, rising sharply to 75.6% after 6 years [41]. In fact, due to its high recurrence, only the 20% of patients maintain their weight loss beyond 5 years after SG [37].

As is known, weight loss is closely related to the reduction of obesity-related comorbidities; therefore, this is an important factor in bariatric patients [42].

Evidence links both suboptimal weight loss and weight regain to lower rates of type 2 diabetes remission, metabolic relapse after SG, and recurrence of comorbidities [35, 43]. In fact, patients who achieved hypertension remission showed greater weight loss 6 to 12 months after surgery than those without remission [44]. Specifically, in the sixth month, patients who experienced remission of comorbidities achieved a percentage of weight loss closer to 59%, against 47% of those who did not show said remission [44]. Moreover, another study indicates that insufficient weight loss during the first-year post-surgery and subsequent weight regain may predict the recurrence of hypertension within 3 years after SG [45]. Furthermore, a weight loss threshold of approximately 20% of total body weight has been proposed as necessary for the remission of type 2 diabetes [46].

Likewise, another study concluded that patients undergoing SG showed total remission of type 2 diabetes and hypercholesterolemia in the first year, at rates of 50% and 40%, respectively. However, after 5 years, these rates declined to 20% and 36.1%, a reduction that has been attributed to weight regain [47]. Similarly, by the fifth year, 26.8% of patients experienced diabetes relapse, which was associated with an average weight regain of 25% and corresponded to a 5.46-fold increase in the likelihood of diabetes recurrence [48].

These findings underscore the importance of both weight loss and long-term weight maintenance to maximise the cardiometabolic benefits of SG, with structured physical exercise playing a central role.

17.3 Physical Activity and Exercise in Bariatric Patients

17.3.1 General Considerations on Physical Exercise

Considering the evidence presented, SG is associated with certain short- and long-term adverse outcomes. Therefore, developing strategies to mitigate these drawbacks is a crucial next step in improving surgical outcomes. In this context, physical activity (PA) and structured exercise emerge as potentially effective tools.

In the last decade, research related to exercise and health has increased. Today, there is much evidence that exercise can provide several benefits to people. Those range from cardio-respiratory and functional capacity to body composition and cardiometabolic parameters. All of them are related to improved life-quality and longevity.

An analysis of the short, medium, and long-term drawbacks associated with SG, in addition to the benefits of physical exercise, reveals its considerable utility for patients undergoing this procedure. For example, it is well-established that incorporating an exercise programme into a caloric restriction regimen improves weight loss [49, 50]. However, in longer-term nutritional interventions (beyond 12 weeks), complementing dietary treatment with an exercise programme has been shown to be particularly effective [51, 52]. Moreover, a systematic review revealed a dose-response relationship, showing a reduction in total body weight of 0.5 kg for each additional 30 min of weekly aerobic exercise [53]. In the same study, it was reported that from 100 min per week of aerobic exercise, an additional fat mass loss of approximately 2 kg was observed, whereas in individuals performing 300 min or more per week, the increase in weight loss reached 4.19 Kg [53].

Another critically important issue is the role of exercise in preventing the loss of FFM and BMD. Indeed, current evidence confirms that combining a nutritional weight loss intervention with resistance training (RT) mitigates the loss of FFM and preserves BMD. Evidence indicates that during nutritional weight loss interventions, RT markedly reduces the loss of lean mass—by up to 93.5%—and BMD [54].

In light of this evidence, it can be concluded that exercise could be used as a multifaceted therapeutic tool that generates significant benefits for patients undergoing SG. Firstly, physical exercise can enhance fat mass loss during caloric restriction, which is particularly beneficial for patients with suboptimal weight loss. Secondly, exercise helps to mitigate the loss of FFM and BMD that typically accompany weight loss [55]. This protective effect is important, especially when weight loss is rapid, as is the case of bariatric surgery.

Given the established benefits of exercise, attention should now be directed towards how exercise programmes can be structured to optimise these effects. This analysis must consider the fundamental principles of training, specifically the type of exercise. The current chapter addresses both resistance and endurance training (ET), as the training modality is key to optimising the results. Although ET has demonstrated superior efficacy to RT alone in reducing fat mass and improving cardiometabolic parameters, several studies and meta-analyses have shown that a combined training regimen yields the greatest benefits. In other words, integrating both modalities within a single programme results in greater reductions in fat mass and more significant improvements in cardiometabolic health than the modalities separately [56, 57].

Beyond the type of exercise, the way in which it is prescribed is quite important for maximising benefits. In this regard, two key variables must be considered: intensity and volume training.

Regarding training volume, it has previously been demonstrated that a higher volume of ET leads to greater reductions in fat mass and total body weight. Conversely, volume in RT is equally vital for the preservation of FFM. Specifically, a high RT volume -defined as at least 10 sets per muscle group per week- has been reported to mitigate the loss of FFM, particularly in female patients [58].

The effects provided by volume need to be complemented by intensity training, both dimensions are synergistic. Intensity has been demonstrated to have great relevance in maximising the benefit of exercise. This is clearly evidenced by several studies [59–61] which demonstrate that training efficacy on maintenance of FFM increases when high intensities, corresponding to 70–80% of one-repetition maximum (1-RM), are achieved. Likewise, to keep levels of BMD, general recommendations adhere to the aforementioned intensity range [55, 62] although there is a study have demonstrated comparable effects using lower intensities (60% 1-RM) [63]. Beyond its effects on FFM and BMD, training intensity has also demonstrated a significant influence on cardiometabolic parameters and body composition.

Specifically, prescribing exercise at intensities of at least 70% of 1-RM can improve VO_2max and reduce fat mass [61].

Finally, it is important to emphasise that the preservation of FFM requires combining RT with adequate protein intake. Various studies indicate that a minimum intake of 1.5 g/kg of body weight is necessary to prevent loss of fat-free mass [61]. However, other research suggests that to promote gains in fat-free mass, protein intake should be set between 1.7 and 1.8 g/kg of body weight [64].

17.3.2 Regular Physical Activity in Patients Undergoing Sleeve Gastrectomy

Before discussing the results and implications of exercise programmes for patients undergoing SG, it is pertinent to highlight certain aspects of their levels of PA. This approach will not only outline the key characteristics of an optimal exercise programme for this population, but will also determine whether strategies are needed to increase their overall PA.

Physical activity can be an essential component to improve surgical outcomes in these patients. In general, patients who undergo SG increase their PA levels after surgery [65]. This increase is typically observed during the first few months after surgery, but tends to decline with time. For example, significant increases in physical activity levels have been reported at 6 months post-surgery, with patients reaching their peak activity levels during this period [66]. Nevertheless, this level of physical activity is frequently not sustained, and a significant decrease is observed at the 12-month follow-up [67, 68].

Regarding the short-term effects of these activity levels, they appear to have little influence on several outcome measures. In fact, increased PA does not appear to have a significant impact on weight loss in these patients. This may be attributed to two primary reasons. First, the strong effect of SG in the initial months overshadows any additional contribution from PA. Second, although patients increase their activity, the levels achieved are generally low (light-intensity) and often fall short of international minimum recommendations ($\geq$150 min/week of moderate-to-vigorous physical activity (MVPA)). Consequently, the intensity and volume of activity are insufficient to generate significant additional short-term weight loss. In this sense, several studies have reported that patients, although they increased their PA, around 76% did not reach the minimal recommendation. Only a 18% and 6% carried out higher than 150 and 300 min of MVPA per week [69]. This trend is also evident in the analysis of daily step counts. One of the most widespread recommendations in physical activity and public health is to achieve 10,000 steps per day. However, studies report that patients who have undergone SG exhibit average daily step counts ranging from 6072 to 7460 post-surgery [69, 70]. As a result, these patients consistently fail to meet this minimum recommended activity level.

Therefore, although increased PA does not appear to generate additional short-term weight loss, its relevance grows in the medium to long term. Positive effects begin to emerge after the first postoperative year. A recent study illustrates this point: at 12 months after surgery, 24.3% of patients with optimal weight loss engaged in exercise, whereas 100% of those with insufficient weight loss reported being physically inactive [39]. This suggests that the benefits of PA on weight management become increasingly significant as time progresses after the surgical intervention. So, in the long-term, higher levels of PA are associated with superior weight outcomes. A six-year follow-up study revealed that the most active patients not only lost more weight but also demonstrated better weight maintenance, whereas inactive patients exhibited a significantly higher rate of weight regain [71]. Similarly, another study concluded that, 5 years post-surgery, the most active patients were three to five times more likely to maintain their achieved weight loss [72].

A deeper analysis of the scientific literature reveals clinically relevant findings. The main conclusion indicates that while light-intensity physical activity provides mild functional and metabolic benefits, performing more than 150 min a week of MVPA prevents weight regain [66, 72, 73]. Furthermore, regular physical activity is associated with an improved metabolic profile and reduced cardiovascular risk. It has also been reported that approximately 30 min of daily moderate-to-vigorous physical activity (MVPA) may prevent long-term weight regain and the recurrence of comorbidities [70]. For example, at 5 years after surgery, the most active patients exhibited a significantly better cardiometabolic profile: none developed type 2 diabetes mellitus, compared to 7.7% in the least active group.

In summary, the impact of PA on weight loss is limited in the short term but becomes significant after the first postoperative year. Key benefits—such as prevention of weight loss and improved outcomes in cases of insufficient weight loss—are observed when patients exceed the threshold of 150 min of MVPA per week. Therefore, PA is fundamental for optimising and maintaining long-term results.

17.4 Impact of Structured Exercise Programmes on Patients Undergoing Sleeve Gastrectomy

Having analysed the general effects of PA, the focus now shifts to the efficacy of supervised exercise programmes. The following section will evaluate how these structured interventions address the surgery-related complications and limitations detailed in previous sections.

17.4.1 Body Mass Composition

The scientific literature consistently indicates that patients enrolled in supervised exercise programmes achieve greater benefits than those undertaking physical activity on their own. For example, a study that applied different exercise programmes to patients undergoing SG and gastric bypass observed that participants in the ET group—who performed 150–200 min of aerobic exercise per week—achieved a fat mass loss that was 5.4 kg greater than that of the control group [74].

Unfortunately, few studies have been conducted specifically on patients who have undergone SG. Therefore, findings from studies on gastric bypass patients will be reported. In this regard, these studies demonstrate that 120 min per week of stationary walking or cycling, or participation in a RT programme, results in additional fat mass loss [75, 76]. Furthermore, one of these studies concluded that a higher volume of ET was associated with greater reductions in total body weight, fat mass, and abdominal fat. Specifically, both total daily energy expenditure and steps per day were significantly correlated with weight loss [75]. The key aspects to highlight from these studies are that ET was performed at moderate intensities, while RT was conducted at intensities between 50% and 75% of one-repetition maximum, with a frequency of 2–3 days per week.

Regarding FFM, available evidence indicates that exercise can attenuate its loss following SG. A key aspect is determining the optimal time to initiate an exercise programme and its ideal duration. To illustrate, a study implemented a combined aerobic and resistance training programme that began on the third postoperative day and continued until the first month after surgery. However, in this case, the exercise programme did not prevent FFM loss [77]. This suggests that, in the very short term (1 month after surgery), an exercise programme may be insufficient to prevent the loss of FFM, likely because the intervention is too brief and the necessary training intensities are not achieved.

In contrast, other studies investigating medium to long-term programmes that implemented higher training intensities have demonstrated positive effects on FFM preservation. In this regard, several key studies will be highlighted. In one investigation, a combined endurance and resistance training programme was implemented between 3 and 6-months after surgery. The results showed that, although there were no statistically significant differences in FFM loss, the experimental group lost only 1.4 kg compared to 2.1 kg in the control group [78].

A notable study implemented an 11-month exercise programme, concluding 12 months after surgery [79]. The protocol consisted of three weekly 35-min resistance training sessions at intensities of 65–80% of 1-RM. The results demonstrated that the exercise group maintained 1.5 kg more FFM than the control group, a statistically significant difference.

Another relevant study, which included patients who underwent SG and gastric bypass, compared the impact of different exercise modalities on body composition in three groups: (1) endurance training, (2) combined training (ET and RT), and (3) a non-exercise control group. The key findings indicated that the control group lost 2.4 kg more FFM than the ET group, a difference that increased to 3.7 kg compared to the combined training group [74]. This result underscores the critical importance of RT for these patients in favour to preserve FFM [79, 80].

Even modalities such as elastic band training have been shown to be effective in maintaining muscle mass [81]. Furthermore, although more research has been conducted on patients with gastric bypass, the evidence confirms that RT programmes can prevent the reduction of FFM [82–84]. For example, it has been observed that just two weekly sessions are sufficient to mitigate this loss, with a difference of 2 kg of FFM lost in the group that did not perform resistance training [84].

From the interpreted synthesis of these studies, it can be deduced that to effectively prevent the reduction of FFM, it is essential to implement exercise programmes that adhere to specific parameters. First, the frequency should consist of a minimum of two weekly resistance training sessions, with three sessions being optimal. Furthermore, programme duration is crucial: a minimum of 12 weeks is required to observe benefits, which become significantly greater when the programme extends to or exceeds 6 months, particularly if maintained during periods of the most rapid weight loss.

Regarding exercise prescription, evidence suggests that superior results are obtained with high intensities, around 75% of 1RM, and a volume comprising six to ten different exercises. It is recommended to perform two to 3 sets of 8–12 repetitions per exercise, prioritising work on large muscle groups.

17.4.2 Bone Mineral Density

Research on the effects of exercise on BMD in bariatric patients remains limited. To our knowledge, only one study has specifically evaluated this relationship, implementing a RT programme at intensities of 65–80% of 1-RM. This study demonstrated that the exercise group exhibited a smaller reduction in BMD compared to the control group [79]. A crucial finding was the role of adherence, as patients who completed over 50% of the sessions exhibited higher BMD levels [79]. To complement these findings, it is worth highlighting a study in patients with gastric bypass that concluded that two weekly sessions of high-intensity RT resulted in a significantly smaller decrease in BMD compared to patients who did not exercise [84].

17.4.3 Cardiometabolic Parameters

Evidence related to cardiometabolic effects suggests that the implementation of an exercise programme after surgery can produce significant benefits [85]. A protocol that has proven effective in treating dyslipidaemia consists of a combined training regimen performed three times a week in one-hour sessions (25 min of RT and 35 min of ET at 50–75% of heart rate reserve). The results demonstrated that the exercise group exhibited higher HDL cholesterol levels and a greater rate of dyslipidaemia resolution compared to the control group (73% vs. 50%) [78].

Other studies also support these findings, indicating that aerobic exercise at 60–70% of maximum heart rate, with a weekly volume of 120 min, can produce additional improvements in insulin sensitivity and glucose effectiveness [86]. Furthermore, focusing on blood pressure, improvements have also been documented with aerobic exercise programmes at 50–70% of peak heart rate, as observed in a study of patients who underwent gastric bypass [87].

17.4.4 Long-Term Effects of Exercise Following Sleeve Gastrectomy

The available medium and long-term evidence confirms that exercise is an effective tool for maintaining weight loss achieved through bariatric surgery. Although the literature in this field remains limited, existing studies provide significant findings. In one investigation that recruited patients between one and three-years post-surgery, an ET programme was implemented at 70–90% of maximum heart rate. The results demonstrated that exercise group achieved a significant reduction in fat mass and waist circumference, alongside a trend towards an increase in FFM [88].

In addition, other studies have implemented an exercise programme in the medium and long term after surgery [89–91]. These studies yield findings of notable clinical relevance. Patients who participated in structured exercise programmes demonstrated significant reductions in total body weight and fat mass, with some studies reporting a trend towards increased FFM. Similarly, other investigations documented improvements in cardiometabolic parameters and a lesser reduction in BMD. These results were achieved through the implementation of combined exercise programmes (ET and RT). The implemented protocols generally followed a frequency of three sessions per week, with intensities ranging from 60–90% of VO_{2max} for ET component and 50–75% of 1-RM for RT.

Finally, it is important to note that other observational studies have yielded relevant data. PA has been demonstrated to be a key factor in maintaining weight loss [92], becoming particularly critical from 18 months after surgery [93]. In fact, 24 months after surgery, 26.8% of patients with weight regain had low PA levels [93].

From these studies, it can be concluded that the implementation of a medium to long-term exercise programme after surgery is highly beneficial to maintain surgery-induced weight loss and prevent the recurrence of comorbidities.

17.5 Conclusions

This chapter has outlined the drawbacks associated with SG and has explored how exercise can contribute to improving the outcomes of this surgical procedure. Yet it should be noted that although the number of studies investigating the effects of exercise programmes in bariatric patients has increased in recent years, there is a lack of experimental research specifically in patients who have undergone SG. Currently, SG is the most frequently performed bariatric procedure worldwide, accounting for 55.4% of all bariatric surgeries [94]. Therefore, to enhance outcomes associated with this surgery, it would be highly advisable to increase the number of studies on this topic.

Despite the limited number of experimental studies, the available scientific evidence allows the extraction of relevant conclusions with a potential direct impact on the outcomes of bariatric surgery. In summary, it is established that during the first postoperative year (short term), the implementation of structured exercise programmes helps prevent the loss of FFM and BMD, while simultaneously enhancing the reduction of fat mass. In the medium and long term, exercise solidifies its role as a fundamental tool for maintaining lost weight and preventing weight loss and the comorbidities' relapses.

It is also important to emphasise that structured and supervised exercise programmes appear to be more impactful than simply increasing general PA levels or providing unsupervised exercise recommendations. For exercise to be effective (beyond the previously discussed aspects of intensity and volume) the programme must be prescribed and supervised by a professional in exercise science, as this significantly improves outcomes [80].

Finally, based on current scientific evidence on the physiological effects of exercise and its application in patients undergoing SG, as well as the practical experience of the authors, a set of exercise guidelines and recommendations will be provided. These are intended to facilitate the implementation of structured exercise programmes for this patient population.

17.5.1 Short-Term Exercise Guidelines and Recommendations (First Postoperative Year)

The main goal of this prescription step is to prioritise resistance training to mitigate the loss of fat-free mass and bone mineral density associated with rapid weight loss.

1. ***Resistance training prescription***
   - *Frequency*: A minimum of 3 days per week.
   - *Muscle Groups*: Focus on large muscle groups.
   - *Intensity*: Begin with very low intensities (~50% of 1RM), especially for exercise-naïve patients. Progressively increase to higher, more effective intensities (~75% of 1RM) for FFM preservation.
   - *Volume & Duration*: Programmes should be long-term. A minimum duration of 3 months is recommended, with greater efficacy observed from 6 months onwards. An effective volume consists of 6–10 exercises, performed for 2–3 sets of 8–12 repetitions each.
2. ***Endurance training prescription***
   - *Volume*: Endurance training provides additional fat mass loss, for which volume is a key determinant. Although 150 min of MVPA weekly is a common recommendation, 120 min per week have proven sufficient. Additional fat loss is associated with higher volumes, becoming particularly effective at ≥300 min per week.
   - *Intensity & progression*: The effective intensity ranges from 40% to 80% of maximum heart rate. Begin at lower intensities and progress gradually. Consider the patients' reduced energy availability due to post-surgical dietary

restrictions when prescribing aerobic intensity. Series or intervallic exercise can be used to facilitate patient adaptation instead of continuous effort.

3. ***Supporting recommendations***
   - *Protein Intake*: Aim for 1.8–1.9 g of protein per kg of body weight. A minimum intake of 1.5 g/kg should be achieved if the higher target is not feasible.
   - *Supervision*: Participate in supervised exercise programmes to maximise safety, adherence, and outcomes.

17.5.2 Medium- and Long-Term Exercise Guidelines and Recommendations (>12–18 Months After Surgery)

The following recommendations represent a progression from the previous short-term. All previously established criteria that are not explicitly modified here should continue to be applied.

1. ***Integrated or concurrent training approach***
   - Both endurance and resistance training are crucial in this phase. Resistance training is essential to maintain FFM and BMD, while endurance is key to maintaining surgery-induced weight loss.
   - The combination of them helps prevent the recurrence of comorbidities.
2. ***Resistance training prescription***
   - *Frequency*: While 2 days per week is sufficient to prevent reductions in BMD and FFM, a frequency of 3 days per week is recommended for optimal benefit.
   - *Volume & Intensity*: A volume of 4 sets per muscle group is sufficient to maintain FFM. Begin training at low intensities (~60% 1RM) and progress to higher intensities. A target of 10 repetitions per set at 75% 1RM is effective, and intensities of up to 80% 1RM can be safely achieved by patients.
3. ***Endurance training prescription***
   - Volume: Performing 150 min of aerobic exercise per week or 30 min of daily MVPA prevents both weight regain and comorbidity recurrence. However, a weekly volume of 200–300 min is recommended.
   - Intensity: Both moderate and high intensities are effective in preventing weight loss and recurrence of comorbidities. However, since high-intensity training can provide additional benefits, it is recommended to begin at moderate intensities and progressively advance to higher levels as tolerated by the patient (55–90% HRmax; 60–90% VO_{2max}).
4. ***Supporting recommendations***
   - *Protein Intake*: Continue to adhere to the protein intake guidelines previously established (1.8–1.9 g/kg, minimum 1.5 g/kg).

- *Supervision*: Exercise should be supervised to ensure correct technique, safety, and adherence.

References

1. Yu W, Chen J, Fan L, Yan C, Zhu L. Cost-effectiveness of laparoscopic sleeve gastrectomy for chinese patients. Obes Surg. 2024;34:2828–34.
2. Jalal MA, Cheng Q, Edye MB. Systematic review and meta-analysis of endoscopic sleeve gastroplasty with comparison to laparoscopic sleeve gastrectomy. Obes Surg. 2020;30:2754–62.
3. McCarty TR, Jirapinyo P, Thompson CC. Effect of sleeve gastrectomy on ghrelin, GLP-1, PYY, and GIP gut hormones a systematic review and meta-analysis. Ann Surg. 2020;272:72–80.
4. Tovar JR, Angel M, Jose C, Jimenez M, Jose M, Gilberto C, Ortiz J, Lorea DS. Long-term follow-up after sleeve gastrectomy versus Roux-en-Y gastric bypass versus one-anastomosis gastric bypass: a prospective randomized comparative study of weight loss and remission of comorbidities. Surg Endosc. 2018;33:401–10.
5. Balasubaramaniam V, Pouwels S. Remission of type 2 diabetes mellitus (T2DM) after sleeve gastrectomy (SG), one-anastomosis gastric bypass (OAGB), and roux-en-Y gastric bypass (RYGB): a systematic review. Medicina (Lithuania). 2023; https://doi.org/10.3390/medicina59050985.
6. Leyaro B, Boakye D, Howie L, Ali A, Carragher R. Associations between type of bariatric surgery and obstructive sleep apnoea, employment outcomes, and body image satisfaction: a systematic review and meta-analysis. Obes Facts. 2024;18:57–71.
7. Barzin M, Khalaj A, Tasdighi E, Samiei Nasr D, Mahdavi M, Banihashem S, Valizadeh M. Sleeve gastrectomy vs gastric bypass in improvement of depressive symptoms following one year from bariatric surgery, Tehran obesity treatment study (TOTS). Obes Res Clin Pract. 2020;14:73–9.
8. Tuli S, Lopez Lopez AP, Nimmala S, Pedreira CC, Singhal V, Bredella MA, Misra M. Two-year study on the impact of sleeve gastrectomy on depressive and anxiety symptoms in adolescents and young adults with moderate to severe obesity. Obes Surg. 2024;34:568–75.
9. Ramos-Bachiller B, López-Gómez JJ, García-Calvo S, Torres-Torres B, Primo-Martín D, Pinto-Fuentes P, Pacheco-Sánchez D, Ladrón de Cegama FU, De Luis DA. Quality of life and psychological changes in bariatric surgery: an observational study. Ann Nutr Metab. 2025;81:22–31.
10. AboKhozima A, Zidan MH, Altabbaa H, et al. The impact of weight loss after bariatric surgeries on the patient's body image, quality of life, and self-esteem. Langenbeck's Arch Surg. 2025; https://doi.org/10.1007/s00423-024-03568-6.
11. Mouawad C, Aoun R, Dahboul H, El Feghali E, Kassar S, Alkassis M, Osseis M, Noun R, Chakhtoura G. Quality of life after laparoscopic sleeve gastrectomy: pre-operative, 1-year and 5-year results. J Minim Access Surg. 2023;19:459–65.
12. Nielsen HJ, Nedrebø BG, Fosså A, et al. Seven-year trajectories of body weight, quality of life and comorbidities following Roux-en-Y gastric bypass and sleeve gastrectomy. Int J Obes. 2022;46:739–49.
13. Poelemeijer YQM, van der Knaap ETW, Marang-van de Mheen PJ, Demirkiran A, Wiezer MJ, Hazebroek EJ, Greve JWM, Liem RSL. Measuring quality of life in bariatric surgery: a multicentre study. Surg Endosc. 2020;34:5522–32.
14. Syn NL, Cummings DE, Wang LZ, et al. Association of metabolic–bariatric surgery with long-term survival in adults with and without diabetes: a one-stage meta-analysis of matched cohort and prospective controlled studies with 174 772 participants. Lancet. 2021;397:1830–41.

15. Migliore E, Brunani A, Ciccone G, et al. Effect of bariatric surgery on survival and hospitalizations in patients with severe obesity. A retrospective cohort study. Nutrients. 2021; https://doi.org/10.3390/nu13093150.
16. Dicker D, Greenland P, Leibowitz M, Hoshen M, Senderey AB, Rasmussen-Torvik LJ, Balicer RD, Reges O. All-cause mortality of patients with and without diabetes following bariatric surgery: comparison to non-surgical matched patients. Obes Surg. 2021;2:755–62.
17. Heymsfield SB, Gonzalez MCC, Shen W, Redman L, Thomas D. Weight loss composition is one-fourth fat-free mass: a critical review and critique of this widely cited rule. Obes Rev. 2014;15:310–21.
18. Prado CM, Phillips SM, Gonzalez MC, Heymsfield SB. Muscle matters: the effects of medically induced weight loss on skeletal muscle. Lancet Diabetes Endocrinol. 2024;12:785–7.
19. Ashtary-Larky D, Ghanavati M, Lamuchi-Deli N, Payami SA, Alavi-Rad S, Boustaninejad M, Afrisham R, Abbasnezhad A, Alipour M. Rapid weight loss vs. slow weight loss: which is more effective on body composition and metabolic risk factors? Int J Endocrinol Metab. 2017; https://doi.org/10.5812/ijem.13249.
20. Kokura Y, Ueshima J, Saino Y, Keisuke M. Enhanced protein intake on maintaining muscle mass, strength, and physical function in adults with overweight/obesity: a systematic review and meta-analysis. Clin Nutr ESPEN. 2024;63:417–26.
21. Nuijten MAH, Eijsvogels TMH, Monpellier VM, Janssen IMC, Hazebroek EJ, Hopman MTE. The magnitude and progress of lean body mass, fat-free mass, and skeletal muscle mass loss following bariatric surgery: a systematic review and meta-analysis. Obes Rev. 2021;23:e13370.
22. Haghighat N, Ashtary-Larky D, Bagheri R, et al. Preservation of fat-free mass in the first year after bariatric surgery: a systematic review and meta-analysis of 122 studies and 10,758 participants. Surg Obes Relat Dis. 2022;18:964–82.
23. Houmard JA, Pories WJ, Dohm GL. Severe obesity: evidence for a deranged metabolic program in skeletal muscle? Exerc Sport Sci Rev. 2013;40:204–10.
24. Jensen J, Rustad PI, Kolnes AJ, Lai YC. The role of skeletal muscle glycogen breakdown for regulation of insulin sensitivity by exercise. Front Physiol. 2011;2:112.
25. Merz KE, Thurmond DC. Role of skeletal muscle in insulin resistance and glucose uptake. Compr Physiol. 2020;10:785–809.
26. Pedersen BK, Febbraio MA. Muscles, exercise and obesity: skeletal muscle as a secretory organ. Nat Rev Endocrinol. 2012;8:457–65.
27. Kim TN, Choi KM. The implications of sarcopenia and sarcopenic obesity on cardiometabolic disease. J Cell Biochem. 2015;116:1171–8.
28. da Silva FBL, Gomes DL, KMB C. Poor diet quality and postoperative time are independent risk factors for weight regain after Roux-en-Y gastric bypass. Nutrition. 2016;32:1–4.
29. Odom J, Zalesin KC, Washington TL, et al. Behavioral predictors of weight regain after bariatric surgery. Obes Surg. 2010;20:349–56.
30. Faria SL, Kelly E, Faria OP. Energy expenditure and weight regain in patients submitted to Roux-en-Y gastric bypass. Obes Surg. 2009;19:856–9.
31. Naseer F, Zhang SD, Miras AD, et al. Metabolic adaptation following gastric bypass surgery: results from a 2-year observational study. Int J Obes. 2024;48:1577–86.
32. Malinici E, Sirbu A, Popa M, Andrei M, Ioacara S, Copaescu C, Fica S. Bone mineral density trends during the first year after laparoscopic sleeve gastrectomy – a cohort study on 241 patients. Obes Surg. 2021;31:4885–92.
33. Maïmoun L, Aouinti S, Puech M, et al. Effect of nutritional deprivation after sleeve gastrectomy on bone mass, Periostin, Sclerostin and Semaphorin 4D: a two-year longitudinal study. Nutrients. 2023; https://doi.org/10.3390/nu15204310.
34. Winckelmann LA, Gribsholt SB, Bødkergaard K, Rejnmark L, Madsen LR, Richelsen B. Risk of fractures following bariatric surgery with Roux-en-Y gastric bypass or sleeve gastrectomy: a Danish population-based cohort study. Eur J Endocrinol. 2024;191:1–8.

35. El Ansari W, Elhag W. Weight regain and insufficient weight loss after bariatric surgery: definitions, prevalence, mechanisms, predictors, prevention and management strategies, and knowledge gaps – a scoping review. Obes Surg. 2021;31:1755–66.
36. Lee JH, Park J-H, Kim SM. Comparison of dietary quality and surgical satisfaction between patients with suboptimal and optimal weight loss after sleeve gastrectomy using food tolerance score and bariatric analysis and reporting outcome system questionnaires. J Metab Bariatric Surg. 2022;11:54.
37. Lind R, Hage K, Ghanem M, Shah M, Vierkant RA, Jawad M, Ghanem OM, Teixeira AF. Long-term outcomes of sleeve gastrectomy: weight recurrence and surgical non-responders. Obes Surg. 2023;33:3028–34.
38. Yamaguchi T, Tani M, Kasama K, Naitoh T, Oshiro T, Inoue K, Seki Y, Imoto H, Kaida S, Matsubayashi J. Reference values for weight loss during 1 year after sleeve gastrectomy: a multicenter retrospective study in Japan. Obes Surg. 2022;32:2672–81.
39. Said R, Fouad A, Said M, Elasmi A. Predictors of insufficient weight loss after sleeve gastrectomy. Egypt J Surg. 2024;43:1377–85.
40. Voorwinde V, Steenhuis IHM, Janssen IMC, Monpellier VM, van Stralen MM. Definitions of long-term weight regain and their associations with clinical outcomes. Obes Surg. 2020;30:527–36.
41. Lauti M, Kularatna M, Hill AG, MacCormick AD. Weight regain following sleeve gastrectomy – a systematic review. Obes Surg. 2016;26:1326–34.
42. Kanbour S, Ageeb RA, Malik RA, Abu-Raddad LJ. Impact of bodyweight loss on type 2 diabetes remission: a systematic review and meta-regression analysis of randomised controlled trials. Lancet Diabetes Endocrinol. 2025;13:294–306.
43. Mizera M, Wysocki M, Bartosiak K, et al. Type 2 diabetes remission 5 years after laparoscopic sleeve gastrectomy: multicenter cohort study. https://doi.org/10.1007/s11695-020-05088-w/ Published.
44. Kumagai H, Sasaki A, Umemura A, Tanahashi Y, Iwasaki T, Ando T, Katagiri H, Nitta H. Predictive factors involving the remission and recurrence of hypertension post-laparoscopic sleeve gastrectomy in Japanese patients with severe obesity. PLoS One. 2024; https://doi.org/10.1371/journal.pone.0314792.
45. Ebadinejad A, Shahshahani M, Hosseinpanah F, Ghazy F, Khalaj A, Mahdavi M, Valizadeh M, Barzin M. Comparison of hypertension remission and relapse after sleeve gastrectomy and one-anastomosis gastric bypass: a prospective cohort study. Hypertens Res. 2023;46:1287–96.
46. Vetter ML, Ritter S, Wadden TA, Sarwer DB. Comparison of bariatric surgical procedures for diabetes remission: efficacy and mechanisms. Diabetes Spectrum. 2012;25:200–10.
47. Golomb I, Ben David M, Glass A, Kolitz T, Keidar A. Long-term metabolic effects of laparoscopic sleeve gastrectomy. JAMA Surg. 2015;150:1051–7.
48. Watanabe Y, Yamaguchi T, Nagayama D, et al. Factors associated with relapse of type 2 diabetes mellitus after laparoscopic sleeve gastrectomy in Japanese subjects: a subgroup analysis of J-SMART study. Obes Facts. 2023;16:119–30.
49. Xie Y, Gu Y, Li Z, He B, Zhang L. Effects of different exercises combined with different dietary interventions on body composition: a systematic review and network meta-analysis. Nutrients. 2024; https://doi.org/10.3390/NU16173007.
50. Cheng CC, Hsu CY, Liu JF. Effects of dietary and exercise intervention on weight loss and body composition in obese postmenopausal women: a systematic review and meta-analysis. Menopause. 2018;25:772–82.
51. Johns DJ, Hartmann-Boyce J, Jebb SA, Aveyard P. Diet or exercise interventions vs combined behavioral weight management programs: a systematic review and meta-analysis of directcom parisons. J Acad Nutr Diet. 2014;114:1557–68.
52. Kazeminasab F, Mahboobi MH, Mohebinejad M, Nojoumi M, Belyani S, Camera DM, Moradi S, Bagheri R. The impact of exercise training plus dietary interventions on ectopic fat in population with overweight/obesity with and without chronic disease: a systematic review, meta-analysis, and metaregression of randomized clinical trials. Curr Dev Nutr. 2025; https://doi.org/10.1016/j.cdnut.2025.104574.

53. Jayedi A, Soltani S, Emadi A, Zargar MS, Najafi A. Aerobic exercise and weight loss in adults: a systematic review and dose-response meta-analysis. JAMA Netw Open. 2024;7:e2452185.
54. Sardeli AV, Komatsu TR, Mori MA, Gáspari AF, Chacon-Mikahil MPT. Resistance training prevents muscle loss induced by caloric restriction in obese elderly individuals: a systematic review and meta-analysis. Nutrients. 2018; https://doi.org/10.3390/NU10040423.
55. Watson SL, Weeks BK, Weis LJ, Horan SA, Beck BR. Heavy resistance training is safe and improves bone, function, and stature in postmenopausal women with low to very low bone mass: novel early findings from the LIFTMOR trial. Osteoporos Int. 2015;26:2889–94.
56. AL-Mhanna SB, Batrakoulis A, Ghazali WSW, et al. Effects of combined aerobic and resistance training on glycemic control, blood pressure, inflammation, cardiorespiratory fitness and quality of life in patients with type 2 diabetes and overweight/obesity: a systematic review and meta-analysis. PeerJ. 2024; https://doi.org/10.7717/PEERJ.17525.
57. Lopez P, Taaffe DR, Galvão DA, Newton RU, Nonemacher ER, Wendt VM, Bassanesi RN, Turella DJP, Rech A. Resistance training effectiveness on body composition and body weight outcomes in individuals with overweight and obesity across the lifespan: a systematic review and meta-analysis. Obes Rev. 2022; https://doi.org/10.1111/OBR.13428.
58. Roth C, Schoenfeld BJ, Behringer M. Lean mass sparing in resistance-trained athletes during caloric restriction: the role of resistance training volume. Eur J Appl Physiol. 2022;122(5):1129–51.
59. Said M, Lamya N, Olfa N, Hamda M. Effects of high-impact aerobics vs. low-impact aerobics and strength training in overweight and obese women. J Sports Med Phys Fitness. 2017;57:278–88.
60. Sanal E, Ardic F, Kirac S. Effects of aerobic or combined aerobic resistance exercise on body composition in overweight and obese adults: gender differences. A randomized intervention study. Eur J Phys Rehabil Med. 2013;49:1–11.
61. Clark JE. Diet, exercise or diet with exercise: comparing the effectiveness of treatment options for weight-loss and changes in fitness for adults (18-65 years old) who are overfat, or obese; systematic review and meta-analysis. J Diabetes Metab Disord. 2015;14:31.
62. Hong AR, Kim SW. Effects of resistance exercise on bone health. Endocrinol Metab. 2018;33:435–44.
63. Kohrt WM, Bloomfield SA, Little KD, Nelson ME, Yingling VR. Physical activity and bone health. Med Sci Sports Exerc. 2004;36:1985–96.
64. Urdampilleta A, Vicente-Salar N, Martínez-Sanz J. Necesidades proteicas de los deportistas y pautas diétetico-nutricionales para la ganancia de masa muscular. Revista Española de Nutrición Humana y Dietética …. 2012;16:25–35.
65. Bond DS, Jakicic JM, Unick JL, Vithiananthan S, Roye GD, Ryder BA, Sax HC, Wing RR. Pre- to postoperative physical activity changes in bariatric surgery patients: self-report vs. objective measures. Obesity (Silver Spring). 2010;18:2395–7.
66. Bullo V, Pavan D, Gobbo S, et al. From surgery to functional capacity: muscle strength modifications in women post sleeve gastrectomy. BMC Sports Sci Med Rehabil. 2024;16(1):118.
67. Bonn SE, Hult M, Spetz K, Eke H, Andersson E, Wirén M, Löf M, Trolle Lagerros Y. Effect of a smartphone application on physical activity and weight loss after bariatric surgery – results from a randomized controlled trial. Obes Surg. 2023;33:2841–50.
68. Bäuerle A, Marsall M, Niedergethmann M, von Feilitzsch MF, Frewer AL, Skoda EM, Pouwels S, Hasenberg T, Teufel M. Adherence to dietary behavior recommendations moderates the effect between time since metabolic and bariatric surgery and percentage Total weight loss. Obes Surg. 2024;34:2930–9.
69. Imhagen A, Karlsson J, Ohlsson-Nevo E, Stenberg E, Jansson S, Hagberg L. Levels of physical activity, enjoyment, self-efficacy for exercise, and social support before and after metabolic and bariatric surgery: a longitudinal prospective observational study. Obes Surg. 2023;33:3899–906.
70. Coan Romagna E, Grutter Lopes K, Menezes Ferrazani Mattos D, Farinatti P, Guilherme Kraemer-Aguiar L. Physical activity level, sedentary time, and weight regain after bariatric surgery in patients without regular medical follow-up: a cross-sectional study. https://doi.org/10.1007/s11695-020-05184-x/Published

71. Hilbert A, Strömer A, Staerk C, et al. Multivariate trajectories of weight and mental health and their prognostic significance 6 years after obesity surgery. Int J Eat Disord. 2025; https://doi.org/10.1002/EAT.24527.
72. Bellicha A, Ciangura C, Roda C, Torcivia A, Aron-Wisnewsky J, Poitou C, Oppert JM. Effect of exercise training after bariatric surgery: a 5-year follow-up study of a randomized controlled trial. PLoS One. 2022; https://doi.org/10.1371/JOURNAL.PONE.0271561.
73. Coen PM, Carnero EA, Goodpaster BH. Exercise and bariatric surgery: an effective therapeutic strategy. Exerc Sport Sci Rev. 2018;46:262.
74. Hassannejad A, Khalaj A, Mansournia MA, Tabesh MR, Alizadeh Z. The effect of aerobic or aerobic-strength exercise on body composition and functional capacity in patients with BMI ≥ 35 after bariatric surgery: a randomized control. Obes Surg. 2017;27:2792–801.
75. Carnero EA, Dubis GS, Hames KC, Jakicic JM, Houmard JA, Coen PM, Goodpaster BH. Randomized trial reveals that physical activity and energy expenditure are associated with weight and body composition after RYGB. Obesity (Silver Spring). 2017;25:1206–16.
76. Oppert JM, Bellicha A, Roda C, Bouillot JL, Torcivia A, Clement K, Poitou C, Ciangura C. Resistance training and protein supplementation increase strength after bariatric surgery: a randomized controlled trial. Obesity. 2018;26:1709–20.
77. Pino-Zuñiga J, Lillo-Urzua P, Olivares-Galvez M, Palacio-Aguero A, Duque JC, Luengas R, Cancino-Lopez J. Adherence to an early exercise plan promotes visceral fat loss in the first month following bariatric surgery. Obes Surg. 2025;35:746–54.
78. Tardif I, Auclair A, Piché ME, Biertho L, Marceau S, Hould FS, Biron S, Lebel S, Lescelleur O, Poirier P. Impact of a 12-week randomized exercise training program on lipid profile in severely obese patients following bariatric surgery. Obes Surg. 2020;30:3030–6.
79. Diniz-Sousa F, Veras L, Boppre G, et al. The effect of an exercise intervention program on bone health after bariatric surgery: a randomized controlled trial. J Bone Miner Res. 2021;36:489–99.
80. Boppre G, Borges LPSL, Diniz-Sousa F, Veras L, Devezas V, Preto J, Santos-Sousa H, da Costa THM, Oliveira J, Fonseca H. Effects of a supervised exercise training on body composition after bariatric surgery: a randomized controlled trial. Obesity. 2023;31:2750–61.
81. Jassil FC, Manning S, Lewis N, et al. Feasibility and impact of a combined supervised exercise and nutritional-behavioral intervention following bariatric surgery: a pilot study. J Obes. 2015; https://doi.org/10.1155/2015/693829.
82. Lehmann S, Lange UG, Oberbach A, et al. The effect of 6 months of structured strength or endurance exercise program on weight loss after gastric bypass surgery in a randomized controlled trial. Langenbeck's Arch Surg. 2025. https://doi.org/10.1007/s00423-025-03731-7.
83. Stegen S, Derave W, Calders P, Van Laethem C, Pattyn P. Physical fitness in morbidly obese patients: effect of gastric bypass surgery and exercise training. Obes Surg. 2011;21:61–70.
84. Campanha-versiani L, Aparecida D, Pereira G, Ribeiro-samora GA, Ramos AV, Fatima M, Diniz HDS, De Marco LA, Marta M, Soares S. The effect of a muscle weight-bearing and aerobic exercise program on the body composition , muscular strength , biochemical markers, and bone mass of obese patients who have undergone gastric bypass surgery. Obes Surg. 2017;27:2129–37.
85. Marcon ER, Baglioni S, Bittencourt L, Lopes CLN, Neumann CR, Trindade MRM. What is the best treatment before bariatric surgery? Exercise, exercise and group therapy, or conventional waiting: a randomized controlled trial. Obes Surg. 2017;27:763–73.
86. Coen PM, Tanner CJ, Helbling NL, et al. Clinical trial demonstrates exercise following bariatric surgery improves insulin sensitivity. J Clin Invest. 2015;125:248–57.
87. Castello V, Simões RP, Bassi D, Catai AM, Arena R, Borghi-Silva A. Impact of aerobic exercise training on heart rate variability and functional capacity in obese women after gastric bypass surgery. Obes Surg. 2011;21:1739–49.
88. Marchesi F, De Sario G, Reggiani V, et al. Road running after gastric bypass for morbid obesity: rationale and results of a new protocol. Obes Surg. 2015;25:1162–70.

89. Herring LY, Stevinson C, Carter P, Biddle SJH, Bowrey D, Sutton C, Davies MJ. The effects of supervised exercise training 12–24 months after bariatric surgery on physical function and body composition: a randomised controlled trial. Int J Obes. 2017;41:909–16.
90. Muschitz C, Kocijan R, Haschka J, et al. The impact of vitamin D, calcium, protein supplementation, and physical exercise on bone metabolism after bariatric surgery: the BABS study. J Bone Miner Res. 2016;31:672–82.
91. Marc-Hernández A, Ruiz-Tovar J, Aracil A, Guillén S, Moya-Ramón M. Effects of a high-intensity exercise program on weight regain and cardio-metabolic profile after 3 years of bariatric surgery: a randomized trial. Sci Rep. 2020; https://doi.org/10.1038/s41598-020-60044-z.
92. Sundgot-Borgen C, Bond DS, Sniehotta FF, Kvalem IL, Hansen BH, Bergh I, Rø, Mala T. Associations of changes in physical activity and sedentary time with weight recurrence after bariatric surgery: a 5-year prospective study. Int J Obes. 2023;47:463–70.
93. Bozdemır H, Usta E, Pehlıv̇ an M. The effect of mediterranean diet adherence and physical activity level on weight loss after laparoscopic sleeve gastrectomy. Obes Surg. 2025; https://doi.org/10.1007/s11695-025-08332-3.
94. Angrisani L, Santonicola A, Iovino P, Ramos A, Shikora S, Kow L. Bariatric surgery survey 2018: similarities and disparities among the 5 IFSO chapters. https://doi.org/10.1007/s11695-020-05207-7/Published.

18 Follow-Up Schemes and Role of the General Practitioner

Laura Cano-Lallave

18.1 Introduction

Importance of Long-Term Follow-Up

Sleeve gastrectomy is an effective intervention for short- and medium-term weight loss; however, it is essential to recognize that lasting improvement requires permanent lifestyle changes [1]. Strict adherence to follow-up during the first year is crucial to prevent complications and ensure that patients achieve sustainable weight loss [1, 2].

The family physician plays a key role in this process, serving as the first point of contact and the primary coordinator of ongoing care. Through regular assessments and proper management of complications, the family physician can guide patients through the challenges of the postoperative period and help improve their long-term health [3].

Patients who undergo bariatric surgery, such as sleeve gastrectomy (SG) or gastric bypass, require lifelong medical follow-up. Continuous monitoring is fundamental to ensure sustained success in weight loss, assess adherence to the postoperative regimen, and detect macro- and micronutrient deficiencies in a timely manner [2, 4].

18.2 Profile of the Post-sleeve Gastrectomy Patient

General Characteristics

Patients undergoing sleeve gastrectomy are typically individuals with morbid obesity or severe overweight, often accompanied by multiple comorbidities.

L. Cano-Lallave (✉)
María Jesús Hereza Health Center, Leganés, Madrid, Spain

J. Ruiz-Tovar (ed.), *Multidisciplinary Management of Sleeve Gastrectomy*,
https://doi.org/10.1007/978-3-032-25644-7_18

They frequently have a history of type 2 diabetes, hypertension, dyslipidemia, sleep apnea, and metabolic syndrome [2, 5].

This population generally has a history of unsuccessful weight-control attempts through other methods, leading to bariatric surgery as a definitive option [4]. As weight decreases, these patients may require medication adjustments or even discontinuation of certain drugs [6, 7].

Evaluation and Management of Comorbid Conditions
The status of comorbidities is routinely assessed at each postoperative visit:

- **Diabetes**: Bariatric surgery effectively treats diabetes. The need for insulin and/or oral hypoglycemic agents must be reassessed at each early postoperative visit. HbA1c is monitored to evaluate disease severity, and diabetes medications are adjusted accordingly [5, 8].
- **Hypertension**: Closely linked to obesity, blood pressure is routinely measured to monitor the patient's response to surgery, and antihypertensive therapy is reviewed [8].
- **Hyperlipidemia**: Serum lipids and cholesterol levels are monitored, with medications adjusted as necessary [5, 8].
- **Sleep Apnea**: A repeat sleep study may be performed 6–12 months post-surgery to reevaluate the need for continuous positive airway pressure (CPAP) [8].
- **Metabolic Deficiencies**: Laboratory assessments—serum calcium, iron, vitamin B12, vitamin D, folic acid, and thiamine—are performed every 6 months for the first 2 years, then annually [7, 8].
- **Gastroesophageal Reflux**: Is common in sleeve gastrectomy patients, and the introduction of medical therapy should be considered [8].
- **Unexplained Abdominal Pain**: This may occur in any patient after intra-abdominal surgery. In patients who have undergone Roux-en-Y gastric bypass (RYGB) and present with unexplained abdominal pain, there should be a low threshold for surgical exploration—often via laparoscopy—to identify hidden internal hernias, intussusception, or small-bowel obstruction, even if physical examination and imaging studies are inconclusive [8].

The procedure affects both the patient's physiology and psychology. Physiologically, the reduced stomach size limits food intake and alters nutrient absorption, which can lead to vitamin and mineral deficiencies if not properly managed. Psychologically, patients may experience a sense of renewal, but they may also face emotional challenges related to changes in their relationship with food and body image [8, 9].

Patient Expectations and Concerns
After surgery, patients often expect rapid weight loss within the first few months. However, they may not anticipate the challenges that come with the necessary lifestyle changes [10]. Food restriction combined with altered digestion can result in nausea, vomiting, and nutrient malabsorption. Psychological adaptation to these

changes is also critical, as some patients may develop eating disorders or an unhealthy relationship with food.

Emotional difficulties related to body image are also common, particularly when expected weight loss is not achieved. In this regard, the family physician must be sensitive to these psychological aspects, providing support and referring patients to specialists when necessary [10, 11].

18.3 Postoperative Follow-Up Phases of Post-sleeve Gastrectomy Care

Follow-up after sleeve gastrectomy should be progressive and tailored to the individual needs of each patient. The process can be divided into three key phases [12]:

Short-Term (First 6 Months)
During the first 6 months, patients require close monitoring to ensure weight loss occurs without major complications. Family physicians should conduct regular assessments to evaluate weight reduction, eating behavior, and early postoperative concerns:

- **Food Aversions**: Following SG, many patients report symptoms of acid reflux. Given the limited stomach volume, reduced gastric motility during healing, and preservation of gastric acid, reflux can occur if meals are consumed too quickly or in excessive amounts. Although common in the early postoperative period, most patients learn to avoid reflux by the 6-month mark [13].
- **Food Intolerances**: Less frequent after SG compared to RYGB, but postoperative intolerances and aversions vary widely between individuals. The most common issues relate to fatty foods and products with high added sugar content. Some patients may also develop lactose intolerance post-surgery, even without prior history [13, 14].

During this phase, emphasis should be placed on controlled food intake and the promotion of healthy habits, particularly a balanced, protein-rich diet while minimizing simple sugars and fats. Nutritional monitoring is essential, as surgery can interfere with nutrient absorption and increase the risk of deficiencies in iron, calcium, vitamin D, and vitamin B12 [15].

Mid-Term (6 Months to 1 Year)
Between 6 months and 1 year, the goal is to evaluate how well patients have adapted to changes in weight and eating habits [16, 17]. Weight loss typically slows after 6 months, and some may experience weight regain if lifestyle changes are not maintained. Ongoing monitoring allows for timely dietary and exercise adjustments [17].

At this stage, laboratory tests to assess liver and kidney function are also recommended, as some patients may develop complications such as malabsorption or malnutrition [18].

Long-Term (Beyond 1 Year)
After the first year, follow-up visits may become less frequent, but continued monitoring remains essential to detect long-term complications. Over time, patients may face conditions such as:

- **Dumping Syndrome**: Primarily associated with gastric bypass and triggered by the intake of sugary foods [19].
- **Marginal Ulcers**: Affect up to 25% of bypass patients, linked to NSAID use, smoking, or aspirin [19].
- **Cholelithiasis**: A common cause of upper abdominal pain after bariatric surgery, driven by changes in bile composition and rapid weight loss. Patients with an intact gallbladder are often prescribed ursodeoxycholic acid (ursodiol) 300 mg orally twice daily for 6 months to prevent gallstone formation [20].
- **Nephrolithiasis**: Reported in both RYGB and SG patients. Increased oxaluria can lead to kidney stones, oxalate nephropathy, and even renal failure. Patients should be advised to limit dietary oxalate intake [21, 22].
- **Depression**: May be preexisting or develop postoperatively. Reduced bioavailability of selective serotonin reuptake inhibitors (SSRIs) after RYGB increases the risk of symptom exacerbation in patients with prior depression [23].
- **Stenosis after SG**: Can cause gastric outlet obstruction, presenting with dysphagia or vomiting. Diagnosis is made with an upper GI study. Endoscopic dilation is often effective, though surgical revision may be required if endoscopic management fails [24].

18.4 The Role of the Family Physician in Follow-Up

First Point of Contact and Care Coordinator
The family physician plays a central role in the follow-up of post-sleeve gastrectomy patients, acting as the first point of contact for any concerns or complications [25]. Through a comprehensive approach, the family physician ensures that patients receive appropriate care and are referred to other specialists when necessary. This follow-up should include regular checkups, ongoing education, and, when indicated, referrals to nutritionists or psychologists [25].

Recommended Follow-Up Assessments and Tests
At each follow-up visit, the family physician should conduct a thorough evaluation. Laboratory testing is essential to monitor nutritional deficiencies and metabolic changes. Recommended tests include [26, 27]:

- **Blood tests** to assess iron, vitamin B12, calcium, vitamin D, and albumin levels.
- **Renal and liver function tests** to identify potential complications related to surgery.
- **Glucose monitoring and lipid profile** to evaluate the control of comorbidities such as diabetes and dyslipidemia.

Comprehensive Approach to Comorbidities

Post-gastrectomy follow-up extends beyond weight control to the management of preexisting comorbidities. The family physician should collaborate with endocrinologists, pulmonologists, and other specialists to optimize care for conditions such as diabetes, hypertension, and sleep apnea. Medication regimens should be continuously adjusted to reflect the patient's new metabolic status after surgery [18].

Surgery is only one part of the treatment. Long-term success depends largely on healthy eating habits, regular physical activity, and psychological support.

Practical recommendations include [8]:

- Encourage hydration, prioritizing water and avoiding carbonated beverages, straws, and caffeinated drinks due to their diuretic effects.
- Discourage the consumption of ultra-processed foods and sugary drinks, which provide empty calories with minimal nutrients.
- Prioritize lean protein sources in the diet.
- Reinforce the importance of daily vitamin and mineral supplementation, emphasizing compliance at every visit.
- Promote regular physical activity, starting with walking. For patients with joint disease, aquatic exercise is recommended.

18.5 Management of Nutritional Complications

Common Nutrient Deficiencies

One of the most frequent complications after sleeve gastrectomy is malnutrition and nutrient deficiencies. This occurs because surgery reduces the stomach's capacity to store and process food, limiting the absorption of essential nutrients [7, 8]. The most common deficiencies include:

- **Iron**—may result in iron-deficiency anemia [4, 5].
- **Vitamin B12**—deficiency leads to fatigue, weakness, and neurological symptoms [4, 13].
- **Vitamin D and Calcium**—deficiencies increase the risk of osteoporosis (28).

Macronutrient Management

In the early postoperative phases, the diet focuses on meeting essential nutrient requirements and ensuring adequate hydration. Once weight stabilizes, patients derive most of their energy needs from dietary sources. At this stage, caloric and macronutrient requirements for sleeve gastrectomy patients do not differ significantly from the general population (Table 18.1) [1].

- **Protein**: Recovery guidelines recommend an intake of 60–80 g per day. For weight maintenance, protein needs can be calculated as 0.8–1.2 g/kg/day, although exact requirements may vary individually. During active weight loss,

Table 18.1 Macronutrient management

Macronutrient	Recommended intake	Rationale
Protein	60–80 g/day 0.8–1.2 g/kg/day for maintenance 1.2 g/kg/day during active weight loss average: 60–120 g/day for long-term lean mass preservation	Prevents muscle loss, supports wound healing, preserves lean body mass
Carbohydrates	~50% of total caloric intake ≥50 g/day early postop ≥130 g/day as diet progresses	Provides primary energy; focus on complex carbs (fruits, vegetables, whole grains), avoid soft breads, rice, pasta early postop (can cause nausea, early satiety)
Fat	20–35% of total caloric intake	Energy source, supports fat-soluble vitamin absorption

1.2 g/kg/day is recommended to preserve lean body mass. On average, 60–120 g/day is required to maintain lean body mass both during weight loss and long term [6, 11].

- **Carbohydrates**: Should provide ~50% of total daily calories. Patients should consume a minimum of 50 g/day early postoperatively, progressing to 130 g/day as tolerance improves. Complex carbohydrates from fruits, vegetables, and whole grains should be emphasized. Foods such as soft breads, rice, or pasta are best avoided in the first months, as they often cause discomfort, early satiety, or nausea [11, 25].
- **Fat**: Should represent 20–35% of daily caloric intake [3, 11].

Micronutrient Management

Micronutrient deficiencies are of particular concern after malabsorptive or combined procedures, due to reduced nutrient intake and altered anatomy bypassing parts of the stomach, duodenum, and/or proximal jejunum [7, 11].

After partial or total gastrectomy, patients must take lifelong vitamin and mineral supplementation (Table 18.2). Bariatric-specific vitamins are often a good option, as they contain nearly all essential micronutrients except calcium. Patients should take one to two bariatric multivitamins daily, depending on the formulation. Over-the-counter multivitamins are acceptable but must be supplemented with additional vitamin D and B12 [9].

Patients who develop symptoms suggestive of deficiency, or who are found to have laboratory-confirmed deficiencies, should receive appropriate repletion [9, 15].

Specific Deficiencies

- **Iron**: One of the most common deficiencies after bariatric surgery, leading to hypochromic microcytic anemia. Iron is primarily absorbed in the duodenum

Table 18.2 Micronutrient supplementation guidelines

Supplement	Dosage & notes
Calcium citrate	1000–1200 mg/day in divided doses (2–3x/day), taken separately from multivitamins
Iron	18 mg/day (men, non-anemic); 45–60 mg/day (women, SG patients)
Vitamin B12	350–1000 mcg/day oral (or parenteral if deficiency persists)
Vitamin D	3000 IU/day to maintain 25(OH)D > 30 ng/mL

and proximal jejunum; bypass procedures worsen this. Additionally, gastric acid normally helps release iron from dietary proteins, but reduced acid production in SG further impairs absorption [3, 12].

  - Men and non-anemic patients should receive at least 18 mg of iron daily via a multivitamin.
  - Menstruating women and SG patients should take 45–60 mg of elemental iron daily.
  - Most multivitamins do not provide sufficient elemental iron, so additional supplementation is often required.

- **Vitamin B12**: Post-SG deficiency prevalence ranges from 4% to 20%. Due to reduced gastric acid and intrinsic factor, absorption is impaired. This can result in permanent pernicious (megaloblastic) anemia, warranting lifelong oral or parenteral supplementation [23, 24].
  - A daily oral dose of 350–1000 mcg of vitamin B12 is recommended.
  - Because body stores last 12–18 months, deficiency typically appears two or more years postoperatively, underscoring the need for annual laboratory monitoring.
- **Vitamin D**: A systematic review and meta-analysis of 18 bariatric studies including 2869 patients found preoperative vitamin D insufficiency (25[OH]D < 30 ng/mL) in 85% of cases, with postoperative rates of 63%. Persistent deficiency reduces calcium and phosphorus absorption, leading to secondary hyperparathyroidism, bone demineralization, osteomalacia, or rickets [26–28].
  - Postoperatively, patients should receive 3000 IU of vitamin D3 daily from all sources to maintain 25(OH)D > 30 ng/mL (75 nmol/L).
- **Calcium**: Absorbed primarily in the duodenum and proximal jejunum, with better absorption in an acidic environment. Reduced gastric acid exposure in SG increases the risk of deficiency. Daily calcium intake (1000–1200 mg) should be achieved through food and supplements. Calcium citrate is preferred over calcium carbonate for better absorption, taken in divided doses of 500–600 mg two or three times daily, separated from multivitamins to maximize absorption [1, 4, 7].

  - Calcium deficiency is associated with metabolic bone disease and secondary hyperparathyroidism. Treatment includes oral and parenteral calcium plus vitamin D supplementation, tailored to disease severity.

References

1. Taveira Azevedo RC, da Silva Teixeira T, et al. Metabolic significance of nutritional treatment before and after bariatric surgery: a systematic review. Int J Nutrol. 2025:1–7.
2. Lim Acosta M, Flores Ruiz C, Zamora Rivera GI, et al. Laparoscopic sleeve gastrectomy: bariatric surgery peak? Int J Med Sci Clin Res Stud. 2022;2:969–71.
3. Tucker ON, Szomstein S, Rosenthal RJ. Nutritional consequences of weight-loss surgery. Med Clin North Am. 2007;91:499–514.
4. Khan MA, Siddiq G, Uneeb M, Khan MS, Yusufi MA, Siddiqi NN. Comparison of micronutrient deficiencies following Roux-en-Y gastric bypass and one-anastomosis gastric bypass. Cureus. 2024;16(10):e71837.
5. Dalcanale L, Oliveira CP, Faintuch J, et al. Long-term nutritional outcome after gastric bypass. Obes Surg. 2010;20:181–7.
6. Adami GF, Campostano A, Cella F, Scopinaro N. Serum leptin concentration in obese patients with binge eating disorder. Int J Obes Relat Metab Disord. 2002;26(8):1125–8.
7. Mechanick JI, Apovian C, Brethauer S, et al. Clinical practice guidelines for perioperative nutrition, metabolic, and nonsurgical support of patients undergoing bariatric procedures—2019 update. Surg Obes Relat Dis. 2020;16:175–247.
8. Andersen JR, Aasprang A, Karlsen TI, et al. Health-related quality of life after bariatric surgery: a systematic review of prospective long-term studies. Surg Obes Relat Dis. 2015;11:466–73.
9. Stenberg E, Dos Reis Falcão LF, O'Kane M, Liem R, Pournaras DJ, Salminen P, Urman RD, Wadhwa A, Gustafsson UO, Thorell A. Guidelines for perioperative care in bariatric surgery: enhanced recovery after surgery (ERAS) society recommendations: a 2021 update. World J Surg. 2022;46(4):729–51. https://doi.org/10.1007/s00268-021-06394-9. Epub 2022 Jan 4. Erratum in: World J Surg. 2022 Apr;46(4):752
10. Monpellier VM, Antoniou EE, Aarts EO, et al. Improvement of health-related quality of life after Roux-en-Y gastric bypass related to weight loss. Obes Surg. 2017;27:1168–76.
11. Mechanick JI, Youdim A, Jones DB, et al. Clinical practice guidelines for the perioperative nutritional, metabolic, and nonsurgical support of the bariatric surgery patient—2013 update. Obesity (Silver Spring). 2013;21(Suppl 1):S1–27.
12. van Rutte PW, Aarts EO, Smulders JF, Nienhuijs SW. Nutrient deficiencies before and after sleeve gastrectomy. Obes Surg. 2014;24:1639–46.
13. Soliman A, Magd Eldin Saleem H, El Meligi A, et al. Optimización de la cirugía metabólica/bariátrica: Declaración de posición de la Asociación Árabe para el Estudio de la Diabetes y el Metabolismo (AASD). Diabetol Metab Syndr. 2025:17–37.
14. Mechanick JI, Apovian C, Brethauer S, et al. Clinical practice guidelines for perioperative nutrition, metabolic, and nonsurgical support of patients undergoing bariatric procedures – 2019 update. Surg Obes Relat Dis. 2020;16:175–247.
15. Aills L, Blankenship J, Buffington C, Furtado M, Parrott J. ASMBS allied health nutritional guidelines for the surgical weight loss patient. Surg Obes Relat Dis. 2008;4:S73–108.
16. King WC, Hsu JY, Belle SH, et al. Pre- to postoperative changes in physical activity: report from the longitudinal assessment of bariatric surgery-2 (LABS-2). Surg Obes Relat Dis. 2012;8:522–32.
17. Wagner J, Roll M, Lautenbach A, Notz S, Plitzko G, Izbicki J, Mann O, Hackert T, Duprée A, Brodersen F, Weigel A. Patients' expectations and perspectives on follow-up care after bariatric surgery in Germany. Obes Surg. 2025;35(6):2174–84. https://doi.org/10.1007/s11695-025-07890-w. Epub 2025 Apr 30. PMID: 40304842; PMCID: PMC12130090
18. Thorell A, MacCormick AD, Awad S, et al. Guidelines for perioperative care in bariatric surgery: ERAS Society recommendations. World J Surg. 2016;40:2065–83.
19. Uy MC, Talingdan-Te MC, Espinosa WZ, et al. Ursodeoxycholic acid in the prevention of gallstone formation after bariatric surgery: a meta-analysis. Obes Surg. 2008;18:1532–8.

20. Laurenius A, Sundbom M, Ottosson J, et al. Incidence of kidney stones after metabolic and bariatric surgery – data from the Scandinavian obesity surgery registry. Obes Surg. 2023;33:1564–72.
21. Parque Alyssa M, Storm DW, Fulmer BR, et al. Estudio prospectivo de los factores de riesgo de nefrolitiasis tras la cirugía de bypass gástrico Roux-en-Y. Rev Urol. 2009;182(5):2334–9.
22. Hamad GG, Helsel JC, Perel JM, et al. The effect of gastric bypass on the pharmacokinetics of serotonin reuptake inhibitors. Am J Psychiatry. 2012;169:256–63.
23. Khan, et al. Comparative effectiveness of laparoscopic sleeve gastrectomy in morbidly obese and super obese patients. Cureus. 2021;13(12)
24. Deslauriers V, Beauchamp A, Garofalo F, et al. Endoscopic management of post-laparoscopic sleeve gastrectomy stenosis. Surg Endosc. 2018;32:601–9.
25. Côté M, et al. Micronutrient status 2 years after bariatric surgery: a prospective nutritional assessment. Front Nutr. 2024;
26. Ferrer R, Pardina E, Rossell J, et al. Hematologic parameters and serum trace elements in morbidly obese patients before and after gastric bypass. Clin Nutr. 2015;34:276–83.
27. Fox A, et al. Vitamin D status after gastric bypass or sleeve gastrectomy over 4 years of follow-up. Obes Surg. 2020;30:1473–81.
28. Sinha MK, Collazo-Clavell ML, Rule A, Milliner DS, Nelson W, Sarr MG, Kumar R, Lieske JC. Hyperoxaluric nephrolithiasis is a complication of roux-en-Y gastric bypass surgery. Kidney Int. 2007;72(1):100–7.

Nursing Involvement in the Postoperative Follow-Up

19

María-Lara Martínez-Gimeno

19.1 Introduction

Vertical sleeve gastrectomy, also known as *gastric sleeve*, is a restrictive bariatric procedure widely used in the treatment of morbid obesity and its associated comorbidities. It is currently the most commonly performed bariatric surgery worldwide, with notable growth in the last decade, accounting for more than 60% of bariatric procedures in countries such as the United States and up to 44% globally [1, 2].

Gastric sleeve surgery is considered a safe and effective procedure, with a lower risk of malabsorption than gastric bypass surgery. However, it requires strict follow-up to ensure sustainable results and prevent postoperative complications [1–3].

19.2 The Enhanced Recovery After Surgery (ERAS) Protocol

Enhanced Recovery After Surgery (ERAS) programs aim to prepare patients for functional recovery, thereby contributing to improved postoperative outcomes. ERAS programs are associated with shorter hospital stays, reduced overall costs, and improved patient satisfaction [4, 5].

The ERAS protocol in bariatric surgery is based on a multidisciplinary and multimodal approach to address the various problems that may arise after surgical treatment. It is a set of standardized measures covering the pre-, intra-, and postoperative periods to accelerate recovery and reduce surgical stress. In gastric sleeve surgery, the focus is on performing a restrictive laparoscopic procedure, with an emphasis on multimodal analgesia, nausea prophylaxis, and early mobilization [6].

M.-L. Martínez-Gimeno (✉)
Department of Health Sciences, EUEF SAN JUAN DE DIOS-Universidad Pontificia Comillas, Madrid, Spain
e-mail: mlmartinez@comillas.edu

J. Ruiz-Tovar (ed.), *Multidisciplinary Management of Sleeve Gastrectomy*,
https://doi.org/10.1007/978-3-032-25644-7_19

Within this multidisciplinary program, nursing care plays a fundamental role in postoperative follow-up, prevention of complications, and health education. Nursing interventions include monitoring vital signs, pain management, early mobilization, prevention of thromboembolism and respiratory complications, as well as supervision of dietary progression and emotional support. In addition, self-care education and coordination with the multidisciplinary team are essential to ensure treatment adherence and improve the patient's quality of life [7].

Scientific evidence indicates that adequate nursing follow-up reduces the incidence of complications and promotes sustained weight loss, whereas a lack of follow-up increases the risk of weight gain and nutritional problems [8–10].

In this chapter, we will focus on nursing follow-up during the immediate postoperative period (24–72 h) as outlined in the ERAS protocol.

19.3 Nursing Care in the Immediate Postoperative Period within the ERAS Program

Postoperative monitoring can be divided into three stages:

- Immediate Postoperative Period (0–24 h):
  - Intensive monitoring in the ICU or resuscitation unit. Monitoring of vital signs.
  - Monitoring of pain, bleeding, and anesthetic tolerance.
  - Control of nausea, vomiting, and abdominal pain.
  - Early mobilization.
- Immediate (1–7 days):
  - Start of liquid diet.
  - Control of nausea, vomiting, and abdominal pain.
  - Prevention of respiratory and thromboembolic complications.
- Late (after discharge):
  - Nutritional education and monitoring of habits.
  - Emotional support and treatment adherence.

In this chapter, we will focus on the period covering the first 24–72 h, i.e., the immediate postoperative period and part of the immediate period.

19.3.1 Monitoring of Vital Signs

The immediate postoperative period following gastric sleeve surgery, specifically the first 24 h, typically occurs in the intensive care unit.

Monitoring vital signs is critical for detecting early complications such as bleeding, gastric leakage, respiratory failure, or hemodynamic changes.

The vital signs to be monitored are [11]:

- **Heart rate (HR)**
  - Persistent tachycardia (>100 bpm) may indicate bleeding or gastric leakage.
- **Blood pressure (BP)**
  - Hypotension may suggest bleeding; likewise, hypertension may be associated with pain or stress.
- **Oxygen saturation (SpO_2)**
  - Continuous monitoring with a pulse oximeter to detect the risk of hypoxemia due to analgesia (opioids), respiratory complications, and/or obesity itself.
- **Temperature**
  - The early presence of slight fever (T > 37 °C and < 38 °C) or fever (T > 38 °C) may indicate an infection or respiratory complications.
- **Pain and level of consciousness**
  - Use scales such as the VAS (Visual Analogue Scale) for pain assessment and the Glasgow Coma Scale (GCS) for alertness assessment to evaluate anesthetic recovery.
- **Respiratory rate (RR)**
  - Monitor for respiratory depression due to anesthesia or pain.
- **Hourly diuresis**
  - An indicator of renal perfusion and fluid balance.
- **Fluid balance and drainage**
  - Monitor the amount and characteristics of drained fluid.

The frequency of monitoring may vary according to different protocols:

- Every 15 min during the first hour after arrival in resuscitation.
- Every 30 min for the next 2 h.
- Every hour until the first 6 h are complete.
- Subsequently, every 4 h if the patient is stable, for a total of 24 h.

It is essential to detect warning signs that allow you to anticipate possible complications:

- Persistent tachycardia (>120 bpm).
- Hypotension not explained by analgesia.
- Sudden decrease in SpO_2.
- Severe uncontrolled abdominal pain.
- Excessive blood loss through drains.

19.3.2 Postoperative Pain Management

Pain management in patients after gastric sleeve surgery is crucial, and current recommendations focus on a multimodal approach that includes [12]:

- Analgesia: an analgesic regimen including **paracetamol and NSAIDs or specific COX-2 inhibitors** is recommended. **Opioids** are reserved for rescue treatment.
- Anesthetic techniques: nerve blocks (**bilateral transverse abdominal plane (TAP) blocks**) and local anesthetic infiltrations.

Proper pain management ensures patient comfort. Nursing care includes: pain monitoring (fifth constant) with standardized assessment using validated scales:

- **Continuous assessment (fifth constant)** using scales such as VAS (Visual Analogue Scale).
- **Safe administration** of prescribed analgesia (usually opioids in the first 24 h, then NSAIDs if indicated).
- **Observation of side effects**: nausea, drowsiness, constipation.
- **Patient education** on non-pharmacological techniques: deep breathing, relaxation.

19.3.3 Prevention of Nausea and Vomiting

Postoperative nausea and vomiting (PONV) are multifactorial. Prevention is essential because it can delay recovery, increase the risk of dehydration, and prolong hospital stay.

Current strategies for the prevention and treatment of PONV include proactive risk assessment (common risk factors include: female gender, non-smoker, history of motion sickness or PONV, and postoperative opioid use). There are scales for detecting the risk of PONV, one of which is the Apfel scale, which considers four variables to classify risk [13]. Table 19.1 shows the scale and its classification.

It is essential to avoid PONV triggers by administering prophylactic antiemetics preoperatively, administering rescue antiemetics postoperatively, and optimizing anesthetic protocols. Minimizing the use of opioids is recommended [14].

Nursing care will focus on:

Table 19.1 PONV risk stratification

Risk factors		Points
Female		1
Use of perioperative opioids		1
Non-smoker		1
History of PONV or motion sickness		1
		Total: 0 to 4
Risk		*Possibility of NVPO*
Low	(0–1 points)	10–20
Medium	(2 points)	40%
High	(3–4 points)	60–80%

- **Continuous monitoring**
  - Monitoring for signs of PONV in the post-operative recovery unit and during the first few hours after surgery.
  - Monitor hydration and fluid balance to prevent dehydration.
- **Safe administration of medication**
  - Verifying prescribed prophylaxis (ondansetron, dexamethasone, droperidol).
  - Record response and adverse effects.
- **Non-pharmacological measures**
  - Encourage the semi-fowler position to reduce abdominal pressure.
  - Apply cold compresses and maintain a calm environment to minimize stimuli that can cause nausea.
- **Patient education**
  - Explain the importance of reporting early symptoms of NVPO.
  - Provide instructions on a progressive postoperative diet (clear liquids → purees → soft solids).
  - Reinforce adherence to medical guidelines and warning signs.
- **Emotional support**
  - Reduce anxiety through active listening and support.
  - Involve the family in care and education.

19.3.4 Early Mobilization

The implementation of enhanced recovery after surgery (ERAS) programs that include early mobilization reduces the length of hospital stay by 18% and decreases the use of postoperative opioids by 61% [5].

This strategy, defined as the progressive initiation of controlled physical activity in the first hours after surgery, aims to reduce complications arising from prolonged rest, improve respiratory function, and accelerate functional recovery [15, 16].

Early mobilization programs during the immediate postoperative period significantly shorten the time to first flatulence, defecation, and oral intake, and decrease the incidence of pain, abdominal distension, and nausea, improving tolerance to oral intake [4].

In the context of gastric sleeve surgery, mobilization should begin as soon as the patient's clinical condition allows, usually within the first 6–8 h after surgery (once the patient is stable and has regained consciousness after anesthesia), following enhanced recovery after surgery (ERAS) protocols [17].

The phases include:

- Postural changes in bed.
- Breathing exercises with a volumetric incentive device.
- Active mobilization of the lower extremities.
- Sitting at the edge of the bed and, subsequently, assisted walking in the hallway.

These actions help prevent respiratory complications, such as atelectasis and pneumonia, as well as deep vein thrombosis, while also maintaining muscle mass and improving the patient's psychological well-being [18].

The role of nursing is fundamental in the safe implementation of early mobilization. Nurses must assess patient tolerance, monitor vital signs before and after activity, educate patients on the importance of movement, and coordinate with physical therapy when necessary [15, 16].

- **Initial assessment:**
  - Assess hemodynamic status, pain, and tolerance before initiating mobilization.
  - Check drains and devices to avoid risks.
- **Patient education:**
  - Explain the benefits and objectives of early mobilization.
  - Teach breathing exercises and safe movements.
- **Progressive interventions**
  - Breathing exercises and passive mobilization in bed.
  - Sitting on the edge of the bed in the early hours.
  - Assisted walking within the first 24–48 h, depending on tolerance.
- **Prevention of complications**
  - Monitor for signs of orthostatic hypotension.
  - Pain control to facilitate mobility.
  - Use of compression stockings is indicated.
- **Recording and monitoring**
  - Document mobilization times, tolerance, and progress.
  - Adjust plan according to patient response.

19.3.5 Nutritional Care

Enhanced Recovery After Surgery (ERAS) protocols have revolutionized perioperative management in bariatric surgery, promoting **early feeding** as a strategy to mitigate the metabolic response to surgical stress, prevent insulin resistance, and enhance functional recovery [19, 20]. Traditionally, reintroduction of the diet was delayed until the onset of peristalsis, but current evidence indicates that early initiation of oral intake is safe and beneficial in patients undergoing gastric sleeve surgery [21].

ERAS principles applied to the immediate postoperative period of gastric sleeve surgery [22]:

- **Early initiation of clear liquids**: generally within the first 6–8 h after surgery, provided the patient is hemodynamically stable and without significant nausea.
- **Structured dietary progression**:

  - **Clear liquid phase** (first 7–10 days): water, sugar-free herbal teas, broths, non-carbonated protein drinks.
  - **Supplementation**: vitamins and minerals from the outset, as clinically indicated.

The implementation of these measures, combined with nutritional education and multidisciplinary follow-up, reduces complications such as vomiting, dehydration, and nutritional deficiencies, while also shortening hospital stays.

Nursing care includes:

- **Continuous nutritional assessment**:
  - Body mass index (BMI), tolerance, and signs of dehydration.
- **Patient education**:
  - Recognizing signs of intolerance and when to seek medical attention.
- **Recording and monitoring**:
  - Weight changes, intake, and gastrointestinal symptoms.

19.3.6 Surgical Wound Care

During the first 24–72 h after gastric sleeve surgery, it is essential to take the following into account as part of nursing care related to the surgical wound [17]:

- **Daily assessment of the surgical wound**: to detect signs of infection (redness, heat, discharge, pain) or bleeding.
- **Maintaining asepsis** when changing dressings.
- **Education on self-care** of the wound in preparation for the transition to the hospitalization area.

19.4 Nursing Care in the Prevention of Complications During the Immediate Postoperative Period of Gastric Sleeve Surgery

19.4.1 Prevention of Respiratory Complications

These are one of the leading causes of morbidity after bariatric surgery, especially in patients with severe obesity, due to decreased residual functional capacity, hypoventilation, and the frequent presence of obstructive sleep apnea [1, 4]. The **Enhanced Recovery After Surgery (ERAS)** protocol incorporates specific measures to reduce the risk of pulmonary complications, optimizing respiratory function, and accelerating postoperative recovery [18].

- **Breathing exercises** with a volumetric incentive device every 2 h.

- **Frequent postural changes** to promote lung expansion.
- **Early mobilization** (sitting up in bed, walking with assistance) from the first 24 h.
- **Monitoring for signs of respiratory distress** or hypoxia.
- **Education on** wound **self-care** in preparation for the transition to the hospitalization area.

19.4.2 Prevention of Venous Thromboembolism

The **ERAS** protocol includes measures to prevent venous thromboembolic disease (VTE) through [19]:

- **Early mobilization**
  - Assisted walking within the first 24 h after surgery.
  - Active exercises in bed if walking is not possible.
- **Pharmacological prophylaxis**
  - Use of **low molecular weight heparins (LMWH)** according to individual risk.
  - Early initiation (6–12 h post-surgery) and duration according to bariatric protocol (7–14 days or more if high risk).
- **Mechanical measures**
  - **Graduated compression stockings** and/or **intermittent pneumatic compression devices** during hospitalization.
- **Perioperative optimization**
  - Avoid prolonged fasting, maintain adequate hydration.
  - Pain control to facilitate early mobilization.
- **Patient education**
  - Explain the importance of mobilization and adherence to pharmacological prophylaxis.
  - Teach how to detect warning signs: calf pain, unilateral edema, sudden dyspnea.

19.5 Conclusion

Nursing care within the ERAS protocol is essential for:

- Reducing respiratory, thromboembolic, and gastrointestinal complications.
- Improve functional recovery and postoperative quality of life.

Early mobilization, multimodal analgesia, prevention of PONV, and nutritional care are pillars of success in the postoperative period of gastric sleeve surgery.

Health education and nursing follow-up are crucial for treatment adherence and sustainable results.

Evidence suggests that integrating the nursing team into postoperative management reduces risks and optimizes both clinical and economic outcomes.

References

1. Howard R, Chao G, Yang J, Thumma J, Chhabra K, Arterburn D, Ryan A, Telem D, Dimick J. Comparative safety of sleeve gastrectomy and gastric bypass up to 5 years after surgery in patients with severe obesity. JAMA Surg. 2021; https://doi.org/10.1001/jamasurg.2021.4981.
2. Clapp B, Wynn M, Martyn C, Foster C, O'Dell M, Tyroch A. Long-term (7 or more years) outcomes of sleeve gastrectomy: a meta-analysis. Surg Obes Relat Dis. 2018;14:6. https://doi.org/10.1016/j.soard.2018.02.027.
3. Carandina S, Zulian V, Nedelcu A, Danan M, Vilallonga R, Nocca D, Nedelcu M. Is it safe to combine a fundoplication to sleeve gastrectomy? Review of literature. Medicina (Kaunas). 2021:57. https://doi.org/10.3390/medicina57040392.
4. Kırtıl İ, Kanan N, Karip AB. Effects of a mobilization program applied to bariatric surgery patients on preventing gastrointestinal complications: a quasi-experimental study. Obes Surg. 2023;33(6):1820–30. https://doi.org/10.1007/s11695-023-06609-z. Epub 2023 Apr 21
5. Sapin A, Hilden P, Cinicolo L, Stein J, Turner A, Pitera R, Yodicei P, Paragi PR. Enhanced recovery after surgery for sleeve gastrectomies: improved patient outcomes. Surg Obes Relat Dis. 2021;17(9):1541–7. https://doi.org/10.1016/j.soard.2021.04.017. Epub 2021 May 3
6. Huh YJ, Kim DJ. Enhanced recovery after surgery in bariatric surgery. J Metab Bariatr Surg. 2021;10(2):47–54. https://doi.org/10.17476/jmbs.2021.10.2.47.
7. Soroceanu RP, Timofte DV, Danila R, Timofeiov S, Livadariu R, Miler AA, et al. The impact of bariatric surgery on quality of life in patients with obesity. J Clin Med. 2023;12(13):4225. https://doi.org/10.3390/jcm12134225.
8. Huk A, Yeryomenko G. Role of nursing interventions in preventing postoperative complications. Inter Collegas. 2025; https://doi.org/10.35339/ic.2025.12.2.huk.
9. Mendes C, Carvalho M, Oliveira L, Rodrigues L, Gregório J. Nurse-led intervention for the management of bariatric surgery patients: a systematic review. Obes Rev. 2023:24. https://doi.org/10.1111/obr.13614.
10. Chen W, Fan X, Hao Y. Nursing care during sleeve gastrectomy. J Surg Anesth Res. 2025; https://doi.org/10.47363/jsar/2025(6)225.
11. Cohen RV, Kermansaravi M, Levinson R, et al. International Federation for the Surgery and Other Therapies for obesity (IFSO) global consensus recommendations for optimizing outcomes after sleeve gastrectomy. Br J Surg. 2025;112(10):znaf188.
12. Debel N, Snijkers E, van de Velde M, Joshi GP, Sauter AR, Freys S, Pogatzki-Zahn E, Dewinter G, on behalf of the PROSPECT working Group of the European Society of Regional Anaesthesia and Pain Therapy (ESRA), Albrecht E, Bugada D, Beloeil H, Bonnet MP, Desai N, Dewinter G, Freys SM, Joshi GP, Kehlet H, Lavand'homme P, Lobo DN, Moka E, Pogatzki-Zahn EM, Raeder J, Rawal N, Sauter AR, Van de Velde M, Wu CL. Pain management for laparoscopic sleeve gastrectomy: an update of the systematic review and procedure-specific postoperative pain management (PROSPECT) recommendations. Eur J Anaesthesiol. 2026;43(1):19–33. https://doi.org/10.1097/EJA.0000000000002296.
13. Acosta-Villegas F, García-López JA, Aguayo-Albasini JL. Management of postoperative nausea and vomiting. Cir Esp. 2010;88(6):369–73. https://doi.org/10.1016/j.ciresp.2010.07.009.
14. Naeem Z, Chen IL, Pryor AD, Docimo S, Gan TJ, Spaniolas K. Antiemetic prophylaxis and anesthetic approaches to reduce postoperative nausea and vomiting in bariatric surgery patients: a systematic review. Obes Surg. 2020;30(8):3188–200. https://doi.org/10.1007/s11695-020-04683-1.

15. Lasheras R, et al. Early mobilization techniques in the postoperative period. Rev Ocronos [Internet]. 2024;7(9):1179. Available at: https://revistamedica.com/analisis-tecnicas-movilizacion-temprana-postoperatorio/[revistamedica.com]
16. Ruiz-Tovar J, et al. Multimodal rehabilitation in bariatric surgery. Cir Esp [Internet]. 2019;97(10):551–9. Available at: https://www.elsevier.es/es-revista-cirugia-espanola-36-articulo-rehabilitacion-multimodal-cirugia-bariatrica-S0009739X19301502[elsevier.es]
17. Stenberg E, Falcão LF, O'Kane M, et al. Guidelines for perioperative care in bariatric surgery: ERAS society recommendations: a 2021 update. World J Surg. 2022;46:729–51. Available at: https://link.springer.com/article/10.1007/s00268-021-06394-9
18. Morón A, et al. Nursing care in bariatric surgery. Rev Sanitaria Investig [Internet]. 2024. Available at: https://revistasanitariadeinvestigacion.com/cuidados-de-enfermeria-en-las-cirugias-bariatricas/
19. Thorell A, MacCormick AD, Awad S, et al. Guidelines for perioperative care in bariatric surgery: enhanced recovery after surgery (ERAS) society recommendations. World J Surg. 2016;40(9):2065–83. Available at: https://perioperativeitaliansociety.org/wp-content/uploads/2017/10/ERABS-2016.pdf
20. Sánchez C, Papapietro V. Perioperative nutrition in surgical protocols for better postoperative recovery (ERAS protocol). Rev Méd Chile. 2017;145(11):1447–56. Available at: https://www.scielo.cl/scielo.php?script=sci_arttext&pid=S0034-98872017001101447
21. ERAS® Society. Guidelines. Available at: https://erassociety.org/guidelines/
22. Mortensen K, Nilsson M, Slim K, et al. Consensus guidelines for enhanced recovery after gastrectomy. Br J Surg. 2014;101(10):1209–29. Available at: https://www.grace-asso.fr/wp-content/uploads/grace-pdf/Sources/Recommandations/eras-guidelines-gastrect_0.pdf

Postoperative Quality of Life 20

Laura Visiers-Jiménez

20.1 Introduction

Obesity is a global public health concern, associated with increased morbidity, mortality, and reduced health-related quality of life (HRQoL).

Sleeve gastrectomy (SG), a popular bariatric procedure, has emerged as a primary surgical intervention for weight loss and metabolic improvement. However, while weight reduction and metabolic outcomes are crucial, postoperative quality of life is an equally vital endpoint that encompasses the physical, emotional, and social dimensions of health.

This chapter explores the concept of HRQoL in the context of bariatric surgery, specifically after SG. We discuss commonly used HRQoL instruments, analyze key findings from the literature, and explore future perspectives in enhancing and personalizing postoperative care.

20.2 Conceptualizing Quality of Life in Bariatric Surgery

Quality of life is a multidimensional concept defined by the World Health Organization (WHO) as an individual's perception of their position in life, within the context of their culture and value systems, and in relation to their goals, expectations, and concerns [1]. In bariatric surgery, HRQoL extends beyond traditional biomedical outcomes and includes physical functioning, mental health, social relationships, self-esteem, and body image.

L. Visiers-Jiménez (✉)
Department of Health Sciences, Comillas Pontifical University, San Juan de Dios School of Nursing and Physical Therapy, Madrid, Spain

San Juan de Dios Foundation, Madrid, Spain
e-mail: lvisiers@comillas.edu

J. Ruiz-Tovar (ed.), *Multidisciplinary Management of Sleeve Gastrectomy*,
https://doi.org/10.1007/978-3-032-25644-7_20

Importantly, HRQoL must be interpreted through the lens of obesity-specific impairments and the dramatic lifestyle changes following surgery. The psychological and social reintegration aspects following massive weight loss are as relevant as the physiological outcomes.

20.3 Assessment Tools for Quality of Life After Sleeve Gastrectomy

Several standardized and validated instruments are employed to assess HRQoL in patients undergoing bariatric surgery. These can be categorized into generic HRQoL instruments, obesity-specific questionnaires, and bariatric surgery-specific tools.

20.3.1 Generic Instruments

Generic tools allow for cross-population comparisons and are not tailored to obesity or surgery. Commonly used tools include:

- *The Gastrointestinal Symptom Rating Scale (GSRS)* is a questionnaire used to assess the presence and severity of various gastrointestinal symptoms, and is used in various clinical settings, including evaluating the gastrointestinal tolerance of treatments or interventions. It's a disease-specific instrument, typically with 15 items that are grouped into five symptom dimensions: Reflux (including heartburn and acid reflux), abdominal pain (covers pain or discomfort in the upper abdomen or stomach), indigestion (including rumbling, bloating, burping, and flatulence), diarrhea (assesses diarrhea, loose stools, and urgent need for defecation), and constipation (covers constipation, hard stools, and incomplete bowel emptying). The GSRS can be administered as a self-administered questionnaire or through an interview. It questions how individuals feel in terms of gastrointestinal problems in the last week and uses a seven-point Likert scale, where 1 represents "no discomfort" and 7 indicates "very severe discomfort". The scores are averaged within each domain and/or all items. The higher the score on the scale, the greater the severity of the symptoms [2].
- *SF-36 (Short Form Health Survey—36 items)*: Evaluates eight domains of health, including physical functioning, role-physical, bodily pain, general health, vitality, social functioning, role-emotional, and mental health. The domains can be analyzed separately or cumulatively as a physical component score (PCS) and a mental component score (MCS). Unlike individual domains, the summary scales (PCS and MCS) were demonstrated to have adequate validity in the population of patients with morbid obesity, and as such, were recom-

mended as primary endpoints in the studies of generic HRQoL after bariatric surgery [3].

- A limitation of the SF-36 is that it does not measure some obesity specific aspects, such as body image and social stigma [4].
- *WHOQOL-BREF (World Health Organization Quality of Life Questionnaire—BREF)***:** It consists of 26 items, which consider different aspects of social relationships, psychological health, physical health, and environment for determining health. The physical health domain consists of several items assessing mobility, daily activities, functional capacity, energy, pain, and sleep, while the psychological domain considers the perceived self-image, negative thoughts, positive attitudes, self-esteem, mindset, learning ability, memory, concentration, and mental state. The social relationships domain looks at personal relationships, social support, and sex life, while the environmental health field covers financial resources, safety, social and health services, the physical living environment, opportunities for learning and personal development, recreation, noise and pollution, and transportation [5, 6].
- It is a shortened form of the WHOQOL-100. Each item on this scale is scored from 1 to 5 for each response, and then they are displayed linearly on a 1–100 scale [1, 5].
- *EQ-5D (EuroQol-5D)*: A brief instrument that consists of three sections [7]:

1. In the first part, the individual must assess their health status at the time of completing the questionnaire, using five health dimensions (mobility, personal care, activities of daily living, pain/discomfort, and anxiety/depression), each with three levels of severity. In each EQ-5D dimension, severity levels are coded as 1 if the response option is "no (I have) problems"; 2 if the response option is "some or moderate problems"; and 3 if the response option is "many problems." The combination of the values from all the dimensions generates 5-digit numbers, with 243 possible combinations (health states) that can be used as profiles.
2. The second part of the EQ-5D is a 20-cm vertical visual analog scale (VAS), with millimeters, ranging from 0 (worst imaginable health) to 100 (best imaginable health). The individual must mark the point on the vertical line that best reflects their current assessment of their overall health status. The VAS provides a complementary score to the descriptive system for self-assessment of an individual's health status. This provides an index that can be used directly or combined with life years to calculate quality-adjusted life years, useful as an indicator of the outcome of interventions and, if costs are also calculated, for cost-effectiveness or cost-utility studies.
3. A third element of the EQ-5D is the index of social values obtained for each health state generated by the instrument.

   The EQ-5D was initially developed to be self-administered, meaning the subject would read, interpret, and respond to the items in a questionnaire. This is the preferred method of administration in clinical studies. However, the instrument can also be administered in a one-on-one interview or via telephone interviews [7].

20.3.2 Obesity-Specific Instruments

This tool captures the unique challenges faced by individuals with obesity:

- *IWQOL-Lite (Impact of Weight on Quality of Life—Lite)*: One of the most widely used instruments developed and validated for use in people with severe obesity. This scale consists of 31 items covering five domains: physical function, self-esteem, sexual life, public distress, and work [8]. Responses were given on a Likert scale from 1 (never true) to 5 (always true). The total score ranged from 0 to 100, with a higher score denoting a better quality of life.

20.3.3 Bariatric-Specific Instruments

Tailored for post-bariatric patients, these address surgical side effects and procedure-specific issues:

- *BAROS (Bariatric Analysis and Reporting Outcome System)*: Validated scoring system based on a combination of physician-reported outcomes (weight loss), changes in medical conditions, and patient-reported outcomes in terms of the quality of life [9]. Points are added or subtracted according to changes in these domains. Points are deducted for complications or reoperation. The total number of points defines the 5 outcome groups (failure, fair, good, very good, and excellent). Weight loss is analyzed by the percentage of total excess weight loss.
- *MA-II (Moorehead-Ardelt Quality of Life Questionnaire II)*: Included in the BAROS, six items are used for measuring a patient's subjective impression of QoL, covering general self-esteem, physical activity, social life, satisfaction concerning work, pleasure related to sexual activity, and eating behavior. Points are added or subtracted based on the patient's responses. The results of this questionnaire are then incorporated into the BAROS to determine the final score [10].
- *BQL (Bariatric Quality of Life Index)*: Designed to evaluate QoL before and after bariatric procedures [11, 12]. It consists of 30 questions divided into two sections. The first section consists of 16 items, assessing non-QoL factors including obesity-related comorbidities, gastrointestinal symptoms that are common after bariatric surgery, and medication intake. The second section consists of 14 items, assessing QoL factors with a five-point Likert scale ranging from 0 to 5 points. The BQL Index score is calculated by adding all the item scores from both sec-

tions, and ranges from 0 to 78 points, with lower scores denoting worse results [13].

20.4 Qualitative Research in Assessing the Psychosocial Impact of Bariatric Surgery

The patient's perspective on the psychosocial outcomes of bariatric surgery can also be investigated using qualitative research methods, as it can provide complementary information by exploring patients' perspectives of outcomes in greater depth to help understand complexities. Previous studies highlighted that the impact of bariatric surgery on physical health and activities of daily living was generally positive. Also reported some psychological benefits, including reduced depression and improved self-confidence; however, they also experienced challenges in establishing a new identity and acquiring new coping strategies to replace food [14].

20.5 Postoperative Quality of Life after Sleeve Gastrectomy: Evidence from Literature

20.5.1 General Trends

Most studies report significant improvements in HRQoL following SG, particularly within the first 12–24 months postoperatively, and then deteriorate again [15]. These improvements align with peak weight loss and metabolic benefits. Improvements are most notable in physical functioning, mobility, and self-esteem.

No gender-based disparities were found in QoL after bariatric surgery [5].

20.5.2 Long-Term Outcomes

Long-term data (5–10 years) are more limited but suggest that bariatric treatment seems to provide a persistent benefit in terms of HRQoL, especially its physical component score. Due to psychological predispositions, some patients appear to be less likely to benefit from bariatric treatment. QoL scores could gradually decline over time (within the initial 5–6 years after bariatric treatment), often paralleling weight regain or the emergence of new symptoms like Gastroesophageal reflux disease (GERD). However, scores generally remain better than baseline [15].

20.5.3 Comparative Studies

When compared to other bariatric procedures, such as Roux-en-Y gastric bypass (RYGB), SG shows comparable early QoL outcomes, though RYGB may show superior long-term stability in certain domains like reflux symptoms and eating satisfaction.

20.5.4 Psychological and Social Dimensions

Improvements in depression and anxiety scores are consistently reported, though not universally. Body image disturbance often persists in a subset of patients, particularly if excess skin is not surgically addressed.

20.5.5 Factors Influencing Postoperative HRQoL

Some of the factors that influence postoperative HRQoL are the weight loss magnitude, the resolution of comorbidities, the patient's psychiatric history, their social support and marital status, and the follow-up adherence.

Highly self-compassionate patients may benefit more from bariatric surgery in terms of their well-being and functioning compared to less self-compassionate patients. Higher preoperative self-compassion was associated with lower postoperative depression, greater quality of life, higher body image satisfaction, and better capability to control one's eating behavior [16].

20.6 Challenges and Limitations in HRQoL Assessment

Despite significant progress, several challenges remain:

- *Heterogeneity in measurement tools*: Comparability across studies is limited due to differing instruments.
- *Subjectivity of HRQoL*: Individual expectations and cultural context play a role in self-reporting.
- *Response bias and dropout*: Postoperative follow-up attrition affects the generalizability of findings.
- *Underrepresentation of minority groups*: Socioeconomic and ethnic disparities are rarely addressed in QoL studies.

20.7 Enhancing Postoperative Quality of Life: Future Perspectives

20.7.1 Integrated, Multidisciplinary Care Models

Long-term improvement in HRQoL requires coordinated care involving psychologists, nutritionists, physical therapists, nurses, and surgeons. Personalized follow-up pathways tailored to patient needs should be emphasized. Providing patients with holistic care would likely further improve the outcomes of bariatric treatment [15]. Providing self-compassion training for bariatric surgery candidates could also improve HRQoL afterwards [16].

Given the importance of HRQoL as a "core" outcome of bariatric surgery, it should be included as part of routinely collected bariatric surgery registry data in the therapeutic approach. It should be measured at baseline (pre-surgery) and followed up long-term post-surgery, so that clinical and HRQoL data can be considered in relation to each other. To reduce response bias, HRQoL measures should be reported directly by patients without interpretation, as they provide valuable data for evaluating the success of surgery beyond clinical evaluation [6, 14].

20.7.2 Digital Health and Remote Monitoring

Long-term success after sleeve gastrectomy depends on continuous lifestyle management, nutritional monitoring, and psychological support.

However, many patients face barriers to consistent follow-up (e.g., distance, cost, clinical access). Digital health technologies, including mobile apps, wearable devices, and telemedicine platforms, can track physical activity, mood, and dietary habits, providing innovative solutions for real-time feedback and timely remote postoperative care interventions [17].

20.7.3 Body Contouring and Cosmetic Surgery

After sleeve gastrectomy, patients often experience massive weight loss, which, while beneficial for health, can result in excess skin and loss of tissue elasticity. This is especially noticeable in the abdomen, arms, thighs, breasts, and face.

To address these changes, body contouring procedures and cosmetic surgery are frequently sought to improve appearance, body image, comfort, self-esteem, sexual satisfaction, and quality of life [18].

20.7.4 Mental Health Screening and Interventions

Mental health plays a critical role in both short- and long-term outcomes after gastrectomy. Patients undergo deep lifestyle, hormonal, and psychological changes that can influence their eating behaviors, body image, mood regulation, risk of maladaptive coping, and quality of life. Preoperative and postoperative psychological evaluations, alongside targeted therapies, can mitigate risks of depression, anxiety, or eating disorders among others [19].

20.7.5 Patient-Centered Outcome Measures

Future research should focus on developing and validating patient-derived HRQoL instruments that reflect individual values, cultural differences, and surgical expectations.

20.8 Conclusion

Sleeve gastrectomy significantly improves the quality of life in most patients, particularly in the short to mid-term postoperative period. The measurement of HRQoL is complex and multifaceted, necessitating standardized yet flexible tools that consider both objective outcomes and subjective experiences. As bariatric surgery evolves from purely weight-centric to patient-centered care, understanding and optimizing HRQoL must remain a central focus of clinical practice and research.

References

1. World Health Organization (WHO). WHOQOL: measuring quality of life [Internet]. 2025 [cited 2025 Oct 28]. Available from: https://www.who.int/tools/whoqol
2. Borhan K, Arslan DE. The effect of gastrointestinal symptoms on the quality of life of patients hospitalized in internal medicine service. Int J Caring Sci. 2024;17(2):951–9.
3. Karlsen TI, Tveitå EK, Natvig GK, Tonstad S, Hjelmesæth J. Validity of the SF-36 in patients with morbid obesity. Obes Facts. 2011;4(5):346–51. https://doi.org/10.1159/000333406.
4. Duval K, Marceau P, Pérusse L, Lacasse Y. An overview of obesity-specific quality of life questionnaires. Obes Rev. 2006;7(4):347–60. https://doi.org/10.1111/j.1467-789X.2006.00244.x.
5. Monga V, Chauhan M. Gender differences in quality of life and depression among post-bariatric surgery patients. Ann Neurosci. 2025:09727531251352630. https://doi.org/10.1177/09727531251352630.
6. Soroceanu RP, Timofte DV, Danila R, Timofeiov S, Livadariu R, Miler AA, et al. The impact of bariatric surgery on quality of life in patients with obesity. J Clin Med. 2023;12(13):4225. https://doi.org/10.3390/jcm12134225.
7. Herdman M, Badia X, Berra S. El EuroQol-5D: una alternativa sencilla para la medición de la calidad de vida relacionada con la salud en atención primaria. Aten Primaria. 2013;28(6):425.
8. Kolotkin RL, Crosby RD, Kosloski KD, Williams GR. Development of a brief measure to assess quality of life in obesity. Obes Res. 2001;9(2):102–11. https://doi.org/10.1038/oby.2001.13.
9. Oria HE, Moorehead MK. Bariatric analysis and reporting outcome system (BAROS). Obes Surg. 1998;8(5):487–99. https://doi.org/10.1381/096089298765554043.
10. Myers JA, Clifford JC, Sarker S, Primeau M, Doninger GL, Shayani V. J Soc Laparoendosc Surg. 2006;10(4):414.
11. Weiner S, Sauerland S, Fein M, Blanco R, Pomhoff I, Weiner RA. The bariatric quality of life (BQL) index: a measure of Well-being in obesity surgery patients. Obes Surg. 2005;15(4):538–45. https://doi.org/10.1381/0960892053723439.
12. Weiner S, Sauerland S, Weiner R, Cyzewski M, Brandt J, Neugebauer E. Validation of the adapted Bariatric Quality of Life Index (BQL) in a prospective study in 446 bariatric patients as one-factor model. Obes Facts. 2009;2(Suppl 1):63. https://doi.org/10.1159/000198263.

13. Jirapinyo P, Dayyeh BKA, Thompson CC. Weight regain after Roux-en-Y gastric bypass has a large negative impact on the bariatric quality of life index. BMJ Open Gastroenterol. 2017;4(1):e000153. https://doi.org/10.1136/bmjgast-2017-000153.
14. Coulman KD, Blazeby JM. Health-related quality of life in bariatric and metabolic surgery. Curr Obes Rep. 2020;9(3):307–14. https://doi.org/10.1007/s13679-020-00392-z.
15. Sierżantowicz R, Ładny JR, Lewko J. Quality of life after bariatric surgery – a systematic review. Int J Environ Res Public Health. 2022;19(15):9078. https://doi.org/10.3390/ijerph19159078.
16. Pyykkö JE, Aydin Ö, Gerdes VE, Acherman YI, Groen AK, van de Laar AW, et al. Psychological functioning and well-being before and after bariatric surgery; what is the benefit of being self-compassionate? Br J Health Psychol. 2022;27(1):96–115. https://doi.org/10.1111/bjhp.12532.
17. Farinella E, Koliakos N, Papakonstantinou D, Breuer N, Pau L, Poras M, et al. The utilisation of digital applications for measuring patient outcomes following bariatric surgery: a systematic review and meta-analysis of comparative studies. Obes Surg. 2024;34(2):635–42. https://doi.org/10.1007/s11695-023-07000-8.
18. Dalaei F, De Vries CE, Poulsen L, Möller S, Kaur MN, Dijkhorst PJ, et al. Body contouring surgery after bariatric surgery improves long-term health-related quality of life and satisfaction with appearance: an international longitudinal cohort study using the BODY-Q. Ann Surg. 2024;279(6):1008–17. https://doi.org/10.1097/SLA.0000000000006244.
19. Albadareen B, AlBadareen A. Is bariatric surgery a crime? A systematic review and meta-analysis of postoperative psychiatric symptoms and eating disorders. Clin Obes. 2025;15(5):e70017. https://doi.org/10.1111/cob.70017.

Economic Impact of Multidisciplinary Management of Sleeve Gastrectomy

21

Alfonso Higueras

Patients with obesity, regardless of the type of intervention performed, the reason for admission, or the surgical protocol applied, generate a significantly higher consumption of resources than the general population [1]. This patient profile demands a very high volume of outpatient, inpatient, and pharmacological services, which can strain the sustainability of the healthcare system [2]. This chapter analyzes bariatric surgeries, and especially sleeve gastrectomy, from the perspective of the economic savings they can produce. These savings derive primarily from the improvement or resolution of comorbidities, making these interventions economically efficient procedures with clear value when performed early, beyond the direct clinical benefits.

In 1995, the FDA (Food and Drug Administration) indicated that the cost of surgery was approximately half the cost of medical treatment for each pound of weight lost [3]. Since then, numerous studies have consistently shown that bariatric surgery is a cost-effective strategy for obesity. It is important to remember that this is a tertiary prevention measure, focused on reducing complications and mitigating the high costs associated with these patients. Most of the literature concludes that surgery involves a higher initial cost but offers better results in terms of weight loss, comorbidity management, survival, and quality of life. Only one study conducted in the United Kingdom in patients with diabetes mellitus showed that, after 5 years, the surgical intervention was more expensive [4], in addition to two studies by Maciejewski ML et al. and Weiner JP et al. that did not identify a clear economic benefit in bariatric surgery programs [5, 6]. However, these authors do highlight economic advantages derived from the improvement of specific obesity-related pathologies, such as diabetes and osteoarthritis [7].

A. Higueras (✉)
Universidad Alfonso X el Sabio: Villanueva de la Canada, Comunidad de Madrid, Madrid, Spain

J. Ruiz-Tovar (ed.), *Multidisciplinary Management of Sleeve Gastrectomy*,
https://doi.org/10.1007/978-3-032-25644-7_21

A significant limitation in interpreting these results is the difficulty of comparing costs between countries. Most available economic analyses come from the United States, whose highly private healthcare system with significantly higher costs differs entirely from the European model based on the universal right to healthcare. Within Europe, there is also considerable variability [8], both in the funding structure and in the number of procedures performed per million inhabitants. For a perspective more aligned with public systems, it is particularly useful to review studies from the United Kingdom, whose National Health Service (NHS) operates under the recommendations of the National Institute for Health and Care Excellence (NICE), whose recommendations are binding at the national level. The NHS classifies bariatric surgery as a cost-effective intervention, setting a maximum threshold of £30,000, while the reference value used by the European Community is considerably lower, at £6289 [9].

Currently, a comparative analysis between GLP-1 receptor agonists and bariatric surgery is needed, including techniques such as sleeve gastrectomy and Roux-en-Y gastric bypass. Although studies present significant limitations, such as variability in clinical practice, individual treatment costs across different insurance systems, and insufficient long-term cost assessments, GLP-1 agonists have been shown to generate cumulative costs related to the time required to reach maximum efficacy, as well as the risk of weight regain after treatment discontinuation [40]. Evidence clearly shows that surgical intervention for obesity is superior to conventional medical treatment. However, surgery requires a considerable initial outlay, leading some authors to question the possibility of recouping this investment during the patient's lifetime [10], an aspect that may be overlooked in the literature due to survival bias. Even so, most economic evaluations agree that the long-term savings generated in both direct costs, such as reduced medication use, and indirect costs, such as work absences associated with obesity, result in a net benefit for surgery, solidifying its status as a cost-effective measure [11, 12]. Several studies even estimate that the cost of the procedure can be recouped within 2–4 years [13, 14], especially in individuals with comorbidities such as diabetes mellitus [15, 16]. According to the analysis by Borisenko et al. [17], Roux-en-Y gastric bypass would be the option with the highest economic return, and its hypothetical replacement with sleeve gastrectomy or another type of bypass would entail a loss in both quality-adjusted life years (QALYs) and economic efficiency [7].

21.1 What Costs Should be Analyzed to Assess the Economic Impact of Sleeve Gastrectomy?

To properly assess the economic impact of surgical obesity treatment, it is essential to first identify the actual cost of the procedures based on the strongest available evidence. This task presents significant challenges, as the associated costs vary widely depending on the healthcare system and funding model. In the United States, for example, published studies show highly disparate figures: Snow et al. estimate a cost of $8090 [18], Sinha et al. place it at $17,400 [19], Medicare data show a cost of $20,948 [20], and Morton et al. describe a cost of up to $25,000 for laparoscopic surgery [21]. In Spain, the analysis by Sánchez-Ramos et al. calculates an average cost of €7468 for bariatric surgery [22], slightly exceeding €10,000 for laparoscopic techniques [4].

Two years after the intervention, surgery directly reduces medication use associated with the most common pathologies, as well as other difficult-to-control costs. In Spain, Rodicio et al. estimate that the savings generated per patient undergoing surgery are around €1822, regardless of pre-existing comorbidities [7]. The conceptual framework to consider regarding costs includes:

- Direct costs (hospitalization, surgery, medication, complications).
- Indirect costs (absenteeism, productivity, disability).
- Long-term costs avoided through improved comorbidity management.
- Intangible costs (pain, quality of life, autonomy).

Furthermore, the economic analysis can be segmented by obesity-related pathologies. For example, the study by Gould et al. [23] shows that the prevalence of hypertension, which reached 46% before surgery, decreases to 10% after the intervention. This data has a significant impact on the National Health System (NHS), given that hypertension accounts for 3.5% of direct healthcare expenditure [24], and that 70% of this cost corresponds to medication [25]. In line with this is the study by Rodicio et al. They calculated annual savings of €734 per patient with obesity and hypertension [7], a figure very similar to official public administration data, which place the annual cost per patient at €1312, of which €894 corresponds specifically to medication costs related to this condition.

In the study by Gould et al. [23], diabetes affected 26% of patients before surgery, reducing this proportion to 4% after the intervention. In the Spanish context, diabetes represents 7% of total NHS healthcare expenditure [26], with 15% of this cost directly related to medication [27]. In the series by Rodicio et al., the annual savings in medication consumption for type 2 diabetes was estimated at €243 per patient with obesity and T2DM [7], figures very close to those reported by the public administration, which calculates an average cost per patient/year of €1770, including €265 of annual pharmaceutical expenditure [28]. Long-term studies (more than 15 years of follow-up) recommend prioritizing bariatric surgery programs in people with diabetes [29], due to the high number of comorbidities and the progressive deterioration of pancreatic function.

Regarding dyslipidemia, data from Gould et al. [23] show a reduction in its prevalence from 23% before surgery to just 3% afterward. In Spain, Rodicio et al. estimated annual savings of €250 in lipid-lowering drugs per patient with obesity and dyslipidemia [7].

As for obstructive sleep apnea-hypopnea syndrome (OSAHS), Rodicio et al. describe a pre-surgical prevalence of 58% and annual savings of €675 in therapeutic devices per patient with obesity and OSAHS [7].

With respect to depression, Rodicio et al. report a prevalence of 40% before surgery, which decreases to 3% after the procedure, with annual savings of €358 in antidepressant use [7]. Other previous studies, published in 2010, estimate savings of up to €1000 per year [30].

For other obesity-related conditions such as cancer, cardiovascular disease, and osteoarticular diseases, economic evidence is limited due to the complexity of their measurement and the heterogeneity of the available data. Even so, a favorable economic impact of bariatric surgery has been observed in all of these conditions.

Indirect costs, including lost workdays, absenteeism, permanent disability, and functional limitations, as well as intangible costs related to pain, discomfort, or suffering, and the additional consumption of healthcare resources, have not been considered in this analysis.

21.2 What Modifications Could Improve the Economic Impact of Sleeve Gastrectomy?

The Portuguese study by Faria et al. [31], which focused particularly on promoting bariatric surgery in young patients and at early stages, showed that from a cost-saving perspective, the benefits are extraordinary, with the intervention described by Snow et al. [18] recouping its costs in less than 22 months.

From another perspective, Nguyen et al. [32] suggested that relaxing access criteria based on the number of comorbidities could reduce annual healthcare spending by $2016. In line with this situation of patients with multiple pathologies, Rodicio et al. [7] calculated annual savings of €2115 for individuals undergoing surgery with five obesity-related comorbidities.

When pharmacological savings are analyzed as justification, the results are also diverse. Some authors indicate that the accumulated pharmaceutical expenditure during the waiting list (average of 22 months) exceeds the cost of the surgical intervention [18], while others have detected an increase in medication expenditure 6 years post-surgery [33]. Most frequently, however, a reduction in pharmacological treatment is observed in most comorbidities, although more complex pathologies such as depression do not always show this trend [34]. On average, surgery reduces the number of medications per patient by two [35]. Other analyses place the point at which pharmaceutical savings exceed the initial cost of surgery at 7 years [32]. Although preventive medication is more intensive in the first months after surgery, it is subsequently reduced and usually limited to vitamins and minerals, representing minimal expenditure.

Given the heterogeneity of patients and the complexity of obesity, it follows that sleeve gastrectomy offers a significant economic benefit due to the reduction in the use of medications and devices. Consequently, it seems reasonable to implement policies aimed at shortening waiting lists and facilitating access to surgery for patients refractory to medical treatment [36, 37]. This recommendation is controversial due to the marked territorial, economic, and political variability in access to this surgery [7]. Minimally invasive sleeve gastrectomy remains the most widely used technique in bariatric and metabolic surgery, and its performance using robotic platforms such as the da Vinci system has progressively increased despite the still limited evidence comparing both approaches. Although robotic surgery presents equivalent results in terms of operative time, postoperative CRP, and 30-day complications, it is associated with a significantly shorter hospital stay, with a higher percentage of discharges on the first night. In economic terms, the total cost of consumables was significantly lower in the robotic group (£2310) compared to the laparoscopic group (£2665), suggesting a direct advantage in material costs. Furthermore, the learning curve for the robot-assisted procedure was relatively short, estimated at 26 cases. Taken together, these findings indicate that fourth-generation robotic sleeve gastrectomy is safe, effective, and potentially advantageous both for its impact on hospital efficiency and for the reduction of direct costs [41].

Most economic studies conclude that bariatric surgery generates long-term savings in both direct and indirect costs, establishing it as a cost-effective intervention [11, 12, 38]. In the Spanish context, it is also considered a relatively low-investment surgery with superior clinical outcomes, so that, although the initial cost is high, it is usually recovered over the patient's lifetime [7, 39]. Only a few studies [5, 6, 10] do not observe significant improvements in overall cost-effectiveness, proposing to segment the patients who benefit the most due to the burden of associated comorbidities.

The main drivers of the economic benefit of sleeve gastrectomy are: (a) the sustained reduction in pharmaceutical spending, especially relevant in diabetes and hypertension; (b) the decrease in avoidable hospitalizations associated with metabolic decompensation; and (c) the gain in QALYs derived from improvements in functionality, quality of life, and survival. This last component, despite not generating a direct accounting savings, substantially increases the total economic value of the intervention.

One of the most striking paradoxes that emerges from this review is that, although bariatric surgery is one of the most cost-effective interventions in modern medicine, it remains underutilized in most European healthcare systems. This imbalance between evidence and actual practice reveals more of an organizational than a clinical problem.

References

1. Mason RJ, Moroney JR, Berne TV. The cost of obesity for nonbariatric inpatient operative procedures in the United States: national cost estimates obese versus nonobese patients. Ann Surg. 2013;258(4):541–51. e553
2. Lobo F. Polıticas publicas para la promocion de la alimentacion saludable y la prevencion de la obesidad. Rev Esp Salud Publica. 2007;81(5):437–41. 256. CHAPTER 22 Economic impact of malabsorptive procedures
3. Martin LF, Tan TL, Horn JR, Bixler EO, Kauffman GL, Becker DA, et al. Comparison of the costs associated with medical and surgical treatment of obesity. Surgery. 1995;118(4):599–606. 606–607
4. Anselmino M, Bammer T, Fernandez Cebrian JM, Daoud F, Romagnoli G, Torres A. Cost-effectiveness and budget impact of obesity surgery in patients with type 2 diabetes in three European countries(II). Obes Surg. 2009;19(11):1542–9.

5. Maciejewski ML, Livingston EH, Smith VA, Kahwati LC, Henderson WG, Arterburn DE. Health expenditures among high-risk patients after gastric bypass and matched controls. Arch Surg. 2012;147(7):633–40.
6. Weiner JP, Goodwin SM, Chang H-Y, Bolen SD, Richards TM, Johns RA, et al. Impact of bariatric surgery on health care costs of obese persons: a 6- year follow-up of surgical and comparison cohorts using health plan data. JAMA Surg. 2013;148(6):555–62.
7. Rodicio JL, Alonso JF, Moreno M, Rizzo A, Turienzo E, Gonzalez JJ, et al. Evaluacion economica del tratamiento quirurgico de la obesidad. Cirugıa Espanola. 2020;98(7):381–8. https://doi.org/10.1016/j.ciresp.2020.01.001.
8. Borisenko O, Colpan Z, Dillemans B, Funch-Jensen P, Hedenbro J, Ahmed AR. Clinical indications, utilization, and funding of bariatric surgery in Europe. Obes Surg. 2015;25(8):1408–16.
9. Clegg A, Colquitt J, Sidhu M, Royle P, Walker A. Clinical and cost effectiveness of surgery for morbid obesity: a systematic review and economic evaluation. Int J Obes. 2003;27(10):1167–77.
10. Wang MC, Guo XH, Zhang YW, Zhang YL, Zhang HH, Zhang YC. Laparoscopic Roux-en-Y gastric bypass versus sleeve gastrectomy for obese patients with type 2 diabetes: a meta-analysis of randomized controlled trials. Am Surg. 2015;81(2):166–71.
11. Paxton JH, Matthews JB. The cost effectiveness of laparoscopic versus open gastric bypass surgery. Obes Surg. 2005;15(1):24–34.
12. Craig BM, Tseng DS. Cost-effectiveness of gastric bypass for severe obesity. Am J Med. 2002;113(6):491–8.
13. Cremieux P-Y, Buchwald H, Shikora SA, Ghosh A, Yang HE, Buessing M. A study on the economic impact of bariatric surgery. Am J Manag Care. 2008;14(9):589–96.
14. Klein S, Ghosh A, Cremieux PY, Eapen S, McGavock TJ. Economic impact of the clinical benefits of bariatric surgery in diabetes patients with BMI 35 kg. Obesity. 2011;19(3):581–7.
15. Ikramuddin S, Klingman D, Swan T, Minshall ME. Cost-effectiveness of Roux-en-Y gastric bypass in type 2 diabetes patients. Am J Manag Care. 2009;15(9):607–15.
16. Hoerger TJ, Zhang P, Segel JE, Kahn HS, Barker LE, Couper S. Cost- effectiveness of bariatric surgery for severely obese adults with diabetes. Diabetes Care. 2010;33(9):1933–9.
17. Borisenko O, Adam D, Funch-Jensen P, Ahmed AR, Zhang R, Colpan Z, et al. Bariatric surgery can lead to net cost savings to health care systems: results from a comprehensive European decision analytic model. Obes Surg. 2015;25(9):1559–68.
18. Snow LL, Weinstein LS, Hannon JK, Lane DR, Ringold FG, Hansen PA, et al. The effect of Roux-en-Y gastric bypass on prescription drug costs. Obes Surg. 2004;14(8):1031–5.
19. Sinha AC, Singh PM, Bhat S. Are we operating too late? Mortality analysis and stochastic simulation of costs associated with bariatric surgery: reconsidering the BMI threshold. Obes Surg. 2015;26(1):219–28.
20. Flum DR, Kwon S, MacLeod K, Wang B, Alfonso-Cristancho R, Garrison LP, et al. The use, safety and cost of bariatric surgery before and after medicare's national coverage decision. Ann Surg. 2011;254(6):860–5.
21. Morton J, Brethauer S, Ponce J, Rosenthal R, Nguyen N. Bariatric surgery reduces national healthcare utilization in the long-term. Surg Obes Relat Dis. 2015;11(6):S3–4.
22. Sanchez-Santos R, Sabench Pereferrer F, Estevez Fernandez S, del Castillo Dejardin D, Vilarrasa N, Frutos Bernal D, et al. Es rentable operar a los obesos morbidos en tiempos de crisis? Analisis coste-beneficio de la cirugıa bariatrica. Cir Esp. 2013;91(8):476–84.
23. Gould JC, Garren MJ, Starling JR. Laparoscopic gastric bypass results in decreased prescription medication costs within 6 months. J Gastrointest Surg. 2004;8(8):983–7.
24. Saez M, Barcelo MA. Coste de la hipertension arterial en Espana. Hipertens Riesgo Vasc. 2012;29(4):145–51.
25. Sicras-Mainar A, Navarro-Artieda R. Coste de la hipertension arterial segun grados de morbilidad en atencion primaria. Med Clınica. 2009;133(8):290–5.
26. Lopez-Bastida J, Boronat M, Moreno JO, Schurer W. Costs, outcomes and challenges for diabetes care in Spain. Glob Health. 2013;9:17.

27. Crespo C, Brosa M, Soria-Juan A, Lopez-Alba A, Lopez-Martınez N, Soria B. Costes directos de la diabetes mellitus y de sus complicaciones en Espana (Estudio SECCAID: Spain estimated cost Ciberdem-Cabimer in Diabetes). Av En Diabetol. 2013;29(6):182–9.
28. Sicras-Mainar A, Navarro-Artieda R. Coste de la hipertension arterial segun grados de morbilidad en atencion primaria [Cost of arterial hypertension according to levels of morbidity in primary care setting]. Med Clin. 2009;133(8):290–5. https://doi.org/10.1016/j.medcli.2009.05.017. Epub 2009 Jul 10. PMID: 19596366
29. Keating C, Neovius M, Sjoholm K, Peltonen M, Narbro K, Eriksson JK, et al. Healthcare costs over 15 years after bariatric surgery for patients with different baseline glucose status: results from the Swedish obese subjects study. Lancet Diabetes Endocrinol. 2015;3(11):855–65.
30. Sicras-Mainar A, Blanca-Tamayo M, Gutierrez-Nicuesa L, Salvatella-Pasant J, Navarro-Artieda R. Impacto de la morbilidad, uso de recursos y costes en el mantenimiento de la remision de la depresion mayor en Espana: estudio longitudinal de ambito poblacional. Gac Sanit. 2010;24(1):13–9.
31. Faria GR, Preto JR, Costa-Maia J. Gastric bypass is a cost-saving procedure: results from a comprehensive Markov model. Obes Surg. 2013;23(4):460–6.
32. Nguyen NT, Varela JE, Sabio A, Naim J, Stamos M, Wilson SE. Reduction in prescription medication costs after laparoscopic gastric bypass. Am Surg. 2006;72(10):853–6.
33. Narbro K, Agren G, Jonsson E, Naslund I, Sjostrom L, Peltonen M, et al. Pharmaceutical costs in obese individuals: comparison with a randomly selected population sample and long-term changes after conventional and surgical treatment: the SOS intervention study. Arch Intern Med. 2002;162(18):2061–9.
34. Gesquiere I, Aron-Wisnewsky J, Foulon V, Haggege S, Van derSchueren B, Augustijns P, et al. Medication cost is significantly reduced afterRoux-en-Y gastric bypass in obese patients. Obes Surg. 2014;24(11):1896–903.
35. Lopes EC, Heineck I, Athaydes G, Meinhardt NG, Souto KEP, Stein AT. Is bariatric surgery effective in reducing comorbidities and drug costs? A systematic review and metaanalysis. Obes Surg. 2015;25(9):1741–9. 258. CHAPTER 22 Economic impact of malabsorptive procedures
36. Christou NV, Efthimiou E. Bariatric surgery waiting times in Canada. Can J Surg J Can Chir. 2009;52(3):229–34.
37. Padwal R, Klarenbach S, Wiebe N, Hazel M, Birch D, Karmali S, et al. Bariatric surgery: a systematic review of the clinical and economic evidence. J Gen Intern Med. 2011;26(10):1183–94.
38. Picot J, Jones J, Colquitt JL, Gospodarevskaya E, Loveman E, Baxter L, et al. The clinical effectiveness and cost-effectiveness of bariatric (weight loss) surgery for obesity: a systematic review and economic evaluation. Health Technol Assess. 2009;13(41):1–190. 215–357
39. Buchwald H, Estok R, Fahrbach K, Banel D, Jensen MD, Pories WJ, et al. Weight and type 2 diabetes after bariatric surbgery: systematic review and meta-analysis. Am J Med. 2009;122(3):248–56.
40. Docimo S Jr, Shah J, Warren G, Ganam S, Sujka J, DuCoin C. A cost comparison of GLP-1 receptor agonists and bariatric surgery: what is the break even point? Surg Endosc. 2024;38(11):6560–5. https://doi.org/10.1007/s00464-024-11191-1. Epub 2024 Sep 16. PMID: 39285034
41. van Boxel GI, Straatman J, Carter NC, Glaysher MA, Fajksova V. Robotic-assisted sleeve gastrectomy: an analysis of cost, peri-operative outcomes and learning curve in a prospective cohort study. J Robot Surg. 2025;19(1):193. https://doi.org/10.1007/s11701-025-02348-8. PMID: 40316868

Part IV

Mechanism of Action of Sleeve Gastrectomy and Challenges

Hormonal and Biochemical Changes After Sleeve Gastrectomy

22

Inés Macías-Gamero

22.1 Introduction

Sleeve gastrectomy (SG) has emerged over the past two decades as the most performed bariatric procedure worldwide [1]. Originally it was thought of as a purely restrictive operation, but its clinical outcomes have consistently exceeded expectations. Patients have been shown to experience rapid improvements in type 2 diabetes, mellitus, dyslipidaemia, hypertension, and systemic inflammation, sometimes preceding significant weight loss [2, 3]. These observations suggest that SG functions not only as a restrictive procedure but also as a metabolic intervention.

The resection of the gastric fundus, a major source of **ghrelin**, alters appetite regulation and energy balance [4]. In addition, the accelerated gastric emptying enhances the secretion of incretin hormones such as **glucagon-like peptide-1 (GLP-1)** and **peptide YY (PYY)**, which further modulate satiety and glucose homeostasis [5]. Beyond hormonal adaptations, SG induces favourable shifts in insulin sensitivity, lipid metabolism, adipokine profiles, and inflammatory markers [2, 6]. But unfortunately, the operation carries a risk of nutritional deficiencies that require careful biochemical monitoring [7, 8].

Understanding the hormonal and biochemical consequences of sleeve gastrectomy is essential to be able to understand its mechanisms of action and to optimise patient care. This chapter reviews the key endocrine and biochemical changes following SG, their clinical implications, and areas of ongoing investigation.

I. Macías-Gamero (✉)
Vascular Pathology Laboratory, Hospital Fundación Jiménez Díaz, Madrid, Spain

J. Ruiz-Tovar (ed.), *Multidisciplinary Management of Sleeve Gastrectomy*,
https://doi.org/10.1007/978-3-032-25644-7_22

22.2 Physiological Basis of Sleeve Gastrectomy

Sleeve gastrectomy involves a **longitudinal resection of approximately 80%** of the stomach (Fig. 22.1), extending from the antrum to the esophagogastric junction, removing the side along the greater curvature. This results in the creation of a tubular gastric remnant with reduced capacity (100–150 mL) [9].

The anatomical modification has several important consequences beyond mechanical restriction. The excision of the gastric fundus eliminates the principal site of ghrelin production, reducing circulating levels of this orexigenic hormone [2, 5]. The altered gastric geometry also accelerates gastric emptying, increasing the early delivery of nutrients to the small intestine and stimulating enteroendocrine L-cells in the distal ileum [2]. This leads to augmented secretion of hormones such as glucagon-like peptide-1 (GLP-1) and peptide YY (PYY), which modulate appetite, insulin release, and satiety (Fig. 22.1) [3].

Additionally, the removal of a large portion of acid-secreting parietal cells affects gastric pH and can have potential downstream effects on nutrient absorption and bile acid metabolism [7]. Changes in gut motility and bile acid circulation further contribute to metabolic improvements, particularly in glucose and lipid homeostasis (Fig. 22.1) [2, 5].

In sum, the physiological alterations induced by sleeve gastrectomy extend beyond the reduction of gastric volume. They establish the foundation for the

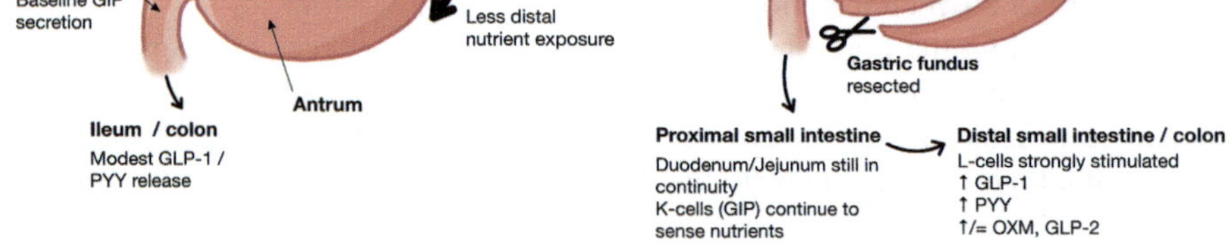

Fig. 22.1 Anatomy and nutrient flow before and after sleeve gastrectomy. The left schematic shows the normal stomach with an intact ghrelin-producing fundus and relatively slower gastric emptying, leading to predominant nutrient exposure of the proximal small intestine (duodenum/jejunum, K-cells; GIP secretion) and only modest stimulation of distal L-cells (GLP-1, PYY). The right schematic illustrates the post–sleeve gastrectomy anatomy, with resection of the fundus (↓ ghrelin) and creation of a narrow tubular stomach. Accelerated gastric emptying results in more rapid delivery of nutrients to the distal ileum and colon, enhancing L-cell stimulation and increasing postprandial GLP-1 and PYY secretion, while the proximal small intestine remains in continuity and GIP-secreting K-cells continue to be stimulated. Oxyntomodulin (OXM) and GLP-2 may also increase postprandially, although evidence in SG is more limited

hormonal and biochemical adaptations that underpin the procedure's efficacy in weight loss and metabolic disease resolution.

22.3 Hormonal Changes

22.3.1 Ghrelin

Ghrelin is an orexigenic hormone (stimulates appetite) secreted primarily by the X/A-like cells located in the gastric fundus. It circulates in two main forms: acylated ghrelin, the biologically active isoform that binds to the growth hormone secretagogue receptor (GHS-R1a), and des-acyl ghrelin, whose physiological role remains less clearly defined. Des-acyl ghrelin was originally considered as an inactive form of ghrelin, but recent studies have proved that it may have diverse biological roles [10, 11]. Beyond its main function in stimulating appetite, ghrelin also has roles in stimulating growth hormone (GH) secretion, enhancing gastric motility, and contributes to energy homeostasis [12].

After sleeve gastrectomy, most studies report a significant reduction in fasting ghrelin levels postoperatively. This is due to the removal of the gastric fundus, which is the major ghrelin source [2, 4]. This decrease is believed to contribute to the early postoperative reduction in hunger and food intake frequently observed after SG [13, 14]. Ghrelin levels may exhibit a partial rebound; however, they generally remain lower than preoperative values even in the long term [4, 14].

In some comparative studies, SG appears to induce a greater reduction in fasting and postprandial ghrelin than **Roux-en-Y gastric bypass (RYGB)**, likely reflecting the more extensive fundic resection, although other cohorts report smaller or inconsistent results between the different procedures [15–18]. Some studies have suggested associations between postoperative ghrelin changes and weight loss after SG, whereas others report that weight loss and metabolic improvement occur largely independently of ghrelin dynamics, indicating that ghrelin is only one of several contributors to the procedure's benefits [14, 18, 19].

However, when interpreting ghrelin levels after SG, we should consider several methodological and physiological nuances. Reported results vary among studies; this is most probably largely due to differences in measurement protocols, such as the timing of the sampling relative to the surgery, fasting versus postprandial conditions, and whether acylated, des-acyl, or total ghrelin concentrations were assessed [18, 19]. It should also be considered that the acylated form of ghrelin is unstable and prone to rapid deacylation ex vivo, making it a requirement to handle samples meticulously and stabilise them to ensure reliable quantification [18, 19]. These methodological inconsistencies can substantially influence reported values and complicate interstudy comparisons [18].

Additionally, while the gastric fundus is the dominant source of ghrelin, smaller amounts are also synthesised in extra-gastric tissues such as the duodenum, pancreas, and hypothalamus [20]. The persistence of these minor sources or even the potential compensatory upregulation in response to the fundic resection may partially attenuate the overall decline on the ghrelin observed after SG [18, 20].

More recent studies have highlighted the importance of considering ghrelin's regulators, particularly **liver-expressed antimicrobial peptide 2 (LEAP2)**. This peptide is an endogenous ghrelin receptor antagonist [21]. Alterations in the ghrelin-LEAP2 axis following bariatric surgery are emerging as a novel area of investigation, with potential implications for understanding long-term appetite control and metabolic adaptation [21–23].

22.3.2 Incretins (GLP-1, GIP)

22.3.2.1 GLP-1 (Glucagon-Like Peptide-1)

Glucagon-like peptide-1 (GLP-1) is a potent incretin hormone secreted predominantly by enteroendocrine **L-cells** located in the distal ileum and colon in response to nutrient stimulation [24]. It carries out multiple physiological actions that contribute to postprandial glucose regulation, including stimulation of glucose-dependent insulin secretion, suppression of glucagon release, and delay of gastric emptying [24]. In addition, GLP-1 enhances satiety and reduces food intake through central mechanisms, making it an important component of the gut–brain axis in energy balance and glucose homeostasis [5, 24].

Following SG, multiple studies and a meta-analysis have shown a substantial increase in postprandial GLP-1 secretion, with higher peak concentrations and greater area under the curve compared with preoperative responses [17, 25, 26]. By contrast, fasting GLP-1 concentrations usually change little or remain inconsistent, and many studies report no significant difference from baseline despite the clearly augmented postprandial response [25]. This exaggerated postprandial GLP-1 secretion appears within days to weeks after surgery, before substantial weight loss has occurred, indicating that it is driven largely by altered gastric emptying, nutrient transit, and more rapid delivery of chyme to the distal small intestine [17, 26].

Enhanced GLP-1 activity is widely considered a central mechanism underlying the rapid improvement in glycaemic control and insulin sensitivity observed after SG [3, 24, 26]. Increased nutrient exposure to the distal gut accelerates L-cell stimulation, thereby amplifying the incretin (GLP-1) response and improving β-cell glucose sensitivity [24–26]. Recent mechanistic work using selective incretin receptor blockade has shown that, after SG, pharmacological GLP-1 receptor antagonism impairs β-cell function and worsens postprandial glucose tolerance, underscoring the importance of endogenous GLP-1 in the postoperative state [27]. Overall, the potentiation of GLP-1 signalling represents one of the key endocrine adaptations contributing to the metabolic efficacy of SG [24, 26, 27].

22.3.2.2 GIP (Glucose-Dependent Insulinotropic Peptide)

Glucose-dependent insulinotropic peptide (GIP), another principal incretin hormone, is secreted by **K-cells** located predominantly in the mucosa of the proximal small intestine, especially the duodenum and jejunum [24, 28]. Like GLP-1, GIP enhances glucose-stimulated insulin secretion, but it responds primarily to nutrient ingestion rich in carbohydrates and fats. Beyond its incretin action, GIP influences lipid metabolism and may modulate adipocyte function and bone remodelling [24, 28].

The impact of SG on circulating GIP concentrations has been less consistent and less extensively characterised than that observed for GLP-1 [25–27]. A systematic review and meta-analysis found no significant overall change in fasting GIP levels after SG, suggesting that basal secretion remains relatively stable despite major changes in gastric anatomy [25]. Other mechanistic studies have identified modest or variable alterations in postprandial GIP responses; however, these effects are generally smaller and less consistent than the robust GLP-1 surge typically observed after metabolic bariatric surgery [26, 27].

Recent work using selective incretin receptor blockade has provided further insight. After SG, pharmacological GIP receptor antagonism reduces β-cell glucose sensitivity and worsens postprandial glucose tolerance, indicating that GIP continues to contribute meaningfully to the incretin effect in the SG setting [27]. Nevertheless, the long-term behaviour of GIP after SG remains incompletely defined, and its contribution to postoperative metabolic improvements appears more modest than that of GLP-1 [24, 25, 27, 28].

Interpretation of GIP dynamics after sleeve gastrectomy (SG) should be cautious. Unlike Roux-en-Y gastric bypass (RYGB), SG leaves the proximal small intestine in continuity, so the duodenum and jejunum remain fully exposed to ingested nutrients [3, 9]. As a result, the main anatomical stimulus for K-cell activation is largely unchanged, which likely explains why reported changes in GIP secretion after SG are generally small or variable compared with the more pronounced GLP-1 responses driven by enhanced distal gut stimulation [3, 9]. In addition, the relative contributions of GLP-1 and GIP to improved glycaemic control and insulin sensitivity after SG are not fully defined. Enhanced GLP-1 secretion is consistently implicated as a major driver of postoperative metabolic benefits, whereas the role of GIP appears more modest and context-dependent, varying with β-cell responsiveness, nutrient composition, and time since surgery [24, 25, 27].

22.3.3 Peptide YY (PYY)

Peptide YY (PYY) is an anorexigenic gut hormone secreted predominantly by enteroendocrine **L-cells** located in the distal small intestine and colon in response to nutrient exposure, particularly to fat and protein, during the postprandial period [29–31]. Circulating PYY exists mainly in two biologically active forms, PYY_{1-36} and PYY_{3-36}; the latter is generated by dipeptidyl peptidase-4 cleavage of PYY_{1-36} and is the principal isoform implicated in appetite regulation [30, 32]. PYY_{3-36} acts primarily via Y_2 receptors in the hypothalamus and brainstem to promote satiety, reduce food intake, and slow gastric emptying, thereby contributing to the regulation of meal size and overall energy balance [29, 32, 33].

After SG, several prospective studies and a systematic review have demonstrated on average significant increases in postprandial PYY concentrations compared with preoperative levels, although the magnitude of this response shows substantial inter-individual and inter-study variability [17, 25, 34]. In many cohorts, these elevations manifest predominantly as higher postprandial peaks rather than consistent changes in fasting concentrations, whereas in others modest fasting changes have also been reported [32, 34, 35]. The elevated PYY response is generally interpreted as a consequence of accelerated nutrient delivery to more distal intestinal segments and enhanced stimulation of L-cells, in line with broader evidence on post-bariatric nutrient handling [31, 35, 36]. This endocrine adaptation is thought to contribute, together with other gut hormones, to the heightened satiety and reduced caloric intake commonly reported after SG [25, 34, 35].

Longer-term follow-ups suggest that an enhanced postprandial PYY response can persist for at least 6–12 months after SG, with some studies indicating maintenance beyond the first postoperative year, although partial attenuation over time has been observed in certain cohorts and in individuals with significant weight regain [25, 35, 37, 38]. Overall, PYY responses after SG frequently remain higher than preoperative values at medium-term follow-up, but the extent and durability of these elevations are variable [35, 36, 38, 39].

The interpretation of PYY dynamics after SG requires consideration of several methodological and physiological factors. Some studies have reported associations between the magnitude of postoperative PYY elevation and clinical outcomes such as weight loss or subjective satiety ratings, supporting a potential mechanistic contribution of PYY to behavioural adaptations and sustained negative energy balance [34, 38]. However, these associations are not universal, and other cohorts show weak or absent correlations [38, 39]. Considerable inter-study heterogeneity arises from differences in experimental design, including timing of sampling (fasting vs postprandial), test-meal composition and caloric load, and assay characteristics (e.g., total vs PYY_{3-36} measurement), all of which can influence the reported magnitude of change [25, 32, 34].

Moreover, PYY does not act in isolation; it shares a common L-cell origin with GLP-1, and research has shown concurrent rises in PYY and GLP-1 after bariatric procedures (including SG) with the two hormones likely acting in tandem to enhance satiety and slow gastric emptying [17, 31, 35]. Nonetheless, the strength of the correlation between PYY and GLP-1 responses varies across studies, and the precise temporal and mechanistic relationships between these peptides are not completely defined, stressing the complexity of enteroendocrine regulation in the post-SG state [25, 34, 36].

22.3.4 Other Gut Hormones

Beyond the major incretin and satiety hormones mentioned above, SG also modulates a broader spectrum of gastrointestinal peptides that participate in digestive regulation and metabolic adaptation. Changes in these hormones are generally more subtle and less consistently characterised than those of GLP-1 or PYY, but they form part of the wider enteroendocrine remodelling observed after bariatric surgery [34–36].

Gastrin Gastrin is secreted primarily by G-cells in the gastric antrum and stimulates gastric acid secretion and mucosal growth, while also contributing to upper gastrointestinal motility and trophic signalling [40].

After SG, postoperative studies show heterogeneous changes in circulating gastrin. In a mixed-meal study, SG was associated with modest increases in postprandial gastrin compared with presurgical values, whereas RYGB tended to reduce postprandial gastrin [41]. A prospective study of gastric biomarkers found no major hypergastrinemia at 1 year after either SG or RYGB, despite anatomical alteration of the stomach [42]. Variability among reports likely reflects differences in antral preservation, acid suppression, and gastric pH, as well as assay timing and meal composition, rather than a uniform effect of SG on gastrin secretion [40–42].

Pancreatic Polypeptide (PP) Pancreatic polypeptide (PP) is secreted by F-cells in the pancreatic islets and exocrine pancreas. It influences appetite, hepatic insulin sensitivity, and pancreatic exocrine secretion, and is strongly regulated by vagal tone [29, 32].

After SG, PP responses show only modest changes: in a study comparing RYGB and SG, fasting PP changed little and post–oral glucose PP profiles were only mildly altered, with no large or consistent differences between procedures [43].

Overall, SG does not appear to produce large, consistent shifts in basal PP, and the small postprandial changes observed have uncertain physiological significance, though they may relate to altered vagal signalling and gastric emptying [34, 43].

Obestatin Obestatin is derived from the same preproghrelin precursor as ghrelin. Early experimental work suggested anorexigenic effects and delayed gastric emptying, but its physiological relevance and receptor remain controversial, and human data are inconsistent [12, 44].

In SG patients, evidence is limited but does *not* support a strong, consistent rise in obestatin:

- In a 6-month LSG cohort, obestatin levels actually decreased postoperatively, whereas ghrelin increased slightly, in the context of ongoing calorie deficit [45].
- Other bariatric cohorts (including mixed procedures) show **small or no changes** in obestatin, and reviews emphasise the lack of robust, reproducible patterns after surgery [44, 46].

Thus, it is more accurate to state that obestatin changes after SG are inconsistent and often small, and there is currently no strong evidence that obestatin plays a major mechanistic role in SG-induced weight loss.

Oxyntomodulin (OXM) Oxyntomodulin (OXM) is co-secreted with GLP-1 and PYY from L-cells in the distal small intestine and colon. It exerts anorectic and glucoregulatory effects by activating both GLP-1 and glucagon receptors, reducing food intake and increasing energy expenditure [24, 32, 47].

Data after SG are sparse, but in broader bariatric cohorts:

- A large study of different bariatric procedures found that among nine gut hormones, postprandial OXM and glicentin showed some of the largest postoperative increases, and early OXM elevations predicted future weight loss [47].
- Reviews of OXM physiology and bariatric surgery suggest that RYGB shows strong OXM rises, while SG appears to produce more modest and variable increases, likely reflecting differences in nutrient delivery and L-cell stimulation [34, 47, 48].

Therefore, it is reasonable, but still somewhat tentative, to view OXM as a potential contributor to appetite suppression and improved glucose metabolism after SG, acting in unison with GLP-1 and PYY [34, 47, 48].

Glucagon-Like Peptide-2 (GLP-2) GLP-2 is another proglucagon-derived peptide released from L-cells, with predominantly trophic effects on the intestinal mucosa: it enhances intestinal growth, increases absorptive capacity, and improves barrier integrity [24, 49, 50].

After bariatric surgery:

- In RYGB, postprandial GLP-2 area under the curve (AUC) increases significantly and correlates with satiety measures [50].
- A dedicated review of GLP-2 in bariatric surgery concludes that GLP-2 is often elevated postprandially after metabolic procedures, but data are heterogeneous and SG-specific evidence is still limited [49].

Some exploratory work suggests similar postprandial GLP-2 increases in mixed RYGB/SG cohorts, although not all studies detect significant changes, and fasting GLP-2 is often unchanged [24, 49–51].

Thus, while GLP-2 may support intestinal adaptation and mucosal health after SG, the strength of evidence is modest and mainly extrapolated from RYGB and small SG subgroups, not large SG-only trials.

Other Peptides Secretin, vasoactive intestinal peptide (VIP), cholecystokinin (CCK), and somatostatin are rarely measured systematically in SG cohorts. Most bariatric studies either omit them or report small, inconsistent changes without clear clinical implications [29, 32, 34].

From general physiology, it is plausible that SG affects their secretion **indirectly**, via altered gastric emptying, luminal pH, bile delivery, and mucosal adaptation, but **direct human evidence after SG is limited** [29, 31, 32]. Consequently, these peptides are best regarded as part of the broader neuroendocrine context rather than as individually well-characterised drivers of SG outcomes.

22.3.5 Adipokines

Because SG induces substantial and durable weight loss, it is accompanied by wide-ranging changes in **adipose-derived hormones (adipokines)** and systemic metabolic markers. These adaptations reflect both the **reduction in fat mass** and **improved insulin sensitivity**, and they extend well beyond the gastrointestinal tract [3, 6, 18, 52].

Leptin Leptin is secreted mainly by white adipose tissue and signals energy sufficiency to the hypothalamus, regulating appetite, energy expenditure, and neuroendocrine axes. Obesity is characterised by **elevated leptin with relative leptin resistance** [29, 53, 54].

After SG:

- Multiple cohorts and meta-analyses show a marked fall in circulating leptin, broadly proportional to the reduction in fat mass [3, 52–54].
- Some analyses suggest that postoperative leptin can be lower than expected for the degree of weight loss, or that the leptin-to-adiponectin ratio (LAR) falls more than predicted, consistent with improved leptin sensitivity, although this is not uniform across all studies [52–54].

Overall, SG **substantially lowers leptin levels**, and this change likely interacts with other satiety signals (GLP-1, PYY, OXM) to support a new metabolic baseline [3, 52–54].

Adiponectin Adiponectin, also produced predominantly by adipocytes, **enhances insulin sensitivity**, promotes fatty-acid oxidation, and exerts anti-inflammatory and anti-atherogenic effects. Obesity is associated with **low adiponectin**, which improves with weight loss [29, 53].

Following SG and other bariatric procedures:

- Meta-analyses and SG cohorts consistently show a **significant rise in circulating adiponectin**, often detectable months after surgery [3, 52, 53].
- This increase correlates with improvements in HOMA-IR, glucose homeostasis, and lipid profiles, indicating a strong association between higher adiponectin and improved cardiometabolic risk [52, 53, 55, 56].

Thus, in contrast to leptin, adiponectin rises after SG, contributing to a more insulin-sensitive and anti-inflammatory adipokine profile and likely participating in early remission or improvement of type 2 diabetes [3, 52, 53, 55, 56].

Resistin, Visfatin, and Other Adipokines For other adipokines, such as **resistin, visfatin, chemerin, and PAI-1**, the evidence is more varied:

- Comprehensive meta-analyses indicate that after bariatric surgery **resistin and visfatin often show small or non-significant net changes**, whereas **PAI-1 and chemerin tend to decrease**, with substantial inter-study heterogeneity [53, 56].
- A focused review of SG and adipokines notes that resistin and visfatin responses differ across cohorts, and for some markers (e.g., visfatin) SG-specific data is sparse [53].

It is therefore accurate to say that adipokine changes beyond leptin and adiponectin are variable, and their independent contribution to SG outcomes remains incompletely defined [53, 54].

Insulin, C-Peptide, and β-Cell Function Profound changes in insulin dynamics and β-cell function occur after SG:

- Mechanistic studies show that, post-SG, **insulin secretion after mixed meals happens earlier and is more physiologic**, with improved β-cell glucose sensitivity [15, 26, 54].
- These improvements are often seen within weeks to months, before major weight loss has occurred, and coincide with marked rises in GLP-1 and PYY and improved hepatic and peripheral insulin sensitivity [15, 25–27, 54].

C-peptide profiles similarly shift towards a **more robust, early postprandial response**, reflecting enhanced β-cell function and reduced insulin resistance [15, 26, 27, 54].

Thus, the postoperative improvement in glucose homeostasis after SG is driven by a **combination** of:

1. Enhanced incretin effect (GLP-1, PYY ± OXM).
2. Improved insulin sensitivity linked to weight loss and adipokine changes (↑ adiponectin, ↓ leptin).
3. Direct changes in β-cell function and hepatic glucose output [3, 15, 52–54].

Ghrelin-LEAP2 Axis Liver-expressed antimicrobial peptide 2 (LEAP2) is an endogenous antagonist and inverse agonist of the ghrelin receptor (GHS-R1a) [21]. LEAP2 and ghrelin exhibit largely opposite regulation with energy balance: LEAP2 tends to be higher in obesity and in the postprandial state, whereas ghrelin is elevated during fasting and weight loss [21–23]. After bariatric surgery, including sleeve gastrectomy, available data suggest that both ghrelin and LEAP2 often decline in parallel with weight loss. That shift in the LEAP2/ghrelin balance and receptor context modulate net ghrelin signalling rather than LEAP2 simply rising to block ghrelin action [21–23]. Overall, the ghrelin–LEAP2 axis represents an emerging area of interest in the metabolic adaptations to bariatric surgery, but its precise contribution to appetite regulation and weight-loss maintenance after sleeve gastrectomy remains to be fully defined [21–23].

Other Endocrine Axes SG-induced weight loss also affects several **non-gastrointestinal hormonal axes**:

- **Sex steroids (especially in men):** After bariatric surgery (including SG), multiple studies and meta-analyses show significant increases in total and free testosterone and sex hormone-binding globulin (SHBG), with hypogonadism frequently improving or resolving. Oestradiol often falls slightly or remains stable, depending on sex and baseline status [53, 55, 57, 58].
- **Thyroid axis:** Sleeve gastrectomy-induced weight loss is also associated with changes in thyroid function. In obese individuals, weight-loss interventions, including SG, typically lead to reductions in TSH and free T3 (FT3), while free T4 (FT4) often remains unchanged [55, 57–59]. These changes are generally interpreted as a reversal of obesity related thyroid axis adaptations and a shift in the energy expenditure set point rather than the development of true hypothyroidism [55, 57–59]. Data on reverse T3 after bariatric surgery are limited and inconsistent, and no clear consensus exists regarding its long-term behaviour, accordingly, strong conclusions about reverse T3 dynamics after SG are not warranted at present [55, 57–59].
- **GH/IGF-1:** Obesity is associated with functional GH deficiency. Weight loss (including after SG) is generally followed by partial normalisation of GH secretion and IGF-1 levels, although SG-specific data are less robust than for sex steroids and thyroid hormones [3, 34, 53].

Together, these endocrine changes reflect a **system-wide rebalancing**. Reducing chronic inflammation and lipidic profile, improving insulin sensitivity, and regulating several obesity-related hormonal disruptions [3, 6, 34, 53–55].

22.4 Biochemical Changes

Sleeve gastrectomy induces profound biochemical adaptations that extend well beyond weight reduction. These include improvements in glucose and lipid metabolism, modulation of inflammatory and immune markers, and changes in micronutrient and vitamin status. While several of these effects are shared across bariatric procedures, others appear more characteristic of SG due to its unique anatomical and hormonal consequences [2, 3, 5, 9].

22.4.1 Glucose Metabolism and Insulin Sensitivity

One of the most striking metabolic outcomes after SG is the rapid improvement in glucose homeostasis, often preceding substantial weight loss. Numerous studies have documented early and sustained reductions in fasting plasma glucose, insulin, and insulin resistance indices such as HOMA-IR, with changes emerging within days to weeks postoperatively [15, 26, 54, 60]. These findings support the presence of weight-independent mechanisms contributing to improved glucose control.

Early enhancement of insulin sensitivity likely reflects a combination of factors. Altered secretion of incretin and satiety hormones (particularly GLP-1 and PYY, together with reduced ghrelin) enhances glucose-dependent insulin secretion, suppresses glucagon, and slows gastric emptying [26, 36, 39]. Changes in bile acid metabolism and gut microbiota after SG also modulate hepatic and peripheral insulin sensitivity through nuclear receptor and GPCR pathways (FXR, TGR5), while the emerging ghrelin-LEAP2 axis may help counteract orexigenic and diabetogenic ghrelin signalling [3, 21, 22]. Collectively, these adaptations promote more physiological postprandial glucose handling and a healthier insulin response pattern [1, 34–36].

As weight loss progresses, longer-term improvements in glycemia are driven by reductions in visceral adiposity, ectopic fat in liver and muscle, and low-grade inflammation. Decreased hepatic and intramyocellular fat improves insulin receptor signalling, while rising adiponectin and falling leptin and resistin further promote insulin sensitivity [3, 5, 52]. Clinically, these changes translate into substantial gains in glycaemic control and, in many patients, partial or complete remission of type 2 diabetes mellitus [2, 27, 35].

Although both SG and RYGB achieve broadly comparable glycaemic improvements, their mechanisms are not identical. In SG, incretin enhancement occurs without intestinal bypass, emphasising the role of altered gastric emptying, nutrient flow, and gut hormone secretion rather than malabsorption [9, 26, 35]. Thus, SG is best understood not only as a restrictive procedure but also as a potent **metabolic intervention** capable of restoring glucose regulation via both immediate hormonal and delayed weight-dependent pathways [2, 3].

Early Data and Metabolomic Insights In non-diabetic patients evaluated as early as 6 days after SG, reductions in fasting glucose and insulin compared with baseline have been reported, suggesting an immediate improvement in basal insulin sensitivity even before substantial weight loss occurs [60]. Short-term Oral Glucose Tolerance Test (OGTT) data also point to some differences compared with RYGB, with slightly less pronounced 120-min glucose reductions after SG in the very early postoperative period, in line with the distinct patterns of nutrient transit and incretin responses observed between the two procedures [26, 35, 60].

Longitudinal cohorts show that postoperative rises in adiponectin and augmented GLP-1/PYY responses are associated with declines in Homeostatic Model Assessment of Insulin Resistance (HOMA-IR) even after adjusting for weight loss, highlighting endocrine mechanisms beyond loss of adipose mass [51, 54]. Metabolomic studies report broad remodelling of energy-related pathways, with changes in glycolysis- and TCA-related metabolites and lipid oxidation profiles compatible with improved mitochondrial efficiency and metabolic flexibility after bariatric surgery, including SG [2, 5, 34]. These systemic shifts support a transition from a metabolically inflexible, glycolysis-biased state towards more efficient oxidative substrate use.

22.4.1.1 Mechanisms and Interpretations

Hepatic Insulin Sensitivity Early improvements in fasting glycemia after SG are largely explained by enhanced hepatic insulin sensitivity. Reductions in liver fat and circulating free fatty acids diminish lipotoxic interference with insulin signalling and decrease hepatic glucose production [3, 5, 26]. Altered portal nutrient and insulin flux, together with increased incretin signalling, further support suppression of gluconeogenesis and normalisation of fasting glucose [3, 5, 26].

Peripheral (Muscle and Adipose) Insulin Sensitivity Improvements in peripheral insulin sensitivity evolve in parallel with reductions in adiposity and systemic inflammation. The loss of dysfunctional adipose tissue decreases the release of pro-inflammatory cytokines and FFAs, mitigating lipotoxic interference with insulin signalling in skeletal muscle and adipose deposits. Enhanced mitochondrial oxidative function and improved substrate utilisation further support glucose uptake and insulin responsiveness at the tissue level. Elevated adiponectin concentrations, which rise progressively after weight loss, exert additional insulin-sensitising effects in muscle and liver, reinforcing these improvements [2, 3, 53].

Role of Gut Hormones and the Enteroinsular Axis SG significantly reshapes the enteroinsular axis. After surgery, postprandial GLP-1 and PYY secretion increases, which boosts glucose-dependent insulin release, reduces glucagon levels, and slows gastric emptying, leading to better postprandial glycaemic control and greater satiety [35, 36]. These changes arise from accelerated nutrient delivery to the distal gut and are further modulated by bile acids and microbiota-derived signals [3, 26, 34]. The rapid onset of glycaemic benefit, often before substantial weight loss, is consistent with these weight-independent endocrine mechanisms.

Metabolomic Shifts and Substrate Flux Metabolomic profiling after bariatric surgery demonstrates widespread shifts in amino acid, lipid, and energy-related metabolites that go hand in hand with improvements in insulin sensitivity and glycaemic control [34, 61]. These include changes in intermediates of glycolysis and the TCA cycle, increased markers of fatty-acid oxidation, and normalisation of branched-chain amino acid profiles, all consistent with enhanced metabolic flexibility and reduced reliance on anaerobic glycolysis [34, 61].

22.4.1.2 Caveats and Complexities

Clinical responses are heterogeneous. Patients with long-standing diabetes, severe baseline insulin resistance, or limited β-cell reserve often experience slower or less complete metabolic improvement than those with preserved insulin secretion [2, 15,

26]. Methodological differences also complicate comparison: studies variously use HOMA-IR, OGTT, IVGTT, or euglycemic clamps, which probe different aspects of insulin sensitivity and secretion [35, 36, 54].

Over the longer term, partial weight regain, adaptive changes in energy expenditure, or attenuation of gut hormone responses can reduce the magnitude of initial improvements [27, 54, 62]. Disentangling weight-dependent from weight-independent mechanisms remains an active area of investigation, and ongoing longitudinal and mechanistic studies will be essential to define the durability and determinants of metabolic remission after SG [2, 3, 26].

22.4.2 Lipid Profile

Bariatric surgery, including SG, is consistently associated with favourable alterations in lipid metabolism. Typical long-term postoperative patterns include reductions in total cholesterol, LDL-cholesterol, and triglycerides, along with increases in HDL-cholesterol, contributing to a lower cardiovascular risk [2, 5, 9]. However, in the very early postoperative period (days to a few weeks), changes in circulating lipids may be modest or variable, reflecting acute catabolic and nutritional shifts during recovery [3, 5, 60].

Evidence from Early and Longitudinal Studies Controlled metabolic studies show that even within the first postoperative weeks, SG can modify lipid parameters, although early changes in HDL, LDL, and triglycerides are often small and sometimes bidirectional, with clearer improvements emerging over months as weight loss and insulin sensitivity improve [3, 60]. Longer-term cohorts and comparative series report significant reductions in atherogenic lipoproteins (LDL, non-HDL cholesterol, triglycerides) and rises in HDL after SG, broadly comparable to those seen after RYGB when matched for weight loss [2, 3, 51].

Metabolomic Insights Lipidomic and metabolomic studies highlight how extensively lipid metabolism is remodelled after surgery. Following bariatric procedures, including SG, multiple lipid species (such as phospholipids, acylcarnitines, and free fatty acids) show marked changes, consistent with enhanced β-oxidation, more efficient mitochondrial lipid use, and reduced lipotoxicity [61]. These changes correlate with improvements in insulin sensitivity and cardiometabolic risk markers, suggesting that qualitative remodelling of the lipidome accompanies quantitative changes in standard lipid panels [61].

Together, this data supports that SG exerts both early and sustained benefits on lipid homeostasis. While many effects are secondary to weight loss and improved insulin sensitivity, others likely arise from direct alterations in hepatic lipid metabolism, bile-acid signalling, and systemic substrate flux induced by the profound endocrine and metabolic reprogramming that follows SG [3, 5, 61].

22.4.2.1 Mechanisms

Improvement in lipid parameters after SG reflects dietary, metabolic, and endocrine contributions. Reduced caloric and fat intake directly lowers substrate availability for hepatic VLDL synthesis, while improved insulin sensitivity decreases hepatic VLDL output and enhances lipoprotein-lipase-mediated triglyceride clearance in peripheral tissues [3, 53].

Loss of ectopic fat in liver and muscle improves intracellular lipid handling, lowering spill-over of FFAs into the circulation and reducing small, dense LDL formation [2, 51]. Altered bile-acid metabolism and signalling via FXR and TGR5 influence cholesterol turnover, hepatic lipid oxidation, and intestinal lipid absorption, further promoting an anti-atherogenic lipid profile [3, 5].

22.4.2.2 Caveats and Nuances

Short-term postoperative catabolism, perioperative fasting, and fluid shifts can transiently disturb lipid measurements, so very early data should be interpreted cautiously [3, 60]. Not all lipid classes behave uniformly; certain phospholipids and sphingolipids exhibit variable trajectories that may differ between individuals and between SG and RYGB [61].

Long-term lipid outcomes are also shaped by diet composition, physical activity, genetics, and adherence to follow-up care. Thus, although SG generally promotes lasting improvements in lipid profiles, the magnitude and durability of these changes vary between patients [2, 53].

22.4.3 Inflammation Markers

Baseline Context Obesity is characterised by chronic, low-grade systemic inflammation, with elevated IL-6, TNF-α, and acute-phase proteins such as C-reactive protein (CRP). Adipose tissue expansion and macrophage recruitment create a cytokine-rich environment that contributes to insulin resistance, endothelial dysfunction, and increased cardiovascular risk [2, 3].

Changes After Surgery Bariatric surgery consistently attenuates this inflammatory burden. A meta-analysis of observational studies showed that bariatric procedures overall reduce CRP and IL-6 levels by about 66% and 27%, respectively, while effects on TNF-α are smaller and more variable [63]. These improvements in inflammatory markers run side by side with gains in metabolic health and reductions in cardiovascular risk factors [53, 54].

SG-specific studies report similar anti-inflammatory trends. In cohorts undergoing SG, significant decreases in CRP and IL-6 typically appear within the first 3–12 months and correlate with reductions in BMI, visceral adiposity, and indices of insulin resistance [6, 51]. Short-term data also show early declines in selected inflammatory cytokines and reciprocal increases in adiponectin after bariatric surgery, supporting a close interplay between weight loss, adipokine changes, and inflammatory resolution [51, 53].

Interestingly, improvements in glycaemia and insulin sensitivity can precede full normalisation of inflammatory markers, suggesting that endocrine and hepatic mechanisms may act more rapidly, whereas remodelling of adipose tissue and immune cell populations evolves over longer time frames [2, 51].

22.4.3.1 Mechanisms and Interpretations

Reduced Adipose Inflammation Weight loss after SG decreases adipocyte hypertrophy and mechanical stress, reducing chemokine-driven recruitment and activation of pro-inflammatory macrophages (M1 phenotype) and T cells. This shift towards a more anti-inflammatory adipose microenvironment lowers systemic IL-6 and TNF-α release and supports improved insulin sensitivity [2, 51].

Lower Systemic Inflammatory Burden Reduced exposure to saturated FFAs and other lipotoxic intermediates dampens TLR- and NF-κB mediated inflammatory signalling. Concurrent improvements in insulin sensitivity reduce oxidative and ER stress, further limiting cytokine production. These changes contribute to improved endothelial function and lower vascular inflammation [2, 51, 63].

Gut–Immune Crosstalk SG-induced changes in gut anatomy, motility, and microbiota can enhance intestinal barrier integrity and reduce circulating LPS, mitigating metabolic endotoxaemia and downstream inflammatory pathways [3, 5]. Bile-acid-FXR/TGR5 signalling also has immunomodulatory effects, influencing cytokine production and macrophage polarisation [3, 5].

Temporal Lag and Heterogeneity Despite substantial improvements, residual low-grade inflammation is common, especially in patients with NAFLD, atherosclerosis, or long-standing obesity [2, 51, 63]. Some markers (e.g., CRP, IL-6) show consistent declines, whereas others (TNF-α, MCP-1, IL-8) exhibit greater inter-study variability. Timing of sampling (immediate postoperative vs months to years), surgical technique, assay methods, and patient heterogeneity all contribute to these differences [6, 51, 63]. Whether reduced inflammation is a primary driver of improved insulin sensitivity or largely a downstream consequence remains an active area of research [2, 53].

22.4.4 Micronutrient and Vitamin Status

Because SG substantially reduces gastric volume and alters gastric physiology, it carries a measurable risk of micronutrient and vitamin deficiencies. Although SG is less malabsorptive than RYGB, its impact on gastric acid production, intrinsic factor secretion, and dietary intake necessitates long-term biochemical surveillance and supplementation [1, 5, 7].

Common Deficiencies and Prevalence The micronutrients most frequently affected after SG are iron, vitamin B_{12}, folate, vitamin D, and calcium. Deficiencies in thiamine, zinc, copper, and fat-soluble vitamins (A, E, K) are less common but well documented, especially in long-term follow-up [1, 7, 8]. Across SG cohorts, within the first postoperative year iron deficiency and anaemia commonly affect roughly a quarter to a third of patients, and vitamin B_{12} and folate deficiencies are reported in approximately 10–20%, though prevalences vary widely between studies depending on baseline status, definitions, and supplementation practices [7, 8]. Longer-term cohort data (up to 6–10 years) show progressive increases in the prevalence of iron, folate, and B_{12} deficiencies after both SG and RYGB, with somewhat different patterns between procedures but persistent risk in SG despite the absence of intestinal bypass [7, 8]. Reviews of anaemia after SG consistently identify iron deficiency as the dominant cause, with vitamin B_{12} and, less often, folate deficiency acting as additional contributors [7, 8].

22.4.4.1 Mechanisms of Deficiency in Sleeve Gastrectomy

Micronutrient deficiencies after SG arise from combined anatomical, physiological, and behavioural factors.

- **Reduced gastric acid and intrinsic factor.** Resection of much of the gastric fundus and body lowers parietal cell mass and gastric acidity, impairing solubilisation of non-heme iron and release of protein-bound vitamin B_{12}, and reducing intrinsic factor secretion needed for ileal B_{12} absorption. Hypochlorhydria also decreases the solubility of calcium and other divalent cations such as magnesium and zinc [1, 5, 7].
- **Reduced intake and dietary restrictions.** Smaller gastric capacity limits overall intake, and intolerance to red meat and some fibrous vegetables or dairy products can reduce iron, B_{12}, and calcium consumption. Early postoperative liquid/pureed diets further restrict micronutrient diversity, so deficiencies can emerge quickly without adequate supplementation [1, 7].
- **Altered transit and digestive dynamics.** Although the absorptive surface is preserved, faster gastric emptying and altered mixing may modestly shorten nutrient contact time in the proximal small intestine, subtly affecting absorption efficiency. Secondary changes in bile acids and gut microbiota may influence absorption of fat-soluble vitamins and trace elements [3, 5].
- **Pre-existing deficiencies in obesity.** Many bariatric candidates already have vitamin D and iron deficiency due to obesity-associated inflammation (elevated hepcidin impairing iron absorption) and sequestration of vitamin D in adipose tissue [7, 8]. Postoperative deficiencies often represent worsening of pre-existing ones rather than entirely new problems.

22.4.4.2 Specific Nutrients

Iron and Anaemia Iron deficiency is among the most common complications after SG, driven by reduced gastric acid–mediated iron solubilisation, lower intake of iron-rich foods, and menstrual losses in women [7, 8]. Postoperative anaemia is often multifactorial, but iron deficiency is usually the primary driver [7, 8].

Vitamin B_{12} (Cobalamin) Although B_{12} deficiency risk is higher after RYGB, SG still carries a clinically relevant risk because of reduced acid and intrinsic factor secretion and the reduction of contact between ingested food and parietal cell-rich gastric mucosa. Untreated B_{12} deficiency can cause megaloblastic anaemia and neurologic complications, so routine supplementation (high-dose oral or intramuscular) is recommended [1, 7, 8].

Folate Folate deficiency is less frequent than iron or B_{12} deficiency and usually reflects low dietary intake rather than impaired intestinal absorption. Because B_{12} and folate metabolism are linked, combined deficiencies can exacerbate anaemia and hyperhomocysteinaemia [7, 8].

Vitamin D, Calcium, and Bone Health Vitamin D insufficiency is very common preoperatively in obesity and often persists after SG without supplementation. Reduced intake of vitamin D and calcium-rich foods, altered fat intake, and low gastric acidity can impair vitamin D and calcium handling, predisposing to secondary hyperparathyroidism and bone mineral loss [5, 7, 8]. Calcium citrate with vitamin D_3 is typically recommended.

Other Micronutrients Trace element deficiencies (zinc, copper, magnesium) and deficits in vitamins A, E, and K are less well characterised after SG but have been reported, particularly in patients with poor adherence to supplements or prolonged vomiting [1, 7, 8]. Copper deficiency, though uncommon, can cause hematologic and neurologic manifestations, highlighting the need for monitoring.

22.4.4.3 Recommendations and Monitoring

Because deficiencies may develop slowly and remain asymptomatic for long periods, **lifelong nutritional surveillance** is essential.

- **Preoperative:** Screening and correction of iron, vitamin D, and B_{12} deficiency are strongly recommended to minimise postoperative risk [1, 7, 8].
- **Postoperative:** Laboratory follow-up (CBC, ferritin/iron studies, B_{12}, folate, 25-OH vitamin D, calcium, PTH, ± trace elements) is usually performed at least annually once stable, and more frequently in the first year or in high-risk patients [1, 2, 5].
- **Supplementation:** Standard care includes a bariatric multivitamin, plus additional iron, vitamin B_{12} (oral/sublingual or parenteral), and calcium with vitamin D; doses are adjusted according to lab results [1, 2, 5, 7]. Specialised bariatric formulations are preferred over generic over-the-counter preparations.

Clinicians should remain alert for clinical signs of deficiency (anaemia, neuropathy, bone pain, alopecia, glossitis), which may precede overt biochemical changes. Even though SG lacks intestinal bypass, the cumulative risk of micronutrient deficiency remains significant, so structured, multidisciplinary follow-up is critical to prevent hematologic, neurologic, and skeletal complications [1, 2, 5, 7, 9].

22.5 Clinical Implications

Sleeve gastrectomy (SG) is now recognised as a metabolic, rather than purely restrictive, procedure, producing marked improvements in glucose and lipid metabolism, systemic inflammation and adipokine profiles in addition to durable weight loss [2, 9]. These changes translate into substantial relief of metabolic syndrome components, high rates of type 2 diabetes remission or major improvement, and reduced need for glucose, blood pressure, and lipid-lowering medications in many patients [2, 15].

Mechanistically, SG improves glycaemic control through both **weight-independent and weight-dependent** pathways. Early after surgery, enhanced GLP-1 and PYY responses, reduced ghrelin, altered bile acid signalling, and changes in adipokines and inflammatory markers contribute to improved β-cell function and insulin sensitivity, often before major weight loss has occurred [15, 25, 34]. With ongoing weight reduction, decreases in visceral and ectopic fat, decline of adipose tissue inflammation, and rising adiponectin further consolidate improvements in insulin resistance and cardiometabolic risk [2, 53, 54].

These metabolic effects have important **cardiovascular implications**. By improving glycemia, blood pressure, lipids, and inflammatory burden, bariatric surgery contributes to lower long-term cardiovascular mortality, and reduced incidence of major cardiovascular events compared with non-surgical care [1, 2, 64].

Clinically, SG must be balanced against **procedure-specific risks and trade-offs**. Compared with RYGB, SG offers similar early improvements in glycaemia and incretin responses, with a lower risk of classic malabsorptive complications but a higher likelihood of persistent or de novo gastroesophageal reflux disease [9, 26, 35]. SG is therefore an attractive first-line metabolic option for many patients with obesity and cardiometabolic disease, whereas RYGB may still be preferred in selected individuals (e.g., severe reflux or more advanced diabetes) after multidisciplinary evaluation [2, 9].

Finally, the **risk of micronutrient deficiency after SG is clinically meaningful**, despite preservation of intestinal continuity. Deficiencies in iron, vitamin B_{12}, folate, vitamin D, and calcium deficiencies accumulate over time, and anaemia and bone loss have been described in long-term series, particularly when supplementation and follow-up are suboptimal [1, 5, 7, 8]. These considerations stress the need for structured, lifelong nutritional surveillance, patient education, and adherence to bariatric-specific supplementation protocols.

22.6 Future Directions and Research Gaps

Several important knowledge gaps remain regarding the metabolic effects of SG.

First, **long-term comparative effectiveness** data for SG versus other bariatric procedures are still limited for hard outcomes such as cardiovascular events, microvascular complications, liver outcomes, and survival. Most studies focus on intermediate markers (weight, HbA1c, lipids) with follow-up of ≤5–10 years and heterogeneous designs [2, 9, 15, 26, 64]. Large, procedure-specific, long-term observational cohorts and pragmatic trials are needed to clarify when SG is sufficient and when more malabsorptive procedures confer additional benefit that justifies their higher nutritional risk.

Second, the **mechanistic underpinnings** of SG are only partly understood. While changes in GLP-1, GIP, PYY, and ghrelin are well documented, the roles of less-studied peptides (e.g., LEAP2, oxyntomodulin, GLP-2), bile acid signalling, and gut microbiota in determining long-term metabolic and weight outcomes are not completely defined [22, 23, 25, 47, 49, 50]. Better integration of hormonal, bile acid, microbiome, adipose tissue, and metabolomic data in longitudinal cohorts will be crucial to identify causal pathways and potential pharmacologic targets that mimic or augment SG's benefits.

Third, **patient-level heterogeneity** in response to SG is substantial. Not all individuals achieve durable diabetes remission, optimal weight loss, or sustained anti-inflammatory changes, and some experience weight regain or recurrence of hyperglycaemia despite apparently similar operations [2, 25, 27, 61, 62, 64]. Predictive models that combine clinical features (e.g., age, diabetes duration, β-cell reserve), behavioural factors, gut-hormone responses, adipokines, and omics-based biomarkers need further validation before routine use for procedure selection or risk stratification.

Fourth, the **optimal long-term nutritional strategy** after SG remains uncertain. Although the need for supplementation is clear, the ideal formulations, doses, and monitoring intervals are not fully standardised and vary among centres and guidelines [1, 5, 7, 8]. Prospective trials comparing supplementation regimens and follow-up intensities could help reduce residual micronutrient deficiency and its aftermath.

Finally, the rapid emergence of **potent incretin-based pharmacotherapies** (GLP-1 receptor agonists, dual GIP/GLP-1 agonists, and newer combinations) raises important questions about how best to **combine or sequence** medical and surgical approaches [24, 32]. Future work should examine whether peri- or postoperative use of such agents can enhance or maintain SG outcomes, mitigate weight regain, or allow less invasive strategies in selected patients, while also defining cost-effectiveness and long-term safety.

22.7 Conclusions

Sleeve gastrectomy is a powerful metabolic intervention that induces far-reaching biochemical and hormonal changes beyond simple gastric restriction. By reshaping the enteroendocrine landscape (notably GLP-1, GIP, PYY, and ghrelin), improving insulin sensitivity, normalising lipid and adipokine profiles, and attenuating chronic low-grade inflammation, SG promotes substantial and often rapid improvements in glucose control, cardiometabolic risk factors, and obesity-related comorbidities [3, 9, 25, 26, 54].

At the same time, SG introduces new long-term challenges, including the risk of cumulative micronutrient deficiencies and bone loss, as well as procedure-specific issues such as gastro-oesophageal reflux and potential weight regain [1, 5, 7, 8, 35]. These risks can be minimised, though not eliminated, through lifelong multidisciplinary follow-up, structured biochemical monitoring, and adherence to tailored supplementation and lifestyle programmes [1, 5, 7, 8].

Overall, current evidence supports SG as a safe, effective, and versatile bariatric-metabolic procedure that offers a favourable balance between metabolic efficacy and nutritional risk for many patients with obesity and related comorbidities [2, 3, 9, 61]. As mechanistic insight deepens and long-term comparative and outcomes data accumulate, SG is likely to be integrated even more precisely into individualised treatment algorithms, potentially in combination with advanced pharmacotherapies. Continued research aimed at clarifying mechanisms, optimising patient selection, and refining postoperative care will be essential to fully realise the metabolic and clinical potential of sleeve gastrectomy.

References

1. Tish S, Corcelles R. The art of sleeve gastrectomy. J Clin Med. 2024;13(7)
2. Poljo A, Kraljevic M, Peterli R, Muller BP, Billeter AT. Role of sleeve gastrectomy in improving metabolic syndrome: an overview. Updat Surg. 2025;77(7):2031–6.
3. Huang R, Ding X, Fu H, Cai Q. Potential mechanisms of sleeve gastrectomy for reducing weight and improving metabolism in patients with obesity. Surg Obes Relat Dis. 2019;15(10):1861–71.
4. Kehagias D, Georgopoulos N, Habeos I, Lampropoulos C, Mulita F, Kehagias I. The role of the gastric fundus in glycemic control. Hormones (Athens). 2023;22(2):151–63.
5. Camastra S, Palumbo M, Santini F. Nutrients handling after bariatric surgery, the role of gastrointestinal adaptation. Eat Weight Disord. 2022;27(2):449–61.
6. Ocakli S, Canlikarakaya F, Dastandir D, Ceylan C, Cinkil NC, Banli O. Anthropometric changes and systemic inflammation after sleeve gastrectomy: do composite markers reflect the change? Obes Surg. 2025;35:4595.
7. Mulita F, Lampropoulos C, Kehagias D, Verras GI, Tchabashvili L, Kaplanis C, et al. Long-term nutritional deficiencies following sleeve gastrectomy: a 6-year single-Centre retrospective study. Prz Menopauzalny. 2021;20(4):170–6.
8. Vieira de Sousa JP, Santos-Sousa H, Vieira S, Nunes R, Nogueiro J, Pereira A, et al. Assessing nutritional deficiencies in bariatric surgery patients: a comparative study of Roux-en-Y gastric bypass versus sleeve gastrectomy. J Pers Med. 2024;14(6)

9. Benaiges D, Mas-Lorenzo A, Goday A, Ramon JM, Chillaron JJ, Pedro-Botet J, et al. Laparoscopic sleeve gastrectomy: more than a restrictive bariatric surgery procedure? World J Gastroenterol. 2015;21(41):11804–14.
10. Delhanty PJ, Neggers SJ, van der Lely AJ. Mechanisms in endocrinology: ghrelin: the differences between acyl- and des-acyl ghrelin. Eur J Endocrinol. 2012;167(5):601–8.
11. Iwakura H, Ensho T, Ueda Y. Desacyl-ghrelin, not just an inactive form of ghrelin? A review of current knowledge on the biological actions of desacyl-ghrelin. Peptides. 2023;167:171050.
12. Bukhari SNA. An insight into the multifunctional role of ghrelin and structure activity relationship studies of ghrelin receptor ligands with clinical trials. Eur J Med Chem. 2022;235:114308.
13. Li X, Aili A, Aipire A, Maimaitiyusupu P, Maimaitiming M, Abudureyimu K. Correlation analysis between the changes in plasma ghrelin level and weight loss after sleeve gastrectomy combined with fundoplication. BMC Surg. 2024;24(1):176.
14. Sethi P, Thillai M, Nain PS, Ahuja A, Aulakh N, Khurana P. Role of hunger hormone "ghrelin" in long-term weight loss following laparoscopic sleeve gastrectomy. Niger J Surg. 2018;24(2):121–4.
15. Mullally JA, Febres GJ, Bessler M, Korner J. Sleeve gastrectomy and Roux-en-Y gastric bypass achieve similar early improvements in Beta-cell function in obese patients with type 2 diabetes. Sci Rep. 2019;9(1):1880.
16. Navarro García MI, González-Costea Martínez R, Torregrosa Pérez N, Romera Barba E, Periago MJ, Vázquez Rojas JL. Fasting ghrelin levels after gastric bypass and vertical sleeve gastrectomy: an analytical cohort study. Endocrinología, Diabetes y Nutrici6n (English ed). 2020;67(2):89–101.
17. Yousseif A, Emmanuel J, Karra E, Millet Q, Elkalaawy M, Jenkinson AD, et al. Differential effects of laparoscopic sleeve gastrectomy and laparoscopic gastric bypass on appetite, circulating acyl-ghrelin, peptide YY3-36 and active GLP-1 levels in non-diabetic humans. Obes Surg. 2014;24(2):241–52.
18. Tuero C, Valenti V, Rotellar F, Landecho MF, Cienfuegos JA, Fruhbeck G. Revisiting the ghrelin changes following bariatric and metabolic surgery. Obes Surg. 2020;30(7):2763–80.
19. Dardzinska JA, Kaska L, Proczko-Stepaniak M, Szymanska-Gnacinska M, Aleksandrowicz-Wrona E, Malgorzewicz S. Fasting and postprandial acyl and desacyl ghrelin and the acyl/desacyl ratio in obese patients before and after different types of bariatric surgery. Wideochir Inne Tech Maloinwazyjne. 2018;13(3):366–75.
20. Ariyasu H. Stomach-derived growth hormone-releasing peptide, ghrelin. J Clin Endocrinol Metabol. 2001;86(10):4753–8.
21. Ge X, Yang H, Bednarek MA, Galon-Tilleman H, Chen P, Chen M, et al. LEAP2 is an endogenous antagonist of the ghrelin receptor. Cell Metab. 2018;27(2):461–9.
22. Sakai K, Nakazato Y, Shiimura Y, Zhang W, Nakazato M. Ghrelin-LEAP2 interactions along the stomach-liver axis. Endocr J. 2025;72(4):341–53.
23. Alic N, Ayaz A. Ghrelin and LEAP2: their interaction effect on appetite regulation and the alterations in their levels following bariatric surgery. Medicina (Kaunas). 2025;61(8)
24. Baggio LL, Drucker DJ. Biology of incretins: GLP-1 and GIP. Gastroenterology. 2007;132(6):2131–57.
25. McCarty TR, Jirapinyo P, Thompson CC. Effect of sleeve gastrectomy on ghrelin, GLP-1, PYY, and GIP gut hormones: a systematic review and meta-analysis. Ann Surg. 2020;272(1):72–80.
26. Nannipieri M, Baldi S, Mari A, Colligiani D, Guarino D, Camastra S, et al. Roux-en-Y gastric bypass and sleeve gastrectomy: mechanisms of diabetes remission and role of gut hormones. J Clin Endocrinol Metab. 2013;98(11):4391–9.
27. Hindso M, Hedback N, Svane MS, Moller A, Martinussen C, Jorgensen NB, et al. The importance of endogenously secreted GLP-1 and GIP for postprandial glucose tolerance and beta-cell function after Roux-en-Y gastric bypass and sleeve gastrectomy surgery. Diabetes. 2023;72(3):336–47.

28. Muller TD, Adriaenssens A, Ahren B, Bluher M, Birkenfeld AL, Campbell JE, et al. Glucose-dependent insulinotropic polypeptide (GIP). Mol Metab. 2025;95:102118.
29. Cummings DE, Overduin J. Gastrointestinal regulation of food intake. J Clin Invest. 2007;117(1):13–23.
30. Chaudhri O, Small C, Bloom S. Gastrointestinal hormones regulating appetite. Philos Trans R Soc Lond Ser B Biol Sci. 2006;361(1471):1187–209.
31. Spreckley E, Murphy KG. The L-cell in nutritional sensing and the regulation of appetite. Front Nutr. 2015;2:23.
32. Steinert RE, Feinle-Bisset C, Asarian L, Horowitz M, Beglinger C, Geary N. Ghrelin, CCK, GLP-1, and PYY(3-36): secretory controls and physiological roles in eating and Glycemia in health, obesity, and after RYGB. Physiol Rev. 2017;97(1):411–63.
33. Nguyen NT, Park JH. Peptide YY in type 2 diabetes: a complementary gut hormone with therapeutic potential beyond GLP-1. Nutrients. 2025;17(21)
34. Papamargaritis D, le Roux CW. Do gut hormones contribute to weight loss and Glycaemic outcomes after bariatric surgery? Nutrients. 2021;13(3)
35. Peterli R, Steinert RE, Woelnerhanssen B, Peters T, Christoffel-Courtin C, Gass M, et al. Metabolic and hormonal changes after laparoscopic Roux-en-Y gastric bypass and sleeve gastrectomy: a randomized, prospective trial. Obes Surg. 2012;22(5):740–8.
36. Svane MS, Bojsen-Moller KN, Martinussen C, Dirksen C, Madsen JL, Reitelseder S, et al. Postprandial nutrient handling and gastrointestinal hormone secretion after Roux-en-Y gastric bypass vs sleeve gastrectomy. Gastroenterology. 2019;156(6):1627–41 e1.
37. Kowalka AM, Alexiadou K, Cuenco J, Clarke RE, Minnion J, Williams EL, et al. The postprandial secretion of peptide YY(1-36) and (3-36) in obesity is differentially increased after gastric bypass versus sleeve gastrectomy. Clin Endocrinol. 2023;99(3):272–84.
38. Lampropoulos C, Mulita F, Alexandrides T, Kehagias D, Kalavrizioti D, Albanopoulos K, et al. Ghrelin, glucagon-like peptide-1, and peptide YY secretion in patients with and without weight regain during long-term follow-up after bariatric surgery: a cross-sectional study. Prz Menopauzalny. 2022;21(2):97–105.
39. Arakawa R, Febres G, Cheng B, Krikhely A, Bessler M, Korner J. Prospective study of gut hormone and metabolic changes after laparoscopic sleeve gastrectomy and Roux-en-Y gastric bypass. PLoS One. 2020;15(7):e0236133.
40. Pérez-Arana G-M, Almorza-Gomar D, Mayo-Ossorio M-A, Ramírez AC, Castro-Santiago M-J, Valverde-Martínez A, et al. Gastrin: a new branch of the gastropancreatic axis that can explain the effect of sleeve gastrectomy on glucose metabolism. J Gastrointest Surg. 2024;28(4):381–8.
41. Grong E, Graeslie H, Munkvold B, Arbo IB, Kulseng BE, Waldum HL, et al. Gastrin secretion after bariatric surgery-response to a protein-rich mixed meal following Roux-En-Y gastric bypass and sleeve gastrectomy: a pilot study in Normoglycemic women. Obes Surg. 2016;26(7):1448–56.
42. Peetsalu A, Kirsimagi U, Sipponen P, Syrjanen K, Riispere Z, Sillakivi T, et al. Serum gastric biomarker levels after sleeve gastrectomy and Roux-en-Y gastric bypass operations: a prospective study with 1-year follow-up. Surg Gastroenterol Oncol. 2019;24(2)
43. Park JM, Chiu CF, Chen SC, Lee WJ, Chen CY. Changes in post-oral glucose challenge pancreatic polypeptide hormone levels following metabolic surgery: a comparison of gastric bypass and sleeve gastrectomy. Neuropeptides. 2020;81:102032.
44. Anastasiou IA, Kounatidis D, Rebelos E, Vallianou NG, Tentolouris A, Tentolouris N, et al. Hormonal alterations in individuals with obesity after metabolic bariatric surgery: a narrative review. Medicina (Kaunas). 2025;61(10)
45. Dogan HYE U, Aslaner A, Cakir T, Oruc MT, Koc U, et al. The impact of laparoscopic sleeve gastrectomy on plasma obestatin and ghrelin levels. Eur Rev Med Pharmacol Sci. 2016;20:2113–22.
46. Zhou D, Jiang X, Ding W, Zhang D, Yang L, Zhen C, et al. Impact of bariatric surgery on ghrelin and obestatin levels in obesity or type 2 diabetes mellitus rat model. J Diabetes Res. 2014;2014:569435.

47. Perakakis N, Kokkinos A, Peradze N, Tentolouris N, Ghaly W, Pilitsi E, et al. Circulating levels of gastrointestinal hormones in response to the most common types of bariatric surgery and predictive value for weight loss over one year: evidence from two independent trials. Metabolism. 2019;101:153997.
48. Mantzoros CS, PN. The role of glicentin and Oxyntomodulin in human metabolism: new evidence and new directions. J Clin Endocrinol Metab. 2020;105(8)
49. Cazzo E, Gestic MA, Utrini MP, Chaim FD, Geloneze B, Pareja JC, et al. Glp-2: a poorly understood mediator enrolled in various bariatric/metabolic surgery-related pathophysiologic mechanisms. Arq Bras Cir Dig. 2016;29(4):272–5.
50. Cazzo E, Pareja JC, Chaim EA, Geloneze B, Barreto MR, Magro DO. GLP-1 and GLP-2 levels are correlated with satiety regulation after Roux-en-Y gastric bypass: results of an exploratory prospective study. Obes Surg. 2017;27(3):703–8.
51. Sebunova N, Stsepetova J, Kullisaar T, Suija K, Ratsep A, Junkin I, et al. Changes in adipokine levels and metabolic profiles following bariatric surgery. BMC Endocr Disord. 2022;22(1):33.
52. Cibickova L, Grega M, Dohnal R, Schovanek J. Effect of laparoscopic sleeve gastrectomy on serum Adipokine levels. Physiol Res. 2023;72(Suppl 2):S165–S72.
53. Askarpour M, Alizadeh S, Hadi A, Symonds ME, Miraghajani M, Sheikhi A, et al. Effect of bariatric surgery on the circulating level of adiponectin, Chemerin, plasminogen activator Inhibitor-1, leptin, Resistin, and Visfatin: a systematic review and meta-analysis. Horm Metab Res. 2020;52(4):207–15.
54. Min T, Prior SL, Churm R, Dunseath G, Barry JD, Stephens JW. Effect of laparoscopic sleeve gastrectomy on static and dynamic measures of glucose homeostasis and Incretin hormone response 4-years post-operatively. Obes Surg. 2020;30(1):46–55.
55. Boonchaya-Anant P, Laichuthai N, Suwannasrisuk P, Houngngam N, Udomsawaengsup S, Snabboon T. Changes in testosterone levels and sex hormone-binding globulin levels in extremely obese men after bariatric surgery. Int J Endocrinol. 2016;2016:1416503.
56. Min T, Prior SL, Dunseath G, Churm R, Barry JD, Stephens JW. Temporal effects of bariatric surgery on Adipokines, inflammation and oxidative stress in subjects with impaired glucose homeostasis at 4 years of follow-up. Obes Surg. 2020;30(5):1712–8.
57. Emami MR, Safabakhsh M, Khorshidi M, Moradi Moghaddam O, Mohammed SH, Zarezadeh M, et al. Effect of bariatric surgery on endogenous sex hormones and sex hormone-binding globulin levels: a systematic review and meta-analysis. Surg Obes Relat Dis. 2021;17(9):1621–36.
58. Kamal M, Aisha HAA, Fahmy MH, Abosayed AK. The impact of laparoscopic sleeve gastrectomy on thyroid functions in Egyptian patients with obesity. J Gastrointest Surg. 2023;27(7):1345–52.
59. Tian Z, Nie Y, Li Z, Wang P, Zhang N, Hei X, et al. Total weight loss induces the alteration in thyroid function after bariatric surgery. Front Endocrinol (Lausanne). 2024;15:1333033.
60. Gudbrandsen OA, Dankel SN, Skumsnes L, Flolo TN, Folkestad OH, Nielsen HJ, et al. Short-term effects of vertical sleeve gastrectomy and Roux-en-Y gastric bypass on glucose homeostasis. Sci Rep. 2019;9(1):14817.
61. Vaz M, Pereira SS, Monteiro MP. Metabolomic signatures after bariatric surgery - a systematic review. Rev Endocr Metab Disord. 2022;23(3):503–19.
62. Calik Basaran N, Dotan I, Dicker D. Post metabolic bariatric surgery weight regain: the importance of GLP-1 levels. Int J Obes. 2025;49(3):412–7.
63. Rao SR. Inflammatory markers and bariatric surgery: a meta-analysis. Inflamm Res. 2012;61(8):789–807.
64. van Veldhuisen SL, Gorter TM, van Woerden G, de Boer RA, Rienstra M, Hazebroek EJ, et al. Bariatric surgery and cardiovascular disease: a systematic review and meta-analysis. Eur Heart J. 2022;43(20):1955–69.

Impact of Microbiota on the Outcomes of Sleeve Gastrectomy

23

Esther Lluch

23.1 Introduction

23.1.1 Severe Obesity and the Gut Microbiome

Severe obesity is a chronic, multifactorial disease associated with metabolic, cardiovascular, and inflammatory complications. It arises from an imbalance between energy intake and expenditure, which are influenced by genetic, behavioural habits, and environmental factors. However, beyond these classical determinants, an increasing body of evidence is identifying the gut microbiota—the dense and diverse microbial ecosystem residing in the human gastrointestinal tract—as a critical regulator of energy metabolism and homeostasis [1, 2].

The gut microbiome is composed of approximately 10^{13}–10^{14} microorganisms, primarily belonging to the phyla *Firmicutes*, *Bacteroidetes*, *Actinobacteria*, and *Proteobacteria*. These microorganisms collectively encode a metabolic capacity that far exceeds that of the human genome, performing essential functions such as the fermentation of indigestible dietary components, the synthesis of vitamins and amino acids, and the production of short-chain fatty acids (SCFAs) such as acetate,

Severe obesity has been consistently associated with gut dysbiosis. Moreover, gastric resection, together with the physiological and functional changes resulting from the procedure, can further modify the composition and activity of the microbiota. These alterations may play a relevant role in shaping postoperative clinical outcomes.

E. Lluch (✉)
Regulatory Affairs Department, Becton Dickinson, Madrid, Spain

J. Ruiz-Tovar (ed.), *Multidisciplinary Management of Sleeve Gastrectomy*,
https://doi.org/10.1007/978-3-032-25644-7_23

propionate, and butyrate [2, 3]. These metabolites serve as substrates for colonocytes, act as signalling molecules in glucose and lipid metabolism, and modulate immune and endocrine functions through G-protein–coupled receptors and epigenetic regulation.

In individuals with obesity, the intestinal microbiome exhibits quantitative and qualitative alterations, including reduced microbial diversity and functional imbalance. These changes extend beyond nutrient metabolism, influencing the immune system, endocrine regulation, and even neural pathways involved in appetite and energy balance [1].

23.1.2 Dysbiosis as a Feature of Obesity

The term dysbiosis refers to a pathological disturbance in the composition, diversity, and metabolic function of the gut microbiota that disrupts the symbiotic relationship between microorganisms and their host. In individuals with obesity, this imbalance is characterized by reduced microbial diversity, a higher *Firmicutes/Bacteroidetes* ratio, and an enrichment of pro-inflammatory and lipopolysaccharide (LPS)-producing taxa, including members of the *Enterobacteriaceae* and *Ruminococcaceae* families [1–3].

This dysbiotic configuration contributes to low-grade endotoxemia, increased gut permeability, and the altered production of microbial metabolites such as short-chain fatty acids (SCFAs) and bile acids [4]. The combined effects of these disturbances promote insulin resistance, fat accumulation, and metabolic dysfunction.

The origin of dysbiosis in obesity is multifactorial. Diets high in saturated fat and refined carbohydrates selectively favour bacteria capable of thriving in energy-dense environments, while reduced fibre intake limits the growth of saccharolytic species producing anti-inflammatory SCFAs. Additional contributors include a sedentary lifestyle, antibiotic exposure, and genetic factors influencing immune–microbial interactions [2, 3].

As a result, dysbiosis in obesity is both a consequence and a driver of metabolic imbalance. It creates a self-perpetuating cycle in which microbial, immunological, and endocrine dysfunctions reinforce one another—ultimately promoting the persistence of the obese phenotype and its associated comorbidities.

23.1.3 Microbiota as a Metabolic Modulator

The human gut microbiota constitutes a highly complex and metabolically active ecosystem, composed of trillions of microorganisms that coexist in a mutualistic relationship with the host. This microbial community collectively forms what is now recognized as a metabolic organ, capable of influencing host physiology at multiple levels—metabolic, endocrine, immune, and even neural [1–3].

The microbiota contributes to fundamental processes such as digestion, nutrient absorption, and energy harvest, while simultaneously producing a vast array of bioactive compounds that function as metabolic and signalling mediators.

One of the microbiota's principal roles is the fermentation of non-digestible dietary polysaccharides and fibres that escape digestion in the upper gastrointestinal tract. This process generates short-chain fatty acids (SCFAs)—mainly acetate, propionate, and butyrate—that serve as energy sources for colonocytes and act as signalling molecules regulating glucose and lipid metabolism [2, 3]. SCFAs influence host physiology through G-protein–coupled receptors (GPR41 and GPR43) and by modulating gene expression via histone deacetylase inhibition, thereby affecting insulin sensitivity, intestinal barrier function, and inflammatory tone.

In addition, the gut microbiota plays a crucial role in the metabolism of bile acids, mediating their deconjugation, dehydroxylation, and transformation into secondary bile acids such as deoxycholic and lithocholic acid. These molecules serve as ligands for the farnesoid X receptor (FXR) and Takeda G-protein–coupled receptor 5 (TGR5), both of which regulate lipid oxidation, glucose homeostasis, and energy expenditure [4, 5]. Through this cross-talk, the microbiota indirectly modulates enterohepatic circulation and contributes to systemic metabolic regulation.

Microbial activity also impacts enteroendocrine signalling. Certain bacterial metabolites stimulate the release of glucagon-like peptide 1 (GLP-1) and peptide YY (PYY) from intestinal L-cells, promoting satiety and improving glycaemic control. Meanwhile, butyrate and other microbial metabolites enhance mucin production and tight-junction integrity, reinforcing mucosal barrier function and preventing the translocation of inflammatory molecules such as lipopolysaccharides (LPS).

Collectively, these interactions illustrate that the gut microbiota operates as a dynamic metabolic interface between the host and the environment. Its balance determines not only nutrient processing but also immune regulation, hormonal communication, and energy storage. Disruption of this equilibrium—through dietary, environmental, or pathological factors—can therefore profoundly influence metabolic health.

Understanding these complex mechanisms establishes the conceptual framework for the analysis of how sleeve gastrectomy surgery (SG) alters the intestinal ecosystem and how microbial adaptations contribute to the procedure's metabolic and clinical outcomes.

23.2 Anatomical and Functional Determinants of Microbiota Remodelling after Sleeve Gastrectomy

Sleeve gastrectomy surgery (SG) not only acts as a restrictive bariatric procedure but also triggers a cascade of anatomical and physiological modifications that extend along the gastrointestinal tract. These changes influence factors such as luminal pH, bile acid metabolism, intestinal transit, and hormonal secretion—all of which create a distinct environment for microbial selection, colonization, and metabolic activity. Understanding these determinants is essential for interpreting the microbial and metabolic shifts observed after surgery.

23.2.1 Anatomical Reconfiguration and Luminal Environment

During SG, approximately 70–80% of the stomach—mainly the fundus and greater curvature—is resected, resulting in a tubular gastric sleeve with a markedly reduced capacity. This anatomical transformation significantly decreases gastric acid secretion due to the loss of parietal cell mass and alters the intragastric pH [2].

The increase in gastric pH weakens the physiological barrier that normally limits bacterial translocation from the upper to the lower gastrointestinal tract. As a result, greater bacterial survival occurs during gastric passage, potentially leading to increased microbial diversity in the small intestine [4].

Moreover, resection of the fundus eliminates a major site of ghrelin production, a hormone implicated in appetite regulation and gastrointestinal motility. The consequent acceleration of gastric emptying modifies the exposure of nutrients to digestive enzymes and alters the physicochemical composition of the chyme reaching the small intestine, which directly affects the availability of substrates for bacterial fermentation [3, 5].

23.2.2 Modifications in Gastrointestinal Transit and Nutrient Flow

The linear shape and reduced compliance of the gastric sleeve promote faster gastric emptying and intestinal transit, reducing the contact time between nutrients and the intestinal mucosa. These mechanical changes modify the distribution of nutrients along the gastrointestinal tract, shifting microbial substrate availability towards more undigested carbohydrates and proteins reaching the distal gut [1, 3].

This altered nutrient flow acts as a selective pressure on microbial communities: slow-fermenting anaerobes, such as certain Firmicutes, may decline, whereas facultative or fibre-degrading taxa, including *Bacteroidetes* and *Akkermansia muciniphila*, can expand [5]. The shift in substrate availability and fermentation kinetics thus initiates an ecological reorganization that favours species associated with improved metabolic efficiency and anti-inflammatory activity.

23.2.3 Bile Acid Metabolism and Microbial Cross-Talk

Bile acids are central mediators in host–microbiota interactions. After SG, changes in gastric capacity, nutrient exposure, and intestinal motility alter the enterohepatic circulation of bile acids. Several studies have shown an increase in circulating secondary bile acids following SG, reflecting enhanced microbial biotransformation and modified intestinal absorption [2, 3].

These metabolites act as signalling molecules through Farnesoid X receptor (FXR) and Takeda G protein-coupled receptor 5 (TGR5), regulating lipid and glucose metabolism. The mutual regulation between bile acids and microbiota forms a bi-directional loop: microbial enzymes such as bile salt hydrolases influence bile composition, while bile acids exert antimicrobial effects that shape microbial communities [3].

Thus, the altered bile acid profile after SG not only supports metabolic improvement but also redefines the ecological landscape of the gut.

23.2.4 Hormonal and Immune Modulation

The endocrine response to SG—marked by decreased ghrelin and increased GLP-1 and PYY—influences not only appetite and glucose homeostasis but also the gastrointestinal milieu [2, 3]. These hormones affect intestinal motility, mucosal secretion, and epithelial turnover, all of which modulate microbial niches and nutrient gradients.

Additionally, SG is associated with a reduction in systemic inflammatory markers and the partial restoration of immune homeostasis. The improved inflammatory profile contributes to the recovery of microbial diversity and the maintenance of mucosal integrity [1, 5]. The interaction between immune regulation and microbial composition represents a crucial component of the surgery's systemic benefits.

23.2.5 Integrated View

The anatomical simplification of the stomach, combined with changes in acid secretion, motility, bile acids, and hormones, reshapes the gut's ecological and metabolic conditions. These modifications collectively promote a microbiota remodelling that favours the taxa involved in SCFA production, bile acid metabolism, and mucosal barrier maintenance.

Hence, the microbiota acts not merely as a passive consequence of surgery but as a dynamic participant in the adaptive process following SG, mediating many of its downstream metabolic effects, as shown in Fig. 23.1.

23.3 Microbiota Composition and Functional Shifts after Sleeve Gastrectomy

Sleeve gastrectomy surgery (SG) results in profound and persistent alterations in the gut microbial community. These changes arise from the combined anatomical, hormonal, and metabolic effects described previously, resulting in a microbial

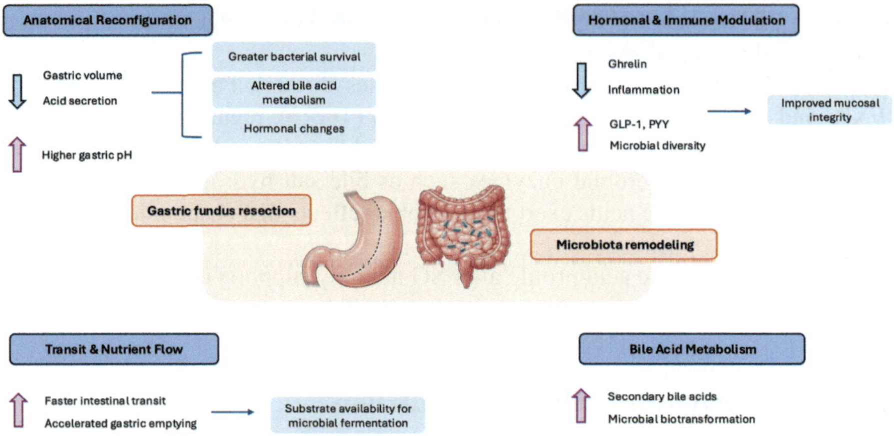

Fig. 23.1 Anatomical and physiological modifications following sleeve gastrectomy surgery and the associated functional adaptations

ecosystem that differs both from the preoperative state and from that of lean, non-operated individuals. An increasing body of evidence is demonstrating that these microbial rearrangements are not transient; rather, they evolve over time and contribute to the metabolic improvements observed after surgery.

23.3.1 Taxonomic Changes and Microbial Diversity

Most studies report a significant increase in microbial diversity within 6–12 months following SG. This contrasts with the low diversity typically observed in severe obesity and is generally interpreted as a marker of restored gut homeostasis.

A consistent finding across human cohorts is a decrease in the *Firmicutes/Bacteroidetes* ratio, a hallmark of dysbiosis in obesity [1, 2]. Following SG, *Bacteroidetes*—particularly genera such as *Bacteroides* and *Alistipes*—tend to proliferate, while *Firmicutes*, including *Clostridium* and *Lactobacillus*, decrease [3, 4].

Another frequently reported change is the enrichment of *Akkermansia muciniphila*, a mucin-degrading bacterium associated with improved mucosal barrier function and anti-inflammatory effects [4]. In some studies, *Proteobacteria* increase transiently after surgery, reflecting a period of microbial adaptation to the new luminal environment [1, 3].

Together, these compositional shifts move the postoperative microbiome towards a "lean-like" phenotype, closer to that observed in metabolically healthy individuals.

23.3.2 Temporal Dynamics of Microbial Adaptation

Longitudinal analyses reveal that microbial restructuring occurs within weeks after SG and continues to evolve over months. Some scientific studies reported early and sustained modifications in community structure up to 9 months postoperatively, while other reports observed that metabolomic profiles gradually aligned with those of healthy controls within a 6-month period [2, 3].

Initially, bacterial diversity may decrease due to surgical stress, perioperative antibiotics, and dietary restriction, but it typically recovers and surpasses baseline values during the intermediate postoperative phase. Over time, the microbiota stabilizes into a new equilibrium shaped by an altered pH, transit, and nutrient flow.

These temporal dynamics suggest that SG initiates a two-phase microbial remodelling process, illustrated in Fig. 23.2:

- An acute adaptive phase (0–3 months), characterized by transient dysbiosis and increased *Proteobacteria*;
- A long-term stabilization phase (6–12 months), marked by higher diversity and functional specialization.

23.3.3 Functional Reprogramming of the Microbial Community

Beyond taxonomy, SG profoundly affects the metabolic potential of the gut microbiota. Metagenomic and metabolomic analyses show an upregulation of microbial pathways involved in:

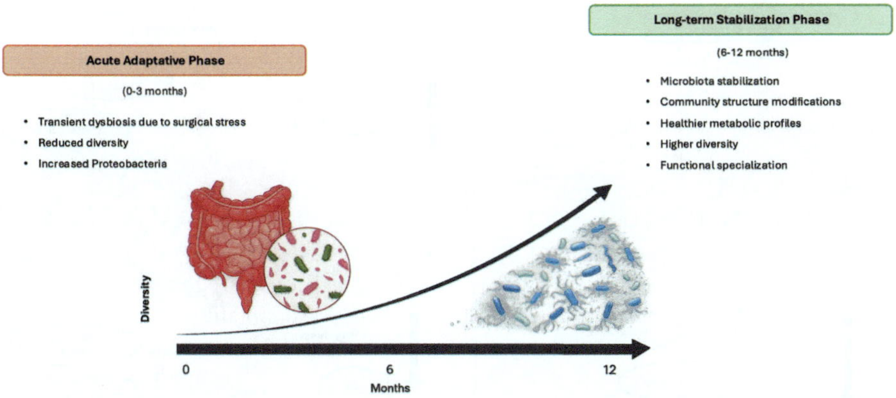

Fig. 23.2 Temporal dynamics of microbial adaptation with two phases of microbiota remodelling process after sleeve gastrectomy

- Short-chain fatty acid (SCFA) synthesis, particularly propionate and acetate, which enhance insulin sensitivity and GLP-1 secretion.
- Bile acid transformation, leading to the increased production of secondary bile acids that modulate host metabolism through FXR and TGR5 receptors.
- Reduction in lipopolysaccharide (LPS) biosynthesis, reflecting decreased endotoxemia and systemic inflammation.

These functional adaptations translate into a metabolically favourable microbiome, capable of producing signalling molecules that reinforce the host's metabolic recovery. Some studies demonstrated that postoperative microbial and metabolite profiles closely resembled those of healthy controls, suggesting a partial normalization of microbial function after SG [2].

Although both SG and Roux-en-Y gastric bypass (RYGB) lead to significant microbial alterations, their magnitude and nature differ. It was found that RYGB produces more abrupt and extensive changes due to intestinal rerouting and the increased exposure of the distal gut to bile acids, while SG induces moderate but persistent microbial reorganization without intestinal bypass [3].

It was further demonstrated that changes in oral and intestinal microbiota were more coordinated after SG, suggesting a more physiological adaptation of the microbial ecosystem [4].

Hence, while both procedures achieve comparable metabolic outcomes, SG maintains a more balanced host-microbiota interaction, potentially reducing the risk of long-term dysbiosis. Together, the microbial shifts induced by SG create a gastrointestinal profile that differs markedly from the patient's preoperative state, as shown in Fig. 23.3.

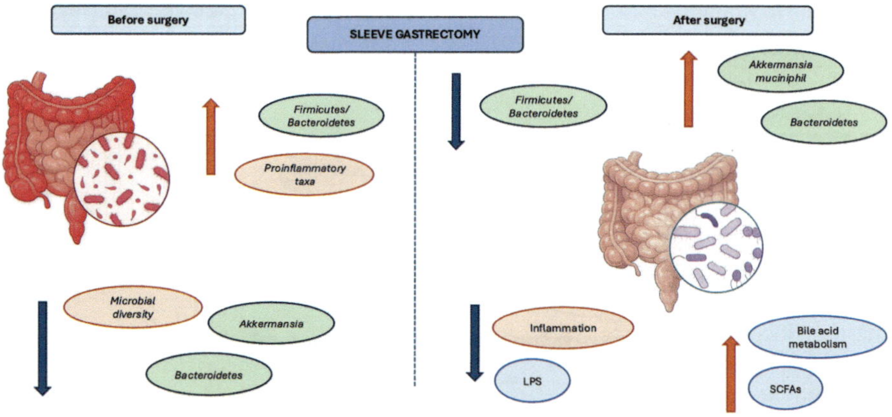

Fig. 23.3 Main microbiota changes after sleeve gastrectomy, including shifts in bacterial diversity and abundance associated with metabolic improvements

23.4 Impact of the Microbiota on the Outcomes of Sleeve Gastrectomy

Microbial remodelling after sleeve gastrectomy surgery (SG) plays an integral role in mediating the surgery's metabolic, gastrointestinal, and psychological outcomes.

The shift towards a more diverse and functionally balanced gut ecosystem enhances nutrient signalling, hormone secretion, and systemic metabolism. Current evidence indicates that the gut microbiota acts not only as a marker of metabolic recovery but as an active effector influencing weight loss, insulin sensitivity, inflammation, and even mental well-being following SG.

23.4.1 Influence on Weight Loss and Metabolic Improvement

The restoration of microbial diversity and the reduction of the *Firmicutes/Bacteroidetes* ratio after SG have been associated with greater postoperative weight loss and improved metabolic markers.

It has been demonstrated that patients who achieved the best glycaemic control and lipid profile improvements exhibited microbiota profiles enriched in *Akkermansia muciniphila* and *Bacteroides*. These taxa are known to support mucosal barrier integrity, bile acid turnover, and short-chain fatty acid (SCFA) production—all essential for glucose and lipid regulation.

Microbiota-derived SCFAs (acetate, propionate, butyrate) modulate hepatic gluconeogenesis, insulin sensitivity, and lipid oxidation through G-protein–coupled receptors (GPR41, GPR43) and the activation of GLP-1 secretion. The improved bile acid composition following SG also influences metabolism via FXR and TGR5 signalling pathways, linking microbial activity with host energy homeostasis [2, 3, 5].

These findings suggest that the microbial reprogramming induced by SG contributes synergistically to the hormonal and biochemical improvements traditionally attributed to the surgery, facilitating long-term metabolic success.

23.4.2 Gut Barrier Function and Inflammation

The improvement in intestinal barrier integrity represents another key mechanism through which microbiota changes influence outcomes.

In obesity, dysbiosis contributes to increased intestinal permeability, allowing for the translocation of lipopolysaccharides (LPS) and activation of proinflammatory pathways. Following SG, the increased abundance of *Akkermansia* and *Bacteroides* correlates with enhanced mucin production and tight-junction restoration, leading to reduced endotoxemia and systemic inflammation.

Some studies reviewed postoperative changes in gastrointestinal permeability, reporting that while transient variations may occur early after surgery, the long-term trend favours improved barrier function and reduced inflammatory signalling.

Consequently, the postoperative microbiota supports an anti-inflammatory state, which is crucial for insulin sensitivity, adipose tissue remodelling, and sustained metabolic recovery [4, 6].

23.4.3 Gastrointestinal Function and Nutrient Absorption

Changes in microbial ecology after sleeve gastrectomy surgery (SG) have significant repercussions on gastrointestinal physiology, digestive efficiency, and nutrient absorption. The anatomical reduction of the stomach and acceleration of gastric emptying modify chyme composition, luminal pH, and bile acid flow, thereby influencing microbial colonization patterns and fermentation dynamics throughout the gut.

Immediately after SG, the rapid alteration in nutrient transit and the selective pressure imposed by the new luminal environment can result in transient dysbiosis. This temporary microbial imbalance, combined with dietary restriction and postoperative antibiotic exposure, often manifests clinically as bloating, constipation, or irregular bowel movements. These symptoms are frequently reported during the first postoperative months and reflect the ongoing adaptation of the intestinal ecosystem to the new digestive physiology.

Furthermore, microbial reorganization affects nutrient absorption and metabolism. Reduced gastric acid production may impair the solubilization and bioavailability of micronutrients such as iron, calcium, and vitamin B_{12}, while shifts in microbial enzymatic activity can alter carbohydrate fermentation and protein putrefaction [2, 3]. The decline in butyrate-producing bacteria may transiently decrease colonic trophic support, although recovery typically occurs as microbial diversity reestablishes. In parallel, the enrichment of the *Akkermansia muciniphila* and *Bacteroides* species promotes mucin turnover and intestinal barrier regeneration, contributing to functional recovery [5].

Evidence also supports the role of microbiota modulation in improving gastrointestinal tolerance after SG. In a randomized, placebo-controlled study, it was demonstrated that patients receiving postoperative probiotic supplementation experienced fewer gastrointestinal symptoms, a more rapid normalization of bowel habits, and a more balanced microbial composition. These benefits are likely mediated by the restoration of commensal populations, increased SCFA production, and the suppression of proinflammatory bacterial taxa.

Over the long term, the microbiota contributes to the optimization of digestive efficiency and reduction in gastrointestinal discomfort by stabilizing fermentation patterns, normalizing bile acid metabolism, and enhancing epithelial nutrient uptake. Hence, targeted microbial strategies—including probiotic, prebiotic, and symbiotic interventions—represent promising adjuncts to facilitate postoperative adaptation, minimize digestive side effects, and improve nutrient utilization in SG patients [6].

23.4.4 Gut-Brain Axis and Psychological Outcomes

Beyond its metabolic and digestive roles, the gut microbiota exerts a profound influence on mental health, emotional regulation, and cognitive function through the gut–brain axis—a bidirectional communication network linking the enteric and central nervous systems via neural, hormonal, and immune pathways.

This system integrates vagal nerve signalling, microbial metabolite production, neurotransmitter synthesis, and immune modulation, enabling intestinal microorganisms to affect stress response, mood, and behaviour [1–3].

Following sleeve gastrectomy surgery (SG), patients often experience notable changes in emotional well-being, which may relate not only to weight loss and hormonal regulation but also to microbiota-mediated neurochemical adaptations.

Microbial metabolites such as short-chain fatty acids (SCFAs)—particularly acetate, propionate, and butyrate—can cross the blood–brain barrier and influence central processes by modulating microglial activity, neuroinflammation, and neurotransmitter turnover.

Additionally, the bacterial metabolism of tryptophan, a precursor of serotonin, yields indole derivatives and kynurenine pathway intermediates that interact with serotonergic and dopaminergic signalling, directly affecting mood and anxiety regulation.

Some studies provided clinical evidence supporting these interactions: in a randomized, double-blind, placebo-controlled pilot study, short-term probiotic supplementation combined with dietary counselling significantly improved depressive symptoms and emotional well-being in post-bariatric patients. The intervention normalized faecal microbial diversity and increased the relative abundance of *Bifidobacterium* and *Lactobacillus* species, taxa known to produce gamma-aminobutyric acid (GABA) and serotonin precursors. These findings suggest that targeted modulation of the microbiota may influence central neurotransmission and stress resilience during postoperative recovery [4, 5].

Although current evidence remains preliminary, these observations underscore the microbiota's potential role in neuropsychological adaptation following metabolic surgery. The restoration of microbial balance may contribute to reduced systemic inflammation, improved vagal signalling, and enhanced serotonin and SCFA-mediated communication between the gut and brain.

Future studies combining microbiome, metabolomic, and neuroimaging analyses are warranted to elucidate the causal pathways underpinning this gut–brain interaction and to determine whether microbiota-targeted therapies can enhance mental health outcomes after SG.

23.4.5 Integrated Mechanistic View

Collectively, as illustrated in Fig. 23.4, the postoperative microbiota contributes to SG outcomes through four interrelated mechanisms:

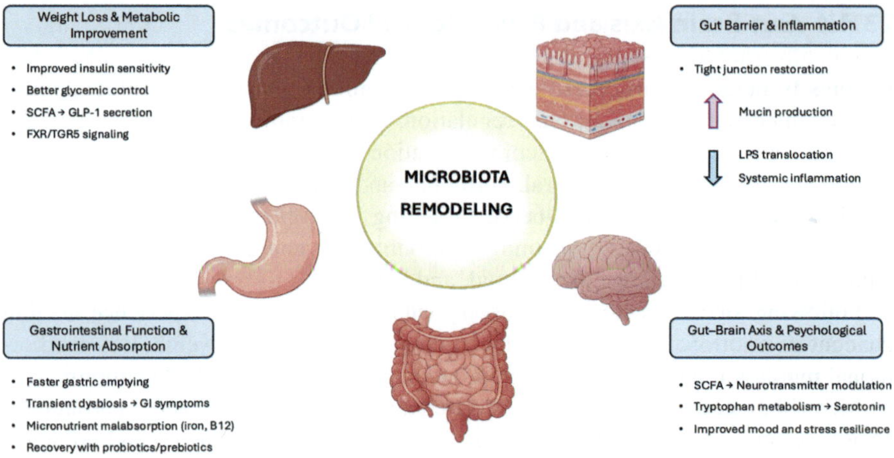

Fig. 23.4 Impact of microbiota remodelling on the outcomes of sleeve gastrectomy, in metabolic system, gut barrier, gastrointestinal function, and gut-brain axis

- Metabolic regulation—enhanced SCFA and bile acid signalling improves insulin sensitivity and lipid metabolism.
- Barrier integrity—restored mucosal protection reduces inflammation and endotoxemia.
- Gastrointestinal function—microbial balance improves motility and nutrient handling.
- Neuroendocrine communication—gut-derived metabolites modulate mood and appetite control.

Thus, microbial recovery acts as both a consequence and catalyst of successful metabolic adaptation, supporting a more holistic understanding of the surgery's effects.

23.5 Therapeutic Perspectives and Research Directions

Although sleeve gastrectomy surgery (SG) induces favourable microbial and metabolic changes, the degree of microbiota recovery and its correlation with long-term outcomes vary among individuals. This inter-patient variability highlights the potential for microbiota-targeted interventions, such as those illustrated in Fig. 23.5, to optimize postoperative adaptation and the durability of weight-loss effects.

23.5.1 Probiotic and Prebiotic Supplementation

Recent studies indicate that probiotic administration can attenuate early postoperative gastrointestinal discomfort and support microbial re-equilibration.

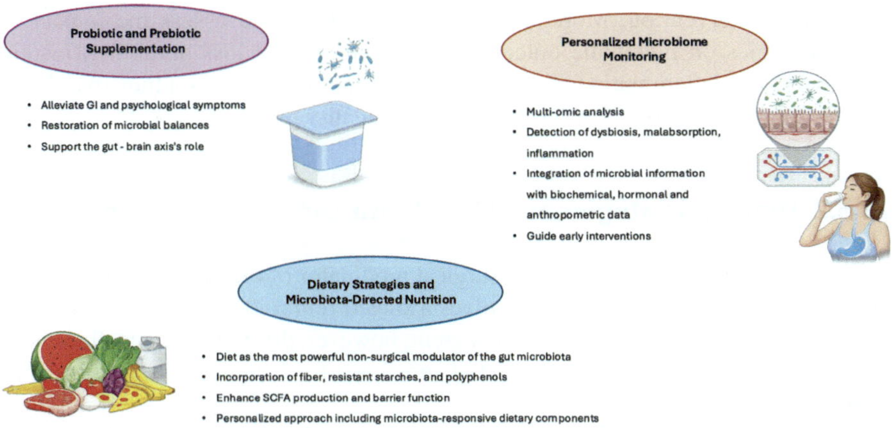

Fig. 23.5 Microbiota-targeted strategies after sleeve gastrectomy, such as probiotic and prebiotic supplementation, dietary strategies, and personalized microbiome monitoring

In a randomized, placebo-controlled trial, it was observed that SG patients receiving *Lactobacillus*- and *Bifidobacterium*-based probiotics experienced fewer symptoms of constipation and bloating compared with controls, suggesting that the restoration of microbial balance facilitates gut motility and tolerance [1].

Similarly, other clinical trials demonstrated that a short-term intervention combining probiotics and dietary counselling significantly improved depressive symptoms and emotional well-being in post-bariatric patients. The observed benefits were associated with an increased abundance of *Bifidobacterium* and *Lactobacillus*, genera known to produce gamma-aminobutyric acid (GABA) and serotonin precursors, supporting the gut–brain axis's role in postoperative neuropsychological recovery.

In addition to probiotics, prebiotic supplementation—the administration of non-digestible food components that selectively stimulate the growth of beneficial microbes—has emerged as a promising adjunct to bariatric surgery. Common prebiotics include inulin, fructo-oligosaccharides (FOS), and galacto-oligosaccharides (GOS), which promote the proliferation of *Bifidobacterium* and *Akkermansia muciniphila* while enhancing the production of short-chain fatty acids (SCFAs) such as butyrate and propionate [3, 4]. These metabolites improve intestinal barrier integrity, regulate glucose and lipid metabolism, and exert anti-inflammatory effects, all of which are particularly relevant in the postoperative metabolic context.

Combining probiotics and prebiotics—forming symbiotic formulations—may offer synergistic effects by recolonizing the gut with beneficial strains and providing them with fermentable substrates for sustained activity. Early studies in bariatric populations suggest that such combinations could accelerate microbial stabilization, support nutrient absorption, and mitigate gastrointestinal and psychological symptoms [1–3].

While current findings are encouraging, large-scale and long-term clinical trials are needed to define the optimal strain selection, prebiotic type, dosage, and duration of intervention. Moreover, future research should assess the impact of these strategies on metabolic outcomes, including weight loss durability, insulin sensitivity, and inflammation markers, to determine their role as adjunctive therapies for improving surgical success and patient quality of life.

23.5.2 Dietary Strategies and Microbiota-Directed Nutrition

Diet remains the most powerful non-surgical modulator of the gut microbiota. After SG, dietary progression typically involves a staged reintroduction of foods with an emphasis on high-protein and low-fat content; however, this regimen may limit fibre and prebiotic intake, which are essential substrates for beneficial bacteria such as *Akkermansia* and *Bacteroides* [3, 4].

Incorporating soluble fibres, resistant starches, and polyphenol-rich foods may promote the production of short-chain fatty acids (SCFAs), enhance barrier function, and counteract dysbiosis.

Nutritional counselling should therefore move beyond macronutrient adequacy to include microbiota-responsive dietary components, supporting a more personalized approach to postoperative nutrition.

23.5.3 Personalized Microbiome Monitoring

Recent advances in metagenomics, metabolomics, and metatranscriptomics now permit a dynamic evaluation of the gut microbiota's composition and function, offering a more integrated view of its role in postoperative recovery. In the context of sleeve gastrectomy (SG), incorporating microbiome monitoring into routine follow-up could help detect persistent dysbiosis, malabsorption, or inflammatory imbalance, enabling early and personalized interventions.

Integrating microbial information with biochemical, hormonal, and anthropometric data provides a more comprehensive framework for risk assessment and clinical decision-making. This multi-omics approach—linking microbial taxa, metabolites, and host metabolic markers—has revealed strong associations between microbiota restoration and improved metabolic outcomes, while persistent microbial alterations correlate with delayed recovery. Longitudinal studies combining sequencing and metabolite profiling have further demonstrated that microbiota adaptation follows a structured trajectory, with early instability followed by long-term stabilization parallel to metabolic improvement.

Such integrative monitoring aligns with enhanced recovery after surgery (ERAS) protocols, supporting a precision medicine approach in which microbial data guide nutritional adjustments, probiotic or prebiotic interventions, and overall postoperative management to optimize surgical success and long-term metabolic health.

23.5.4 Research Challenges and Future Directions

Despite major advances, several knowledge gaps remain:

- Causality: Current studies largely demonstrate associations rather than causal links between microbial shifts and clinical outcomes. Longitudinal and mechanistic models, including germ-free or fecal-transplant experiments, are required.
- Standardization: Differences in sampling sites, sequencing methods, and dietary control complicate comparisons between studies [3, 5].
- Long-term effects: Most analyses are limited to the first postoperative year. The durability of microbial and metabolic changes beyond this period remains unclear.
- Combinatorial therapies: Future work should evaluate the synergistic effects of bariatric surgery + microbiota modulation (e.g., probiotics, bile-acid analogues, GLP-1 agonists) on metabolic remission.

Progress in these areas will consolidate the microbiota as a therapeutic target and predictive biomarker for postoperative outcomes.

23.6 Conclusions

Sleeve gastrectomy surgery (SG) exerts its therapeutic effects through a complex interplay between anatomical modification, hormonal adaptation, and microbial remodelling.

Beyond mechanical restriction and caloric reduction, the surgery fundamentally reconfigures the gastrointestinal environment—altering the luminal pH, bile acid metabolism, transit time, and enteroendocrine signalling—which collectively reshape the gut microbiota.

Postoperatively, the microbial ecosystem undergoes a transition characterized by increased diversity, a reduced *Firmicutes/Bacteroidetes* ratio, and enrichment of metabolically beneficial taxa such as *Akkermansia muciniphila*, *Bacteroides*, and *Alistipes*.

These shifts enhance the microbial production of short-chain fatty acids (SCFAs) and secondary bile acids, metabolites that modulate insulin sensitivity, lipid metabolism, and inflammation. Consequently, the microbiota emerges not only as a marker but as a mediator of metabolic recovery following SG.

Furthermore, microbial restoration contributes to improved intestinal barrier integrity, reduced systemic inflammation, and enhanced neuroendocrine regulation, supporting both metabolic and psychological well-being.

Preliminary interventional studies suggest that probiotic and dietary modulation may reinforce these benefits, reducing gastrointestinal symptoms and improving mood in postoperative patients.

Although causal relationships remain to be fully elucidated, these findings highlight the therapeutic potential of microbiota-centred approaches as adjuncts to bariatric surgery.

Looking forward, integrating microbiome science into metabolic surgery represents a critical step towards precision medicine.

Personalized microbiota profiling, dietary optimization, and probiotic strategies could enable clinicians to predict and enhance surgical outcomes, minimize complications, and sustain long-term metabolic health.

In this context, the gut microbiota should be viewed not as a passive bystander, but as a dynamic biological partner in the success of sleeve gastrectomy surgery.

References

1. Coimbra VOR, Crovesy L, Ribeiro-Alves M, Faller ALK, Mattos F, Rosado EL. Gut microbiota profile in adults undergoing bariatric surgery: a systematic review. Nutrients. 2022;14(23):4979. https://doi.org/10.3390/nu14234979.
2. Ahmad AF, Caparrós-Martín JA, Lee S, O'Gara F, Yeap BB, Green DJ, et al. Gut microbiome and associated metabolites following bariatric surgery and comparison to healthy controls. Microorganisms. 2023;11(5):1126. https://doi.org/10.3390/microorganisms11051126.
3. Dang JT, Mocanu V, Park H, Laffin M, Hotte N, Karmali S, et al. Roux-en-Y gastric bypass and sleeve gastrectomy induce substantial and persistent changes in microbial communities and metabolic pathways. Gut Microbes. 2022;14(1):2050636. https://doi.org/10.1080/19490976.2022.2050636.
4. Stefura T, Zapała B, Gosiewski T, Skomarovska O, Pędziwiatr M, Major P. Changes in the composition of oral and intestinal microbiota after sleeve gastrectomy and Roux-en-Y gastric bypass and their impact on outcomes of bariatric surgery. Obes Surg. 2022;32(5):1439–50. https://doi.org/10.1007/s11695-022-05954-9.
5. Komorniak N, Kaczmarczyk M, Łoniewski I, Martynova-Van Kley A, Nalian A, Wroński M, et al. Analysis of the efficacy of diet and short-term probiotic intervention on depressive symptoms in patients after bariatric surgery: a randomized double-blind placebo-controlled pilot study. Nutrients. 2023;15(23):4905. https://doi.org/10.3390/nu15234905.
6. Dowgiałło-Gornowicz N, Mysiorska D, Sosnowska-Turek E, Botulińska A, Lech P. Initial study on the impact of probiotics on postoperative gastrointestinal symptoms and gut microbiota after sleeve gastrectomy: a placebo-controlled study. Nutrients. 2024;16(20):3498. https://doi.org/10.3390/nu16203498.

Enhanced Recovery After Surgery (ERAS) Protocols

24

Jaime Ruiz-Tovar

24.1 Introduction

Recent improvements in perioperative care for bariatric patients, the optimization of surgical techniques, advances in the instruments available, and the standardization of bariatric surgery programs have led to a decrease in the morbidity and mortality rates of these procedures. All of this has led to an exponential increase in laparoscopic bariatric surgery year after year, with vertical gastrectomy, Roux-en-Y gastric bypass, and one-anastomosis gastric bypass being the most commonly performed procedures worldwide [1].

Given the increase in the prevalence of obesity and its associated diseases, and the economic cost associated with its therapeutic management, bariatric surgery has proven to be not only the most clinically effective method for achieving long-term improvement in these pathologies, but also a cost-effective procedure with low complication rates, despite being a population group at high surgical risk. Sleeve gastrectomy has become the most widely performed technique in the world as it is a simpler procedure than other techniques, with a low complication rate, a shorter learning curve, and excellent results in weight loss and improvement of associated comorbidities [1, 2].

Operating time, surgical equipment, healthcare personnel costs, and hospital stays are expensive and limited resources, so improving the logistics of surgical procedures increases productivity and quality of care [3].

The concept of enhanced recovery after surgery (ERAS) was described by Kehlet in 1997. ERAS programs have been widely developed in colorectal surgery, demonstrating that perioperative care leads to earlier recovery and shorter hospital stays, associated with improved patient well-being. Although the content of different

J. Ruiz-Tovar (✉)
Department of Biomedicine and Health Sciences, Alfonso X University, Madrid, Spain

J. Ruiz-Tovar (ed.), *Multidisciplinary Management of Sleeve Gastrectomy*,
https://doi.org/10.1007/978-3-032-25644-7_24

ERAS programs may vary, there are points that are common to all, such as a minimally invasive approach whenever possible, the administration of short-acting anesthetic drugs, optimal pain control, prophylaxis of postoperative nausea and vomiting, and aggressive postoperative rehabilitation, including early ambulation and reintroduction of oral feeding. The rationale for using these measures is to reduce the body's response to perioperative stress, allowing for early restoration of organ function and, as a result, better and faster patient recovery [4–6]. The key to these programs is a multimodal approach, involving several specialists working on different fronts but with a common goal, which allows for a synergistic effect of the different measures adopted.

24.2 Special Features of ERAS Protocols in Sleeve Gastrectomy

As with all ERAS protocols, and those for sleeve gastrectomy are no exception, a multidisciplinary approach involving different specialists (surgeons, anesthesiologists, endocrinologists, rehabilitation specialists, specialized nursing staff, etc.) is key to the success of these programs. But beyond the participation of healthcare professionals, patient involvement is essential. Therefore, it is important to inform the patient preoperatively about the different stages they will go through before, during, and after the operation, creating realistic expectations about pain management, mobilization, nutrition, and hospital stay. Well-informed patients have been shown to be more accepting of the measures put in place. Working on the basis of established protocols has been shown to improve the reproducibility of the procedure, leaving less room for error and increasing the speed with which the various measures are implemented [1, 7, 9].

To date, most ERAS protocols published in the literature have been based on individual programs at certain institutions [3, 5–10]. In Spain, the Spanish Multimodal Rehabilitation Group (GERM) developed the first national ERAS protocol for bariatric surgery in 2014, focusing mainly on sleeve gastrectomy and Roux-en-Y gastric bypass [11]. Since then, updates have been made every 2 years. Based on this protocol, the Clinical Pathway in Bariatric Surgery was subsequently developed, endorsed by the GERM, the Spanish Society for Obesity Surgery (SECO), and the Spanish Association of Surgeons (AEC) [12].

The ERAS protocol in bariatric surgery, which is entirely applicable to patients undergoing sleeve gastrectomy, has many similarities with any other protocol for other types of surgery. However, given the special characteristics of these patients, there are certain peculiarities that differentiate them from other protocols.

Before surgery, providing detailed information to the patient, optimizing comorbidities, and assessing nutritional status are common protocols for other types of surgery. Within nutritional optimization, patients with severe obesity often present a different type of malnutrition. Their optimization requires intraoperative weight loss of around 10% of their body weight, but ensuring sufficient intake of protein and other macro- and micronutrients. Therefore, balanced diets of 800 kcal/day are prescribed for 2–4 weeks prior to surgery, preferably with commercial formulas, which homogenize caloric intake and ensure a sufficient amount of nutrients are ingested [13].

Likewise, the prevalence of SAHS (sleep apnea-hypopnea syndrome) and OHS (obesity hypoventilation syndrome) among patients indicated for bariatric surgery is 76–96%, but only 15–20% are diagnosed. If OHS is diagnosed and CPAP is indicated, it is essential to use it for at least 4–6 weeks before the operation, as it reduces the incidence of cardiopulmonary complications [11, 12].

It was traditionally thought that patients with severe obesity had delayed gastric emptying and that it was therefore advisable to establish a long preoperative fasting period to avoid bronchoaspiration during the anesthetic intubation process. However, there is now sufficient scientific evidence to disprove the benefits of prolonged fasting. A Cochrane review concludes that avoiding prolonged fasting not only reduces postoperative insulin resistance but also shortens the hospital stay. Therefore, in sleeve gastrectomy, a 6-h fasting period for solids is also recommended, but carbohydrate-enriched drinks may be consumed up to 2 h before anesthetic induction [12].

On the contrary, the RICA (intensified recovery in abdominal surgery) [14], published by the Spanish Ministry of Health, includes among its recommendations that short-acting anxiolytics may interfere with the onset of recovery of mobility and intake capacity, without affecting the length of hospital stay, and may therefore be used to facilitate regional anesthesia techniques when indicated. There is no evidence in this regard in patients undergoing sleeve gastrectomy, but given the increased risk of respiratory depression in these patients, it is recommended to avoid the use of anxiolytics preoperatively [12].

Among intraoperative measures, the importance of multimodal analgesia should be highlighted. There is clear scientific evidence of the superiority of epidural analgesia used in open abdominal surgery, both in terms of analgesic quality and lower rates of postoperative complications. However, epidural analgesia in laparoscopic surgery has not been shown to reduce hospital stay or promote early recovery of intestinal function. Given that sleeve gastrectomy is performed primarily by laparoscopic approach, despite the better analgesic profile, epidural analgesia is not recommended as a routine analgesic method due to the risk-benefit ratio of the technique [12]. Although the Clinical Pathway for Obesity Surgery does not recommend the routine use of local anesthetic infiltration of trocar wounds, considering that there is insufficient evidence to show that it improves immediate postoperative pain after laparoscopy, our group has published studies that have shown that its efficacy may be comparable to that obtained with epidural analgesia [15]. However, two recent studies by our group found that transverse abdominal plane block, guided by laparoscopy to minimize the distortion caused by the adipose tissue in these patients during ultrasound-guided puncture, achieved a greater analgesic effect than port infiltration [16, 17]. A recent meta-analysis has shown that transverse abdominal plane block reduces postoperative pain and opioid consumption in laparoscopic bariatric surgery [18].

Among the postoperative measures, early mobilization with sitting up 6 h after surgery and starting oral fluid intake at the same time are consistent with the measures recommended for other procedures. The use of CPAP is recommended in patients with SAHS who have been adapted to its use preoperatively, starting on the first night after surgery. Far from increasing the risk of anastomotic leakage due to increased pressure from inspired air, in patients well adapted to its use, it improves tissue oxygenation and reduces the risk of dehiscence. Regarding dietary progression, patients undergoing sleeve gastrectomy need to consume a liquid diet for at least 2–4 weeks after surgery [12].

Recently, the use of analytical markers, mainly acute phase reactants (C-reactive protein, procalcitonin, etc.), has become increasingly valuable for the early diagnosis of complications and, as a result, their use prior to patient discharge is becoming more widespread. It has been shown that the greatest prognostic value is when their levels are monitored in several determinations, and a decrease in them is observed once the peak has been reached. This can be very useful for surgeries with average hospital stays of 4–5 days, such as colorectal surgery. However, in sleeve gastrectomy, which allows hospital stays of 24–48 h, monitoring analytical values does not make sense. Nevertheless, it has been observed that single C-reactive protein and procalcitonin values above a threshold 24 h after surgery may be predictive of complications. Therefore, their determination may be helpful, along with other clinical parameters, prior to making the decision to discharge the patient [19, 20].

The discharge criteria for patients undergoing sleeve gastrectomy are the same as for other procedures: no surgical complications or fever, pain controlled with oral analgesia, full ambulation, and patient acceptance [11]. Upon discharge, it is recommended to continue antithrombotic prophylaxis for 3–4 weeks with low molecular weight heparins. Likewise, nutritional recommendations include a low-calorie, high-protein liquid diet, divided into several doses. A telephone check-up with the patient 48 h after hospital discharge is advisable, and the patient should attend an in-person consultation 15 days after the procedure [11].

24.3 Results of the Implementation of ERAS Protocols in Sleeve Gastrectomy

Bamgbade et al. [21] conducted an observational study, analyzing 406 patients who underwent bariatric surgery over a period of 4 years. They reported an intraoperative complication rate of 0.5% and a postoperative complication rate of 3.4%, of which 60% occurred during the first 24 h after surgery. After applying the ERAS protocol, they observed a decrease in the average hospital stay from 2 to 1 day. They concluded that for the correct implementation of these protocols, a learning curve of 100 patients is necessary, establishing the decrease in hospital stay as an indicator of experience. They also argued that most patients can be discharged 24 h after surgery.

Geubbels et al. [10] conducted a retrospective study analyzing the implementation of an ERAS protocol in unselected patients in a high-volume surgical hospital in the Netherlands. They defined the ERAS protocol as the removal of tubes, the use of multimodal analgesia, and early ambulation. They observed that hospital stays decreased with the application of the ERAS protocol, while the complication rate remained unchanged. The readmission rate also remained unchanged, although a greater number of Clavien-Dindo Classification grade I-IVa complications occurred outside the hospital setting, although this did not result in a worse outcome for patients.

Similarly, other groups have also reported hospital stays of less than 24 h, and some authors even argue that bariatric surgery could become an outpatient procedure [22]. Evidence in the literature shows that most complications occur during the first postoperative day and that most complications leading to readmission could not have been prevented by a longer hospital stay [1].

24.3.1 Results of the Implementation of the Spanish Enhanced Recovery Protocol in Bariatric Surgery

Following the ERAS protocol in bariatric surgery developed within the GERM, we conducted a first multicenter pilot study on sleeve gastrectomy and Roux-en-Y gastric bypass to evaluate the implementation of the protocol and its results [23]. A total of 125 patients were included in three Spanish hospitals between January and June 2015. We analyzed compliance with the protocol, morbidity and mortality, hospital stay, and readmission rates. The bariatric procedures performed were 68 Roux-en-Y gastric bypasses (54.4%) and 57 sleeve gastrectomies (45.6%). All procedures were performed laparoscopically, except for one case that required conversion (0.8%). The median postoperative pain, quantified using a visual analog scale, 24 h after surgery was 20 mm (range 0–50 mm). Postoperative nausea and vomiting occurred in 5.6%, complications in 4.8%; the reoperation rate was 4%, and mortality 0.8%. The median hospital stay was 2 days, and the readmission rate was 2.4%. Compliance with all protocol items was achieved in 78.4% of patients. There were no significant differences between the two bariatric techniques.

The morbidity and mortality rates in this study were similar to those described by other groups following ERAS protocols and bariatric surgery quality standards [5, 10]. The main difference between the results of this pilot study and those described by other groups is the length of hospital stay. As mentioned above, some groups describe stays of 24 h and even the possibility of performing outpatient surgery. In our study, the median length of stay was 2 days, but no patient was discharged within 24 h of surgery. To date, we still have concerns about the occurrence of complications away from a hospital setting, which could lead to a fatal outcome. The systematic review by Elliott et al. concluded that there is still insufficient evidence to justify such early hospital discharge [1].

After observing the safety of the implementation of the national ERAS protocol, we sought to determine the benefits of its implementation by comparing it with conventional care. To do this, we conducted a prospective multicenter study including 233 consecutive patients undergoing bariatric surgery, including sleeve gastrectomy and Roux-en-Y gastric bypass, following the national ERAS protocol. We compared it with a historical cohort of 286 patients who underwent bariatric procedures in the same centers and followed a conventional care protocol. As in the previous study, we evaluated compliance with the different items of the protocol, morbidity and mortality, hospital stay, and readmission rate [24]. There were no significant differences between groups in the rate of complications, mortality, and readmission. Postoperative pain and hospital stay were lower in patients who complied with the ERAS protocol. Overall compliance with the protocol was 80%, with the items with the lowest compliance being the preoperative diet (89.6%), goal-directed fluid therapy (80%), opioid-free analgesia (96.7%), the start of oral intake 6 h after surgery (88%), and early mobilization 6 h after surgery (89.6%).

In addition to less postoperative pain in the ERAS group, there was also a reduction in acute phase reactant values (white blood cell count and C-reactive protein). These data reflected that ERAS protocols reduce the perioperative stress response associated with surgical aggression. It has been hypothesized that the different items included in the protocol tend to cause a certain degree of immunomodulation, reducing the immune response, decreasing tissue damage, and ultimately minimizing postoperative pain [25].

The reduction in hospital stay could have been achieved without the need to apply an ERAS protocol, simply by forcing early discharge, but in our opinion, the lower perception of pain is associated with a feeling of higher quality of life in the patient, which increases their satisfaction with the procedure. With good pain control, the patient readily accepts early hospital discharge. Therefore, the shorter hospital stay is simply the result of good pain control. One of the main objectives of ERAS protocols is to reduce the impact of surgical aggression and thus promote post-surgical recovery. The main symptom reflecting surgical aggression is pain. With the aim of reducing the incidence and severity of pain, ERAS protocols include a multimodal approach to pain management. Multimodal analgesia consists of the use of two or more drugs with different mechanisms of action to maximize the analgesic effect and reduce the risk of adverse effects. In addition, these protocols advocate the use of non-opioid analgesia, as opioids contribute to increased nausea and vomiting, postoperative ileus, and delayed ambulation [25]. As our results show, multimodal analgesia performed in the ERAS group contributes to a significant reduction in postoperative pain.

When protocols such as this one are applied, the goal should be full compliance with all the measures outlined. However, full compliance is often very difficult to achieve. In this study [24], full compliance was, in our opinion, high (80%). Nevertheless, compliance varied across the different components. The elements of the protocol with the lowest compliance were early oral fluid administration and goal-directed fluid therapy. The reason for this different compliance rate compared to the protocol could be the taste of the oral fluid, patient refusal due to fear of complications, and lack of availability or training with the devices. Previous studies conducted by GERM on the implementation of the colorectal surgery protocol showed that the weaknesses were the same as in the present study. Implementation could probably be improved by involving and training all professionals who care for patients and by identifying these patients with signs at the bedside [26–28].

As mentioned above, the implementation of goal-directed fluid administration had the lowest implementation rate (80%), probably due to the economic burden associated with the use of the necessary devices, but also because some anesthesiologists are not accustomed to using these devices. The goal of intraoperative fluid administration is to maintain adequate circulating volume, avoiding volume overload and aiming for a perioperative balance of 0. Fluid administration based on patient weight tends to be higher than necessary, and this is especially relevant in patients undergoing sleeve gastrectomy, as increased fluid requirements are not directly correlated with patient weight. In several studies analyzing this method, target-directed fluid administration has been associated with a reduction in postoperative complications, mortality, and hospital stay. Excessive fluid administration causes fluid extravasation into the intestinal wall, lungs, and lower extremities, leading to postoperative ileus, pulmonary edema and atelectasis, and lower extremity edema, which affects ambulation, respectively. Many other complications can arise from these problems [29–31].

References

1. Elliott JA, Patel VM, Kirresh A, et al. Fast-track laparoscopic bariatric surgery: a systematic review. Updat Surg. 2013;65:85–94.
2. Ashrafian H. Bariatric surgery: can we afford to do it or deny doing it? Frontline Gastroenterol. 2011;2:82–9.
3. Dogan K, Kraaij L, Aarts EO, et al. Fast-track bariatric surgery improves perioperative care and logistics compared to conventional care. Obes Surg. 2015;25:28–35.
4. Wilmore DW, Kehlet H. Management of patients in fast track surgery. BJM. 2001;322:473–6.
5. Teeuwen PH, Bleichrodt RP, Strik C, et al. Enhanced recovery after surgery (ERAS) versus conventional postoperative care in colorectal surgery. J Gastrointest Surg. 2010;14:88–95.
6. Spanjersberg WR, Reurings J, Keus F, et al. Fast track surgery versus conventional recovery strategies for colorectal surgery. Cochrane Database Syst Rev. 2011;2:CD007635.
7. Jacobsen HJ, Bergland A, Raeder J, et al. High-volume bariatric surgery in a single center: safety, quality, cost-efficacy and teaching aspects in 2000 consecutive patients. Obes Surg. 2012;22:158–66.
8. Lemanu DP, Srinivasa S, Singh PP. Optimizing perioperative care in bariatric surgery patients. Obes Surg. 2012;22:979–90.
9. Bergland A, Gislason H, Raeder J. Fast-track surgery for bariatric laparoscopic gastric bypass with focus on anesthesia and perioperative care. Experience with 500 cases. Acta Anaesthesiol Scand. 2008;52:1394–9.
10. Geubbels N, Bruin SC, Acherman YIZ, et al. Fast track care for gastric bypass patients decreases length of stay without increasing complications in an unselected patient cohort. Obes Surg. 2014;24:390–6.
11. https://www.grupogerm.es/protocolos-zaragoza-2016/ (Acceso 06/02/2021).
12. Martín García-Almenta E, Ruiz-Tovar J, Sánchez Santos R. Vía Clínica de cirugía bariátrica 2017. Madrid: Im3diA comunicación SL; 2017. ISBN: 978-84-697-7104-4
13. Ruiz-Tovar J, Zubiaga L, Diez M, et al. Preoperative regular diet of 900 kcal/d versus balanced energy high-protein formula ver- sus immunonutrition formula: effect on preoperative weight loss and postoperative pain, complications and analytical acute phase reactants after laparoscopic sleeve gastrectomy. Obes Surg. 2016;26(6):1221–7.
14. https://portal.guiasalud.es/opbe/via-clinica-recuperacion-intensificada-cirugia-abdominal-rica/

15. Ruiz-Tovar J, Muñoz JL, Gonzalez J, et al. Postoperative pain after laparoscopic sleeve gastrectomy: comparison of three analgesic schemes (isolated intravenous analgesia, epidural analgesia associated with intravenous analgesia and port-sites infiltration with bupivacaine associated with intravenous analgesia). Surg Endosc. 2017;31:1–6.
16. Ruiz-Tovar J, Gonzalez G, Sarmiento A, Carbajo MA, Ortiz-de-Solorzano J, Castro MJ, Jimenez JM, Zubiaga L. Analgesic effect of postoperative laparoscopic-guided transversus abdominis plane (TAP) block, associated with preoperative port-site infiltration, within an enhanced recovery after surgery protocol in one-anastomosis gastric bypass: a prospective randomized clinical trial. Surg Endosc. 2020;34:5455–60.
17. Ruiz-Tovar J, García A, Ferrigni C, Gonzalez J, Levano-Linares C, Jimenez-Fuertes M, Llavero C, Duran M. Laparoscopic-guided transversus abdominis plane (TAP) block as part of multimodal analgesia in laparoscopic roux-en-Y gastric bypass within an enhanced recovery after surgery (ERAS) program: a prospective randomized clinical trial. Obes Surg. 2018;28:3374–9.
18. Hamid HKS, Ahmed AY, Saber AA, Emile SH, Ibrahim M, Ruiz-Tovar J. Transversus abdominis plane block using a short-acting local anesthetic reduces pain and opioid consumption after laparoscopic bariatric. Surgery: a meta-analysis. Surg Obes Relat Dis. 2020;16:1349–57.
19. Ruiz-Tovar J, Muñoz JL, Gonzalez J, García A, Ferrigni C, Jiménez M, Duran M. C-reactive protein, fibrinogen and procalcitonin as early markers of staple line leaks after laparoscopic sleeve gastrectomy in morbidly obese patients within an enhanced recovery after surgery (ERAS) program. Surg Endosc. 2017;31:5283–8.
20. Muñoz JL, Ruiz-Tovar J, Miranda E, Berrio DL, Moya P, Gutierrez M, Flores T, Pico C, Perez A. C-reactive protein and procalcitonin as early markers of septic complications after laparoscopic sleeve gastrectomy in morbidly obese patients within an enhanced recovery after surgery program. J Am Coll Surg. 2016;222:831–7.
21. Bamgbade OA, Adeogun BO, Abbas K. Fast-track laparoscopic gastric bypass surgery: outcomes and lessons from a bariatric surgery service in the United Kingdom. Obes Surg. 2012;22:398–402.
22. Raeder J. Bariatric procedures as day/short stay surgery: it is possible and reasonable? Curr Opin Anaesthesiol. 2007;20:508–12.
23. Ruiz-Tovar J, Royo P, Muñoz JL, et al. Implementation of the Spanish National Enhanced Recovery Program (ERAS) in bariatric surgery: a pilot study. Surg Laparosc Endosc Percutan Tech. 2016;26:439–43.
24. Ruiz-Tovar J, Muñoz JL, Royo P, et al. Implementation of the Spanish ERAS program in bariatric surgery. Minim Invasive Ther Allied Technol. 2018;27:365–72.
25. American Society of Anesthesiologists Task Force on Acute Pain Management. Practice guidelines for acute pain management in the perioperative setting: an updated report by the American Society of Anesthesiologists Task Force on acute pain management. Anesthesiology. 2012;116:248–73.
26. Ramırez JM, Blasco JA, Roig JV, et al. Enhanced recovery in colorectal surgery: a multicentre study. BMC Surg. 2011;11:19.
27. Arroyo A, Ramirez JM, Callejo D, et al. Influence of size and complexity of the hospitals in an enhanced recovery programme for colorectal resection. Int J Color Dis. 2012;27:1637–44.
28. Esteban F, Cerdan FJ, Garcia-Alonso M, et al. A multicentre comparison of a fast track or conventional postoperative protocol following laparoscopic or open elective surgery for colorectal cancer surgery. Color Dis. 2014;16:134–40.
29. Jain AK, Dutta A. Stroke volume variation as a guide to fluid administration in morbidly obese patients undergoing laparoscopic bariatric surgery. Obes Surg. 2010;20:709–15.
30. Poso T, Kesek D, Aroch R, et al. Morbid obesity and optimization of preoperative fluid therapy. Obes Surg. 2013;23:1799–805.
31. Arulkumaran N, Corredor C, Hamilton MA, et al. Cardiac complications associated with goal-directed therapy in high-risk surgical patients: a meta-analysis. Br J Anaesth. 2014;112:466–659.

Sleeve Gastrectomy in Pediatric and Adolescent Population

25

María-Cristina Martín-Crespo-Blanco

Abbreviations

BMD	Bone Mineral Density
BMI	Body Mass Index
LSG	Laparoscopic Sleeve Gastrectomy
WHO	World Health Organization
RYGB	Roux-en-Y Gastric Bypass

25.1 Introduction

Childhood and adolescent obesity has become a global public health problem. The World Health Organization (WHO) has defined it as the pandemic of the twenty-first century. Around 30% of the world's pediatric population suffers from overweight and about 10% from obesity [1]. In Europe there are regional differences, with a prevalence range between 10% and 25% [2]. In the United States, 19% of children and adolescents suffer from obesity, and 6.1% from severe obesity [3].

Lindsay Jaacks has proposed a conceptual model explaining the evolution of this health problem. For this purpose, they define four consecutive phases, shown in Table 25.1.

Its health consequences are noticeable from childhood, affecting the endocrine, respiratory, cardiovascular, musculoskeletal, and psychosocial systems, and posing a high risk of complications when undergoing some medical or surgical procedures.

M.-C. Martín-Crespo-Blanco (✉)
Universidad Pontificia Comillas Escuela Universitaria de Enfermería y Fisioterapia "San Juan de Dios", Madrid, Spain
e-mail: mmartinc@comillas.edu

J. Ruiz-Tovar (ed.), *Multidisciplinary Management of Sleeve Gastrectomy*, https://doi.org/10.1007/978-3-032-25644-7_25

Table 25.1 Lindsay Jaacks's evolutionary model of obesity

Stages	Characteristics
First	Higher prevalence of obesity in women, in higher social classes, and in adults.
Second	Rapid increase in adults with prevalence over 20%, in children rising up to 10%. Affects all social groups equally.
Third	Rise among lower social classes and stabilization among women and children of high social classes, except in Asia where it continues increasing.
Fourth	The prevalence begins to decline, especially among children.

Table 25.2 Major comorbidities of pediatric-adolescent severe obesity

System	Comorbidity
Cardiovascular	Hypertension; dyslipidemia
Endocrine	Type 2 diabetes mellitus; insulin resistance; polycystic ovary syndrome
Gastrointestinal	Gastroesophageal reflux; gallstones; fatty liver
Musculoskeletal	Femoral head epiphysiolysis; tibia vara
Neurological	Idiopathic intracranial hypertension
Respiratory	Asthma; obstructive sleep apnea
Psychological	Depression; anxiety; low self-esteem; eating disorders

Often during adulthood, individuals suffer from various pathologies that began during childhood and adolescence [5].

From a therapeutic viewpoint, interventions are implemented to change lifestyle habits—such as a balanced diet and increased physical activity. This approach has proven effective as a primary prevention measure, but in cases of severe obesity the results are very limited. Pharmacological products have also been used, but they too have not achieved a significant decrease in Body Mass Index (BMI) [3, 6]. In these cases, bariatric surgery is emerging as an increasingly used effective therapeutic option in carefully selected adolescents to achieve substantial weight loss, which in turn can improve associated comorbidities [3, 7].

25.2 Comorbidities of Severe Obesity

Understanding comorbidities is a requirement to ensure the effectiveness of bariatric surgery in adolescents, as it improves postoperative management and follow-up—a key phase to achieving surgical success.

Severe obesity during childhood and adolescence impacts almost all bodily systems, generating comorbidities affecting the physical, mental, and social health of this population.

The main comorbidities occurring in each system are summarized in Table 25.2 [5]:

Table 25.3 Selection criteria for candidates according to international scientific societies

Guideline	BMI and comorbidities	Additional requirements
ASMBS (2018)	BMI ≥ 35 kg/m^2 with major comorbidities BMI ≥ 40 kg/m^2 with minor comorbidities	Failure of at least 6 months of lifestyle modification (diet and physical exercise) together with the ability to provide informed consent
ESPGHAN (2015)	BMI ≥ 40 kg/m^{2}with severe comorbidities BMI ≥ 50 kg/m^2 with mild comorbidities	Completion of skeletal and sexual maturity, and commitment to postoperative multidisciplinary follow-up
NICE (updated)	BMI ≥ 35 kg/m^2 with comorbidities BMI ≥ 40 kg/m^2 with no requirement for comorbidities	Updated indications reflecting those of ASMBS Evaluation by an experienced multidisciplinary team

25.3 Selection Criteria

The selection criteria for candidates for bariatric surgery have been defined based on BMI and the presence of comorbidities. However, there are additional requirements that must also be considered. There is no international consensus for selecting adolescent candidates, as differences exist among the main international scientific societies, which can be seen in Table 25.3.

25.3.1 Contraindications

Meeting the inclusion criteria is not sufficient. It is equally important not to present any contraindication for surgery. In such cases, the candidate must be assessed by a multidisciplinary team to ensure suitability [7, 8]:

- Active substance abuse within the past year.
- Medical contraindication to surgery after risk assessment.
- Current pregnancy or planned pregnancy within the next 12–18 months.
- Uncontrolled psychiatric disorders that may interfere with adherence to postoperative recommendations: active psychosis, untreated severe depression, and recent suicide attempt.
- Presence of a treatable medical cause for obesity.
- Inability to understand the procedure and commit to long-term follow-up.
- Patients unable to care for themselves and lacking adequate family or social support.

Additionally, there are two relative contraindications:

- Eating disorder not being managed by a healthcare professional.
- Crohn's disease.

25.4 Multidisciplinary Evaluation

This multidisciplinary evaluation process is carried out to ensure the long-term success of bariatric surgery. To achieve this, it is necessary to identify all potential risks that may arise in the postoperative period. It is also the time to provide health education to the patient and family regarding the surgical process, the realistic outcomes they can expect, and the obligation to maintain permanent lifestyle changes after surgery.

25.4.1 Components of the Evaluation

The evaluation is conducted by a team composed of pediatricians, surgeons, nutritionists, and psychologists or psychiatrists to provide a comprehensive assessment, where each professional evaluates different key aspects [3, 9].

- **Medical Evaluation**

A physical examination and thorough review of the medical history are performed to diagnose, document, and stage all existing comorbidities such as hypertension, dyslipidemia, diabetes mellitus, and sleep apnea, as some are associated with decreased postoperative weight loss [10]. Blood tests and imaging studies are requested to obtain a complete picture of the patient's health status.

- **Nutritional Evaluation**

This component is crucial for identifying and correcting pre-existing nutritional deficiencies. For example, vitamin D deficiency is extremely common in individuals with obesity. Additionally, an intensive educational process is initiated regarding the profound dietary changes required after surgery, including diet progression, the importance of hydration, and critically, the lifelong need for vitamin and mineral supplementation [3].

- **Psychosocial Evaluation**

The adolescent's mental health is assessed, including the presence of depression, anxiety, history of self-harm, and eating disorders. In addition, the patient's maturity, capacity for autonomous decision-making, and level of family support are evaluated factors that are essential for adherence to the complex regimen of postoperative follow-up [5].

25.4.2 Informed Decision-Making

After completing the necessary evaluation to select suitable candidates who may benefit from surgery, it is the adolescent and their family who must make the final decision. They must receive all relevant information and understand that the operation is only one part of the process, which does not end in the postoperative period and involves the need for medication and long-term lifestyle changes. In fact, 35% of candidates considered suitable ultimately decline the intervention and opt instead for medical treatment [10].

25.5 Clinical Outcomes

Bariatric surgery is the most effective intervention for treating severe obesity in adolescents, as it not only reduces BMI but also improves associated comorbidities and enhances the quality of life of these young patients.

25.5.1 Weight Loss

Numerous studies have evaluated the effectiveness of bariatric surgery in adolescents regarding long-term weight loss and BMI reduction. Long-term weight loss is approximately 25%, and BMI reduction is around 14 kg/m^2 [6, 11, 12].

A registry conducted in Australia shows differences in outcomes depending on the surgical technique used, with a 26.5% reduction in total body weight 5 years after sleeve gastrectomy (LSG) and 30.73% after Roux-en-Y gastric bypass (RYGB) [7].

25.5.2 Impact on Metabolic Comorbidities

Bariatric surgery in adolescents also impacts the improvement and even resolution of several metabolic comorbidities. This represents one of the most important effects of surgery, as its effectiveness in this regard is greater than that observed in adults.

25.5.2.1 Type 2 Diabetes

Remission of type 2 diabetes after surgery in adolescents is around 86%. When compared with adults, who show a remission rate of 53%, this demonstrates significantly greater effectiveness when the intervention is performed at younger ages

[12]. After 5 years of follow-up, 61% of adolescents were able to discontinue oral antidiabetic medications [6].

25.5.2.2 Lipid, Liver, and Inflammatory Profile

Significant improvement also occurs in multiple metabolic biomarkers:

- **Lipids:** Significant reduction in total cholesterol (−10 mg/dL), LDL cholesterol (−14.6 mg/dL), and triglycerides (−33.3 mg/dL), along with a protective increase in HDL cholesterol (+8.0 mg/dL).
- **Pancreatic Function:** Insulin resistance, measured by the HOMA-IR index, decreased markedly (−4.1), as did C-peptide levels (−1.8 ng/mL), indicating substantial improvement in pancreatic function.
- **Liver Function:** Improvement in hepatic transaminases (ALT −14.4 U/L, AST −5.4 U/L), reflecting reduced inflammation and hepatic steatosis.
- **Systemic Inflammation:** Pro-inflammatory cytokines—hallmarks of obesity—were significantly reduced, including IL-6 (−12.2 pg/mL) and TNF-α (−54 pg/mL) [11].

25.6 Main Surgical Procedures

The two most commonly used surgical techniques in adolescents are sleeve gastrectomy and Roux-en-Y gastric bypass.

- **Sleeve Gastrectomy (LSG)**

This is the most frequently performed procedure worldwide [4]. It consists of resecting approximately 80% of the stomach, creating a narrow gastric tube or sleeve. It is primarily a restrictive technique, although it also induces hormonal effects.

- **Roux-en-Y Gastric Bypass (RYGB)**

This procedure involves creating a small gastric pouch and rerouting the small intestine to bypass part of the stomach and duodenum. This technique combines restriction with malabsorption, allowing greater weight loss than LSG. However, it also carries a higher risk of malabsorption of certain nutrients [8].

25.7 Risks and Complications

Bariatric surgery provides unquestionable benefits, both in terms of BMI and in the comorbidities of severe obesity. However, it is not a surgery free of risks and complications, both short- and long-term, which may be worsened by low adherence to medication and long-term follow-up.

Table 25.4 Main short- and long-term complications of bariatric surgery

Short-term complications	Long-term complications
Intra-abdominal bleeding	Anastomotic stenosis (higher incidence in RYGB)
Fistula	Bile reflux
Intestinal obstruction (higher incidence in RYGB)	Marginal ulcer (higher incidence in RYGB)
	Malabsorption and malnutrition
	Dumping syndrome (only in RYGB)

25.7.1 Short- and Long-Term Postoperative Complications

The main complications during the first 3 months after surgery do not exceed 4%, and mortality is very low, estimated at 0.02% [6].All complications are shown in Table 25.4.

25.7.2 Long-Term Nutritional Deficiencies

The alteration of gastrointestinal anatomy results in a reduction of the small intestine, which interferes with the absorption of essential vitamins and minerals. The most common deficiencies include [3]:

- Iron, which may lead to iron-deficiency anemia.
- Vitamin B12 and folate, crucial for neurological function and red blood cell production.
- Vitamin D and calcium, fundamental for bone health.
- Hypoalbuminemia (low blood protein levels), especially in the first months.

These deficiencies are often worsened due to low adherence to medical treatment with supplements. One study revealed that only 31% of adolescents reported regular daily intake of their supplements, showing the need for long-term follow-up and reinforcement interventions to improve medication adherence [8].

25.7.3 Bone Health

An important long-term complication is the effect on bone health in an adolescent population—an age at which one of the most significant periods of musculoskeletal development occurs.

A longitudinal study conducted in adolescents showed that those who underwent the intervention presented lower bone mineral density (BMD) compared to those with the same BMI who did not undergo surgery. Additionally, the time elapsed since surgery had a negative effect, as a progressive deterioration of bone mass occurred over time. This effect was more pronounced in patients with gastric bypass

(RYGB), but regardless of the surgical technique performed, trabecular bone BMD decreases over time [13].

This progressive deterioration underscores the critical risk posed by poor adherence to calcium and vitamin D supplementation, a documented problem in this population [8].

25.7.4 Other Long-Term Risks

It is estimated that around 4% of patients require a subsequent intervention, mainly due to two reasons: weight regain or the need to resolve complications such as stenosis or reflux [6]. Likewise, there is also evidence of an increased risk of alcohol or other substance dependence after bariatric surgery [5].

Early detection of complications and proper management of these risks highlight the need for rigorous and continuous postoperative follow-up as a fundamental pillar of long-term care.

25.8 Postoperative Follow-Up

Postoperative follow-up must be multidisciplinary. Three main areas are monitored: nutrition, bone health, and mental health. Follow-up is necessary for all patients who undergo bariatric surgery, but it is especially important in adolescents in order to prevent long-term complications and ensure a healthy adulthood.

25.8.1 Multidisciplinary Follow-Up Protocol

It focuses on conducting periodic evaluations of three fundamental pillars for maintaining health [5].

- **Nutrition:** The aim is to monitor levels of vitamin D, B9, and B12. Minerals such as iron and calcium are also monitored. Depending on the evolution of these values, the doses of the corresponding supplements are adjusted.
- **Bone Health:** Due to the effect of bariatric surgery on BMD, periodic densitometry tests are performed to detect early bone mass loss.
- **Mental Health:** Lifestyle changes and body image changes may lead to the appearance of mental health problems such as anxiety and depression, which in some cases were already present and may worsen due to the stress of surgery. This makes psychological and psychiatric support necessary for adolescents, so their emotional state can be assessed and preventive measures implemented.

25.8.2 Long-Term Adherence

The main problem after bariatric surgery is loss to follow-up, which greatly affects long-term outcomes. While the 12-month follow-up rate within a follow-up program was 94%, this dropped to 56% at 24 months [8].

Different strategies have been designed to improve follow-up rates, including telenursing, whose main benefit has been empowering patients to manage their recovery process, as well as increasing feelings of calm and safety by facilitating access to a professional who monitors their progress and provides individualized care [15].

25.8.3 Adjuvant Pharmacological Therapies

Another new line of follow-up considers the use of adjuvant pharmacological therapy, such as GLP-1 analogs. The introduction of these drugs has been shown to be a safe option that increases weight loss while reducing emotional overeating [14].

The classic follow-up based on the three pillars—mental health, bone health, and nutritional health—combined with interventions to improve adherence and adjuvant pharmacological therapies constitutes an area of research aimed at improving bariatric surgery outcomes.

25.9 Ethical and Psychosocial Aspects

The clinical outcomes of bariatric surgery are unquestionable. However, in adolescence, it raises ethical considerations, particularly regarding two issues: the adolescent's autonomy, still in development, and the impact of this surgery on body image at a life stage that is psychosocially vulnerable.

25.9.1 Ethics and Informed Consent

Truly informed consent in adolescents is difficult to ensure, as cognitive development and autonomy are not determined solely by age. Therefore, adequate psychological evaluation is required to assess the adolescent's capacity for decision-making. It is essential to ensure that the risks of surgery, the need for adherence to postoperative follow-up, and the lifelong commitment to lifestyle change are fully understood. Likewise, existing alternatives must also be presented [6].

25.9.2 Psychosocial Outcomes

The weight-loss outcomes of bariatric surgery have a major impact on the psychosocial life of adolescents, with both positive and challenging results.

- **Quality of Life:** Some activities that were not possible before surgery become attainable afterward. This directly enhances self-esteem and social participation, therefore improving quality of life [8].
- **Mental Health:** Surgery may worsen pre-existing mental health problems or trigger new ones, such as anxiety and depression, requiring continuous treatment independent of these issues, which negatively affect quality of life [5].
- **Eating Behavior:** Anxiety-driven uncontrolled eating is common in this population. Although it tends to improve due to physiological and hormonal changes caused by surgery, medical treatment may still be required [5].
- **Fertility:** Weight loss improves the hormonal profile. In adolescents with polycystic ovary syndrome, it may lead to a rapid increase in fertility. Postoperative follow-up must also include contraceptive counseling to prevent unplanned pregnancies during this period, as the nutritional and metabolic changes experienced by the mother could also affect fetal development [16].

25.10 Research Directions

The field of bariatric surgery in adolescence is in constant evolution. Research aims to achieve greater effectiveness of surgical techniques, individualized treatment, and understanding of very long-term outcomes. Ultimately, the goal is to optimize results while minimizing risks.

The main current lines of research include:

1. **Optimization of Combined Treatment:**

   The arrival of highly effective obesity medications, such as GLP-1 analogs, has opened a new era. Research now faces the challenge of determining protocols that define the ideal timing for their early introduction in the postoperative period to achieve optimal weight recovery and metabolic outcomes, both in the short and long term [5, 13].
2. **Direct Comparison of Surgical Techniques:**

   Although extensive data comparing LSG and RYGB in adults exist, evidence in adolescents is both scarce and urgently needed. It is essential to assess the effects of both techniques on the most significant outcomes of adolescent bariatric surgery that may influence long-term health. Studies are required to evaluate the impact on bone health, the prevalence of nutritional deficiencies, and the need for revision surgeries due to complications such as strictures or reflux. This will help determine the most appropriate procedure to achieve optimal outcomes in a population particularly vulnerable to long-term consequences [8].
3. **Very Long-Term Outcome Studies:**

   Most existing data are limited to 5–10 years of follow-up. It is imperative to establish lifelong registries and cohorts to fully understand the impact of an intervention performed during adolescence. Key questions include adult fracture risk, fertility and pregnancy outcomes, and psychosocial and professional development over the decades [4, 6, 11, 16].

4. **Improving Follow-Up Adherence:**
   The high rate of long-term loss to follow-up makes it necessary to investigate new care protocols, such as telehealth, particularly suited to adolescents, who are accustomed to technology. These strategies show good acceptance, but high-quality research is still needed to evaluate their long-term impact on adolescents' health—not only on their satisfaction [15].

These research directions are essential to refine clinical guidelines, optimize patient care, and ensure the best possible outcomes for future generations of young people undergoing this transformative intervention.

25.11 Conclusions

In summary, bariatric surgery has been established as the most effective treatment for severe obesity in adolescents when lifestyle-based medical interventions have failed. This intervention offers transformative benefits, including substantial and sustained weight loss, as well as notable resolution of associated metabolic and cardiovascular comorbidities. However, these benefits must be carefully weighed against long-term risks, primarily chronic nutritional deficiencies and potential deterioration of bone health.

The success of bariatric surgery in this psychosocially vulnerable population does not depend solely on the surgical technique performed; it fundamentally relies on meticulous patient selection through a multidisciplinary evaluation that determines the adolescent's decision-making capacity and commitment to postoperative follow-up—essential for ensuring a healthy transition into adulthood [3].

References

1. World Health Organization. Obesity and overweight. [Internet]. Available from: https://www.who.int/features/factfiles/obesity/es/. Accessed 15 Nov 2025
2. World Health Organization. NCD-RisC. BMI. [Internet]. Available from: https://www.ncdrisc.org/overweight-prevalence-map-ado.html. Accessed 15 Nov 2025
3. Calcaterra V, Cena H, Pelizzo G, Porri D, Regalbuto C, Vinci F, et al. Bariatric surgery in adolescents: to do or not to do? Children (Basel). 2021;8(6):453.
4. Jaacks LM, Vandevijvere S, Pan A, McGowan CJ, Wallace C, Imamura F, Mozaffarian D, Swinburn B, Ezzati M. The obesity transition: stages of the global epidemic Lancet Diabetes Endocrinol 2019 7(3):231–240. doi:https://doi.org/10.1016/S2213-8587(19)30026-9. Epub 2019 Jan 28. PMID: 30704950; PMCID: PMC7360432.
5. Herrera R, Lurbe E. A holistic perspective of the comorbidities in childhood obesity. An Pediatr. 2024;101:344–50.
6. Janson A, Järvholm K, Sjögren L, Dahlgren J, Beamish AJ, Gronowitz E, et al. Metabolic and bariatric surgery in adolescents: for whom, when, and how? Horm Res Paediatr. 2023;96(6):609–19.
7. Brown WA, Brown DL, Holland JF, Campbell A, Cottrell J, Ahern S, et al. Metabolic bariatric surgery generates substantial, sustained weight loss and health improvement in a real-world setting. ANZ J Surg. 2025;95:895–903.

8. Guadalupe Rodríguez A, Andrade Berrones VE. Bariatric surgery: an interdisciplinary approach. Pontificia Universidad Católica del Ecuador; 2024.
9. Brandt S, Lennerz BS, Wiegand S, Schirmer M, Kleger P, Weyhreter H, et al. Twelve-month outcomes after metabolic and bariatric surgery among youths participating in a structured preparation and follow-up program: results of the youth with extreme obesity study. Obes Facts. 2023;16(6):708–20.
10. Swertfeger D, Kim A, Sexmith H, Moreno-Fernandez ME, Davidson WS, Helmrath M, et al. Pre-surgery health influences outcomes following vertical sleeve gastrectomy in adolescents. Obesity (Silver Spring). 2024;32(6):1187–97.
11. Mitra AT, Wing O, Das B, Fakih-Gomez N, Khwaja H, Parmar C, et al. Impact of metabolic and bariatric surgery on the paediatric & adolescent metabolome: a systematic review and meta-analysis. Sci Rep. 2025;
12. Inge TH, Courcoulas AP, Jenkins TM, Michalsky MP, Brandt ML, Xanthakos SA, et al. Five-year outcomes of gastric bypass in adolescents as compared with adults. N Engl J Med. 2019;380(22):2136–45.
13. Wasserman H, Jenkins T, Inge T, Ryder J, Michalsky M, Sisley S, et al. Bone mineral density 5 to 11 years after metabolic and bariatric surgery in adolescents with severe obesity compared to peers. Res Square. 2023; https://doi.org/10.21203/rs.3.rs-3345103/v1.
14. Vidmar AP, Vu MH, Martin MJ, Kim AG, Abel S, Weitzner M, et al. Early reinitiation of obesity pharmacotherapy post laparoscopic sleeve gastrectomy in youth: a retrospective cohort study. Obes Surg. 2025;35:406–18.
15. Arnaert A, Girard A, Craciunas S, Shang Z, Ahmad H, Debe Z, Demyttenaere S. Patients' experiences of telenursing follow-up care after bariatric surgery. J Clin Nurs. 2022;31(7–8):985–94. https://doi.org/10.1111/jocn.15955. Epub 2021 Jul 9
16. Maggard MA, Yermilov I, Li Z, Maglione M, Newberry S, Suttorp M, Hilton L, Santry HP, Morton JM, Livingston EH, Shekelle PG. Pregnancy and fertility following bariatric surgery: a systematic review. JAMA. 2008;300(19):2286–96. https://doi.org/10.1001/jama.2008.641.

Sleeve Gastrectomy in the Elderly

26

Jesús Muñoz-Muñoz

26.1 Introduction

Obesity prevalence among those over 60 has risen globally due to aging and lifestyle changes [1]. Obesity affects 30–40% of older adults in Europe and North America, with severe obesity affecting up to 10%. In 2017–2018, 42.8% of US adults over 60 were obese [1], and Canadian data confirm a similar figure of 29.3% in the 60–79 age group [2].

Obesity management in this age group is challenging, with lifestyle and pharmacological interventions often failing long-term [3]. In recent years, bariatric surgery (BS) has emerged as the most effective treatment for morbid obesity and its metabolic complications, offering superior durability compared to non-surgical approaches [4]. Among the available procedures, laparoscopic sleeve gastrectomy (SG) has become the most frequently performed bariatric operation worldwide due to its technical simplicity, satisfactory safety profile, and metabolic efficacy [5].

However, the extension of BS to elderly candidates has been subject to debate. Age was historically considered a relative contraindication due to reduced physiological reserve, multimorbidity, and increased surgical risk [2, 5]. Evidence now indicates that, although SG is generally safe in carefully selected older adults, weight loss outcomes are consistently less pronounced than in younger patients, and the risk of perioperative complications, particularly bleeding, anastomotic leak, and pulmonary complications, remains higher [2, 3]. A multicenter study in patients over 65 years showed acceptable morbidity (≈7%) and no perioperative mortality, but noted that intraperitoneal bleeding was the most common complication [2].

SG in patients over 60 yields clinically meaningful improvements in hypertension, dyslipidemia, and sleep apnea, despite lower efficacy than in younger

J. Muñoz-Muñoz (✉)
Comillas Pontifical University, Madrid, Spain
e-mail: jmunozm@comillas.edu

J. Ruiz-Tovar (ed.), *Multidisciplinary Management of Sleeve Gastrectomy*,
https://doi.org/10.1007/978-3-032-25644-7_26

individuals [3]. SG surgical risk is elevated in elderly subjects, and its effectiveness is poorer compared to younger adults. Frailty, sarcopenia, cognitive status, and cardiopulmonary reserve should be considered in evaluating older candidates for SG [3, 5].

The chapter analyzes evidence on SG for elderly patients with severe obesity, reviewing epidemiology, selection criteria, outcomes, and complications.

26.2 Indications and Patient Selection in the Elderly

The classical criteria for BS are well established: a body mass index $\geq$40 kg/m^2, or $\geq$ 35 kg/m^2 in the presence of obesity-related comorbidities such as type 2 diabetes mellitus, hypertension, dyslipidemia, or obstructive sleep apnea [6]. These indications remain valid in older populations; however, chronological age alone cannot be used as the sole criterion when evaluating candidacy for SG. Instead, patient selection must be individualized and incorporate geriatric-specific assessments [5, 7].

Frailty represents a multidimensional syndrome characterized by diminished strength, endurance, and physiological function, rendering older adults more vulnerable to stressors such as surgery. It is an independent predictor of postoperative complications and mortality across surgical disciplines [8]. Instruments such as the Fried Frailty Index, Clinical Frailty Scale, or Edmonton Frail Scale can be employed to quantify frailty and guide risk stratification. Patients with moderate to severe frailty generally experience worse outcomes. They may derive limited benefit from bariatric surgery, whereas robust elderly candidates demonstrate surgical results more comparable to those of younger adults [5].

Older candidates often present with multiple chronic conditions, including cardiovascular disease, chronic kidney disease, pulmonary disorders, and long-standing diabetes. These comorbidities increase perioperative risk and can diminish the likelihood of achieving complete remission postoperatively [2, 9]. Nevertheless, even partial improvement in disease control may lead to significant gains in quality of life and functional independence. The presence of well-controlled comorbidities should not necessarily preclude surgery, but decompensated disease or advanced organ dysfunction may serve as contraindications.

Elderly patients frequently suffer from sarcopenic obesity, a condition in which excess fat mass coexists with reduced muscle mass and strength [6, 10]. This phenotype is associated with impaired recovery, higher risk of falls, and poorer long-term outcomes after SG. Preoperative nutritional evaluation should include assessment of protein intake, micronutrient levels, and muscle function. Optimizing nutrition, implementing resistance exercise programs, and ensuring adequate vitamin and mineral supplementation are essential in the prehabilitation phase [11].

Cognitive impairment, depression, and social isolation are more prevalent among older adults and may affect adherence to postoperative regimens, including dietary restrictions, physical activity, and lifelong supplementation. A comprehensive psychological and cognitive assessment is critical to ensure that patients can comply with the demands of bariatric follow-up [5]. In selected cases, the involvement of caregivers or family members in perioperative education and support can enhance adherence and safety [11].

For elderly patients, BS focuses on enhancing quality of life and decreasing disability, rather than extending lifespan [9]. Life expectancy and surgical risk are considered, with healthier patients projected to survive at least 10 years, potentially benefiting most [7, 11].

A formal geriatric assessment provides a holistic view of the patient's physiological reserve, comorbidity profile, cognitive status, and psychosocial environment. Such evaluation should include frailty screening, cardiopulmonary risk assessment, nutritional and functional testing, and medication review to minimize polypharmacy-related risks [5, 8]. The integration of geriatricians into multidisciplinary bariatric teams ensures safer selection and better perioperative outcomes.

In summary, while standard body mass index thresholds guide the eligibility for bariatric surgery, patient selection in the elderly must account for frailty, comorbidity burden, nutritional reserve, cognitive and psychosocial status, and anticipated life expectancy. Individualized decision-making, supported by comprehensive geriatric assessment, is critical for identifying those older adults who can safely benefit from SG.

26.3 Surgical Outcomes in Elderly Patients

The efficacy and safety of SG in elderly patients has been increasingly studied in the past decade, as the demand for bariatric procedures in this age group rises. Although the outcomes are generally favorable, elderly patients tend to experience lower weight loss and comorbidity remission compared to younger cohorts, while showing slightly higher perioperative risks [2, 5, 7].

26.3.1 Weight Loss Outcomes

Elderly patients achieve substantial reductions in body weight following SG; however, the magnitude of weight loss is consistently lower compared to that of younger adults [5, 10]. Reported excess weight loss ranges between 50% and 60% at 12–24 months in patients over 60, compared with 65–75% in younger cohorts [5, 7]. Total weight loss averages 20–25% in elderly patients, which, although more modest, remains clinically meaningful [11]. Several factors contribute to these differences:

- Reduced basal metabolic rate and lower lean muscle mass with aging.
- Lower levels of physical activity and rehabilitation potential.
- Longer duration of obesity and associated comorbidities, limiting metabolic reversibility.

Nevertheless, even moderate weight reduction has a substantial impact on mobility, pain reduction, and cardiovascular risk in older adults [11].

26.3.2 Comorbidity Remission

SG leads to significant improvement in obesity-related comorbidities in elderly patients:

- **Type 2 Diabetes Mellitus:** Remission rates range from 40% to 55%, compared with 60–70% in younger populations [2, 5]. While complete remission is less common, improved glycemic control and reduced need for medication are consistently reported.
- **Hypertension and Dyslipidemia:** Improvement occurs in 50–65% of cases, with a similar rate across age groups, although complete resolution is less frequent in the elderly [7, 10].
- **Obstructive Sleep Apnea:** Resolution or marked improvement occurs in approximately half of elderly patients, reducing cardiovascular and cognitive risk [10].
- **Musculoskeletal Pain and Osteoarthritis:** Even modest weight loss alleviates joint stress, improving mobility and reducing analgesic requirements [11].

26.3.3 Comparative Outcomes: Elderly vs Younger

Meta-analyses indicate that elderly patients benefit from SG; however, outcomes are attenuated compared to those of younger adults. Pereira et al. reported that patients ≥60 years lost 8–10% less excess weight loss and had slightly lower remission rates of type 2 diabetes mellitus, but morbidity remained acceptable [7]. Nevo et al. observed similar safety and complication rates between elderly and younger patients, but with significantly lower weight loss in the older group [5]. Comparison of percentage excess weight loss at 1–2 years after SG, elderly patients (≥60 years) show lower excess weight loss compared to younger cohorts (<60 years), as shown in Table 26.1 [3]:

Table 26.1 Comparative outcomes after sleeve gastrectomy in younger vs elderly patients from [3], licensed under CC-BY 4.0

Outcome	Younger (<60 yrs)	Elderly (≥60 yrs)
% excess weight loss (1–2 years)	65–70%	50–60%
Diabetes remission	60–70%	40–55%
Hypertension improvement	55–65%	50–60%
OSA resolution	60–70%	50–60%

26.3.4 Long-Term Durability

Long-term data in elderly patients remain limited. Available follow-up data, up to 5 years, suggest the maintenance of significant weight reduction and improvement in comorbidities, although some regain is common [2, 11]. Nutritional deficiencies (iron, vitamin B12, and vitamin D) and sarcopenia require vigilant monitoring, as they may be more detrimental in the elderly [12].

26.4 Risks and Complications

Although SG is considered a technically more straightforward and less aggressive bariatric procedure than gastric bypass or biliopancreatic diversion, surgical risk remains a central concern in elderly patients. With advancing age, the reduced physiological reserve, higher prevalence of comorbidities, and presence of frailty contribute to an increased vulnerability to perioperative and long-term complications [2, 5, 7].

26.4.1 Perioperative Mortality and Morbidity

Several large series and meta-analyses report that elderly patients undergoing SG have slightly higher rates of early morbidity and mortality compared with younger cohorts. Thirty-day mortality is estimated between 0.3% and 0.6% in older patients, compared with <0.3% in younger groups [2, 3]. Early complication rates range from 7% to 10%, most frequently bleeding, staple line leaks, pulmonary complications, and cardiovascular events [5, 11]. Despite these risks, perioperative mortality after SG in the elderly is comparable to that of other standard elective procedures, such as knee arthroplasty [2].

26.4.2 Postoperative Mortality and Morbidity

Intraperitoneal bleeding is the most frequent severe early complication in elderly SG patients, with rates of 2–3% [2]. Risk factors include hypertension, anticoagulant therapy, and inadequate hemostasis.

Between 1% and 2% of elderly patients reported a staple line leak, which is slightly higher than in younger cohorts [7, 11]. Leaks are associated with prolonged hospital stay, sepsis, and need for re-intervention. Early recognition and prompt multidisciplinary management are crucial.

Advanced age is associated with diminished pulmonary function and a higher prevalence of chronic obstructive pulmonary disease, sleep apnea, and cardiovascular disease. Postoperative pneumonia, pulmonary embolism, arrhythmias, and myocardial infarction occur more frequently in the elderly compared with younger adults [2, 13]. Prophylactic measures such as incentive spirometry, early mobilization, and appropriate anticoagulation are essential.

Nutritional deficiencies after SG in elderly patients deserve special attention:

- **Iron, vitamin B12, and vitamin D deficiency** are common due to reduced gastric acid production, altered absorption, and dietary restrictions [7, 14].
- **Sarcopenia and protein malnutrition** may be exacerbated by rapid postoperative weight loss, increasing the risk of frailty, falls, and fractures [9].
- **Bone health:** Accelerated bone loss and higher incidence of osteoporosis-related fractures have been reported, particularly in postmenopausal women. Long-term supplementation and regular monitoring are mandatory [14].

SG is associated with de novo or worsened gastroesophageal reflux disease (GERD) in up to 30% of patients [5]. In the elderly, the prevalence of hiatal hernia and esophageal dysmotility increases the risk of postoperative reflux. Severe or refractory GERD may necessitate conversion to gastric bypass, which carries a higher surgical risk in this age group [13].

Revisional surgery rates in elderly SG patients are higher than in younger populations, mainly due to inadequate weight loss, severe GERD, or complications requiring re-intervention [3, 11]. Readmission rates are also elevated, often related to dehydration, nutritional deficits, or surgical site complications [14].

While SG provides durable weight reduction and comorbidity improvement, elderly patients remain at higher risk of late adverse outcomes [2, 11, 14]:

- Progressive frailty and sarcopenia due to altered body composition.
- Nutritional deficiencies leading to anemia, fatigue, and osteoporosis.
- Need for revisional surgery, although technically challenging and associated with increased risk.

26.5 Quality of Life and Functional Outcomes

Beyond metabolic and weight-related outcomes, one of the most relevant benefits of SG in the elderly population is the improvement in quality of life, functional independence, and psychosocial well-being. While the absolute magnitude of weight loss may be less than in younger cohorts, older patients often report significant improvements in daily functioning and overall health perception [3, 5].

Obesity in elderly patients is strongly associated with mobility limitations, joint pain, and increased dependency. Following SG, most patients report enhanced ability to perform activities of daily living and improved mobility [7]. Even modest reductions in body weight translate into decreased mechanical load on weight-bearing joints, alleviating symptoms of osteoarthritis and reducing the need for analgesics [11]. In addition, improved cardiorespiratory fitness and better control of comorbidities, such as obstructive sleep apnea and hypertension, support greater endurance and physical autonomy [15].

Frailty is a critical determinant of postoperative outcomes in the elderly. Studies show that bariatric surgery, including SG, can attenuate frailty by reducing inflammation, improving nutritional intake, and enhancing physical performance. Gains in gait speed, balance, and muscle strength have been documented, especially when postoperative management includes structured physiotherapy and nutritional support. As a result, many elderly patients shift from frail or pre-frail states to more robust functional categories, reducing the risk of hospitalization and long-term care dependency [16].

Beyond physical health, SG exerts a positive effect on psychosocial domains. Elderly patients often experience improved body image, self-esteem, and reduced symptoms of depression and social isolation [3, 11]. Better sleep quality and increased participation in social activities have been reported, leading to enhanced overall life satisfaction. These improvements are particularly relevant for older adults, where psychosocial health has a strong influence on healthy aging and cognitive resilience.

Quality of life assessments using standardized instruments, such as the Bariatric Analysis and Reporting Outcome System or SF-36, consistently demonstrate significant improvements after SG in the elderly [7, 15]. Physical function, vitality, and general health domains show the greatest gains, though improvements in mental health are also evident. Importantly, these benefits appear durable, persisting for several years after surgery, even in the presence of partial weight regain [16].

For older adults, the value of SG extends beyond survival and remission of comorbidities. Restoration of independence, reduction in disability, and preservation of dignity are often the outcomes most valued by patients [3, 5]. From a geriatric perspective, BS should be considered not only as a metabolic intervention but also as a tool to enhance the quality of aging, supporting autonomy and participation in daily life.

26.6 Multidisciplinary Management

Successful outcomes after SG in elderly patients rely not only on surgical technique but also on comprehensive multidisciplinary care. Given the complexity of aging physiology, multimorbidity, and psychosocial factors, an integrated team approach is essential to maximize benefits, reduce complications, and support long-term adherence [6, 8].

26.6.1 Preoperative Assessment and Optimization

A thorough preoperative evaluation is crucial in elderly candidates, extending beyond standard bariatric assessment. It should include:

- **Geriatric evaluation:** Assessment of frailty, cognitive status, functional reserve, and risk of postoperative delirium. Tools such as the Clinical Frailty Scale and Edmonton Frail Scale provide objective measures to guide selection [6, 8].
- **Cardiopulmonary assessment:** Echocardiography, stress testing, and pulmonary function testing are indicated, when necessary, as cardiovascular and respiratory diseases are common in this population [17].
- **Nutritional and body composition analysis:** Screening for sarcopenia, micronutrient deficiencies, and protein malnutrition, with tailored supplementation and prehabilitation when needed [7, 18].
- **Medication review:** Polypharmacy is common among older adults; deprescribing non-essential medications and adjusting anticoagulants or antihypertensives may lower perioperative risk [17].

26.6.2 Role of the Multidisciplinary Team

Optimal management requires the coordinated involvement of different specialists:

- **Surgeon:** Selects the most appropriate bariatric procedure, balancing risks and benefits in the context of comorbidities and patient goals [6].
- **Geriatrician:** Provides holistic assessment, manages frailty, and ensures alignment of surgical goals with life expectancy and quality of life [8].
- **Nutritionist/Dietitian:** Designs individualized pre- and postoperative nutrition plans, with emphasis on protein intake, prevention of sarcopenia, and correction of deficiencies [7, 19].
- **Psychologist/Psychiatrist:** Evaluates cognitive function, depression, and eating behaviors, ensuring readiness for lifestyle changes and adherence to follow-up [6, 19].
- **Physiotherapist:** Implements prehabilitation to improve mobility and respiratory capacity and prescribes tailored exercise programs after surgery [18].
- **Specialized nurses:** Coordinate perioperative care, patient education, supplementation monitoring, and early detection of complications [19].

26.6.3 Perioperative and Immediate Postoperative Care

Elderly patients benefit from enhanced recovery protocols (ERAS) adapted to bariatric surgery, including [13, 18]:

- Minimally invasive techniques to reduce surgical trauma.
- Early mobilization and respiratory physiotherapy to prevent pulmonary complications.
- Careful fluid management to avoid cardiac overload.
- Analgesic regimens that minimize opioids to lower the risk of delirium and constipation.

26.6.4 Long-Term Follow-Up

Continuous multidisciplinary follow-up is essential to maintain weight loss and prevent complications:

- **Nutritional monitoring:** Regular assessment of micronutrients (iron, vitamin B12, vitamin D, calcium), with supplementation as needed [7, 19].
- **Bone health and sarcopenia prevention:** Periodic bone density testing, resistance training, and adequate protein intake to mitigate osteoporosis and muscle loss [8].
- **Psychological support:** Counseling for depression, anxiety, or maladaptive eating patterns, which may arise in postoperative adaptation [16].
- **Social and caregiver involvement:** Elderly patients may require family or community support to adhere to follow-up and supplementation [16].

26.7 Conclusion

SG has consolidated its role as the most widely performed bariatric procedure worldwide due to its relative technical simplicity, favorable safety profile, and efficacy in achieving sustained weight loss and comorbidity improvement. In elderly patients, the available evidence demonstrates that SG can be performed safely with acceptable morbidity and mortality rates, if candidates are carefully selected and optimized preoperatively.

Although the magnitude of weight loss and the rates of comorbidity remission are generally lower compared with younger populations, the clinical impact of SG in older adults remains substantial. Improvements in functional independence, mobility, quality of life, and psychological well-being often represent outcomes of equal or greater relevance than absolute reductions in body weight. Importantly, these benefits are achieved despite the presence of frailty, multimorbidity, and age-related physiological changes, underscoring the value of SG as a tool not only for weight management but also for enhancing the quality of aging.

Nonetheless, the elderly population remains at increased risk of perioperative and long-term complications, including bleeding, staple line leak, pulmonary events, nutritional deficiencies, and exacerbation of sarcopenia or bone loss. These risks underscore the importance of a structured preoperative evaluation, comprehensive geriatric assessment, and long-term multidisciplinary follow-up.

From an ethical standpoint, decisions regarding SG in the elderly must be grounded in shared decision-making, balancing potential surgical risks against expected gains in autonomy, quality of life, and survival. For many patients, the principal goal is not maximal weight reduction but rather the restoration of independence and dignity in daily living.

In conclusion, SG in elderly patients is a safe and effective option when indications and contraindications are carefully considered and when management is provided within a multidisciplinary framework. Future research should focus on long-term outcomes, frailty-based selection algorithms, and interventions to reduce sarcopenia and bone loss, thereby further refining patient selection and enhancing results in this vulnerable yet growing population.

References

1. Hales CM, Carroll MD, Fryar CD, Ogden CL. Prevalence of Obesity and Severe Obesity Among Adults: United States, 2017 2018.
2. Mokwenye VC, Ochuba JN, Fasoro OS, Nwokolo AS, Osula O, Sowunmi MO, et al. Trends in obesity among canadian adults: a population-level database analysis. Springer; 2025.
3. Fernández-Ananín S, Ballester E, Gonzalo B, Codina C, Miñambres I, Pérez A, et al. Is sleeve gastrectomy as effective in older patients as in younger patients? A comparative analysis of weight loss, related comorbidities, and medication requirements. Springer; 2022. p. 1909.
4. Kermansaravi M, Vitiello A, Valizadeh R, Shahmiri SS, Musella M. Comparing the safety and efficacy of sleeve gastrectomy versus Roux-en-Y gastric bypass in elderly (>60 years) with severe obesity: an umbrella systematic review and meta-analysis. Ovid Technologies (Wolters Kluwer Health); 2023. p. 3541.
5. Nevo N, Eldar SM, Lessing Y, Sabo E, Nachmany I, Hazzan D. Sleeve Gastrectomy in the Elderly. S. Karger AG; 2025. p. 502.
6. Villareal DT, Apovian CM, Kushner RF, Klein S. Obesity in older adults: technical review and position statement of the American Society for Nutrition and NAASO. The Obesity Society. p. 1–5.
7. Pereira AF, Santa-Cruz F, Coutinho LR, Vieira-De-Melo MCPT, Hinrichsen EA, Siqueira LT, et al. Impact of bariatric surgery in elderly patients with obesity. FapUNIFESP (SciELO); 2022.
8. Fried LP, Tangen CM, Walston J, Newman AB, Hirsch C, Gottdiener J, et al. Frailty in Older Adults: Evidence for a Phenotype.
9. Susmallian S, Raziel A, Barnea R, Paran H. Bariatric surgery in older adults. Ovid Technologies (Wolters Kluwer Health); 2019.
10. Jensen GL, Friedmann JM. Obesity is associated with functional decline in community-dwelling rural older persons.
11. Arolfo S, Salzano A, Dogliotti S, Solerio D, Olandese F, Morino M. Bariatric surgery in over 60 years old patients: is it worth it? Springer; 2021. p. 1501.
12. Faria G, Pestana D, Preto J, Guimarães JT, Taveira-Gomes A, Calhau C. Age and weight loss after bariatric surgery: cause or consequence? Springer; 2014. p. 824.
13. Dowgiałło-Wnukiewicz N, Janik MR, Lech P, Major P, Pędziwiatr M, Kowalewski PK, et al. Outcomes of sleeve gastrectomy in patients older than 60 years: a multicenter matched case-control study. Wideochir Inne Tech Maloinwazyjne. 2019:123.
14. Stenberg E, Cao Y, Szabo E, Näslund E, Näslund I, Ottosson J. Risk prediction model for severe postoperative complication in bariatric surgery. Springer; 2018. p. 1869.
15. Søvik TT, Aasheim ET, Taha O, Fagerland MW, Bjo S, Kristinsson J, et al. Weight loss, cardiovascular risk factors, and quality of life after gastric bypass and duodenal switch a randomized trial.
16. Raoof M, Szabo E, Karlsson J, Näslund E, Cao Y, Näslund I. Improvements of health-related quality of life 5 years after gastric bypass. In: What is important besides weight loss? A study from Scandinavian Obesity Surgery Register. Elsevier BV; 2020. p. 1249.
17. Angrisani L, Formisano G, Santonicola A, Hasani A, Vitiello A. Bariatric surgery worldwide. Springer; 2017. p. 19.
18. Thorell A, Maccormick AD, Awad S, Reynolds N, Roulin D, Demartines N, et al. Guidelines for perioperative care in bariatric surgery: enhanced recovery after surgery (ERAS) society recommendations. Wiley; 2016. p. 2065.

19. Mechanick JI, Apovian C, Brethauer S, Garvey WT, Joffe AM, Kim J, et al. Clinical practice guidelines for the perioperative nutrition, metabolic, and nonsurgical support of patients undergoing bariatric procedures—2019 update: cosponsored by American Association of Clinical Endocrinologists/American College of Endocrinology, The Obesity Society, American Society For Metabolic & Bariatric Surgery, Obesity Medicine Association, and American Society of Anesthesiologists, vol. 2019. Elsevier BV. p. 1.

Nissen Sleeve: A Modified Procedure for Treating Severe Obesity and Gastroesophageal Reflux Disease

27

María Rodríguez-Ortega

27.1 Introduction

Sleeve gastrectomy (SG) is the most commonly performed bariatric procedure worldwide, offering significant weight loss and remission of obesity-related diseases [1]. However, SG is associated with a high risk of gastroesophageal reflux disease (GERD), which is already more common in obese patients.

After SG, two-thirds of previously asymptomatic patients experience pathological changes in pH monitoring, although according to the series only one-third need pharmacological treatment to control symptoms [2].

The origin of GERD after GS is multifactorial. Possible causes include motor disturbances of the lower esophageal sphincter (LES), usually in the form of transient relaxations after ingestion [3], possibly related to anatomical changes after GS, such as alteration of the angle of His [4].

In 2016, Nocca and colleagues proposed a combined procedure involving GS and Nissen fundoplication (Nissen sleeve gastrectomy [NSG]). This combined technique addresses GERD while preserving the advantages of GS in terms of weight loss and remission of obesity-related comorbidities. NSG results in sustained weight loss, significant improvement in GERD, and a low complication rate during a 5-year follow-up [5–7].

M. Rodríguez-Ortega (✉)
San Juan de Dios School of Nursing and Physical Therapy, Comillas Pontifical University, Madrid, Spain
e-mail: mrortega@comillas.edu

J. Ruiz-Tovar (ed.), *Multidisciplinary Management of Sleeve Gastrectomy*,
https://doi.org/10.1007/978-3-032-25644-7_27

27.2 Indications

NSG is indicated in patients with obesity associated with GERD, particularly those with a hiatal hernia, where Roux-en-Y gastric bypass (RYGB) is not indicated or preferred [8]. It is also considered for patients with pre-existing Nissen fundoplication who require weight loss surgery [9].

Studies consistently report significant improvement in GERD symptoms following NSG.

A prospective analysis of 34 patients with a mean preoperative BMI of 40.3 kg/m^2 [7] found that GERD symptom severity decreased from a median score of 8 to 1 ($P < 0.001$), with 97.1% achieving GERD remission postoperatively and a significant decrease in obesity-associated comorbidities (type 2 diabetes and hypertension) following weight loss at 1 year. Similarly, in a cohort study [8] of 70 patients undergoing NSG, in which 76% of patients had preoperative esophageal syndromes, only one patient remained symptomatic at 1 year follow-up. Another study involving 28 patients found complete resolution of GERD symptoms in 25 patients and improvement in the remaining 3 [10].

27.3 Technique

The Nissen sleeve technique is performed laparoscopically and involves an initial dissection and reduction within the abdominal cavity of any potential hiatal hernia, followed by closure of the esophageal hiatus [5]. A 360-degree fundus plication (Nissen) is then created to create a valve effect. The fundoplication should be short, typically 3 cm, and is configured with the anterior and superior part of the fundus 4 cm from the angle of His to maintain a small, functional gastric fundus and ensure proper passage of food. The wraparound valve is fixed to the anterior part of the esophagus [5, 10]. Calibration with a probe is recommended [6].

After creation of the Nissen valve and dissection of the greater curvature, a sleeve gastrectomy is performed in a standard fashion. The stapling process is performed using a linear stapler, from the antrum to the valve, generally reinforcing the staple line with absorbable sutures and checking for tightness with dyes [6, 11].

Important technical details include avoiding thermal injury during gastric vessel dissection and gentle handling of the fundus during fundoplication, avoiding double stapling during sleeve creation [11, 12]. A control test with mobilization of a stent through the fundoplication is recommended at the end of the procedure.

27.4 Complications

While NSG is considered a safe technique, it is technically more challenging than standard SG [5]. Early postoperative complications in the largest series studied to date, which consisted of a cohort of 365 patients, mostly women, included acute fundoplication perforation (1.6%), intra-abdominal bleeding (1.4%), and mild dysphagia (4.4%). This study concludes that after the initial learning curve and additional technical modifications, the Nissen sleeve appears to be a safe surgical technique with an acceptable rate of early postoperative complications [13].

In isolation, one study reports a rare but potentially life-threatening complication after N-SG, sheath necrosis, which required immediate surgical intervention [14].

27.5 Results and Comparison with Other Techniques

The short-term results of NSG in relation to weight loss are promising.

A study of 34 patients showed a mean percentage total weight loss (%TWL) of 23% at 6 months and 30.3% at 12 months postoperatively [7]. Another study with a small series of 5 patients undergoing NSG reported a mean excess weight loss of 33.9% at 6 months [9].

In a medium-term retrospective study comparing sleeve gastrectomy with Nissen fundoplication (SGNF) and sleeve gastrectomy with Toupet fundoplication (SGTF) in 51 obese patients, a Nissen wrap was performed if adequate gastric fundus mobility allowed a 360° wrap without tension; otherwise, a Toupet wrap (posterior 270°) was performed. Regarding GERD, no significant differences were found in the mean % TWL at 3–5 years (25.77% for SGNF vs. 28.16% for SGTF, $P = 0.475$) [15]. Both groups showed significant decreases in GERD-Q scores from baseline ($P < 0.001$), with GERD remission in 75.0% (SGNF) and 72.7% (SGTF) of patients ($P = 0.846$).

A systematic review and meta-analysis comparing Nissen fundoplication and Toupet fundoplication, not associated with bariatric surgery, for GERD found that Toupet fundoplication was associated with less postoperative dysphagia and bloating, while both were equally effective in controlling reflux symptoms in the short and long term [16, 17]. On the other hand, a meta-analysis of 13 randomized controlled trials also indicated that Toupet fundoplication had a lower incidence of dysphagia compared with Nissen fundoplication, with comparable long-term results for other GERD-related symptoms [18]. These findings are relevant to the fundoplication component of Nissen sleeve procedures.

Regarding Barrett's esophagus, a bicentric retrospective study involving 692 patients undergoing NSG reported that 64.1% of patients with confirmed Barrett's esophagus (BE) showed regression at 2 years of follow-up, and no new-onset BE was observed in 234 patients who underwent follow-up endoscopy within 2 years, concluding that NSG is associated with cure of known BE in approximately two-thirds of patients at 2 years of follow-up [19].

While long-term (more than 5 years) studies specifically on Nissen sleeve gastrectomy are limited, some studies on conventional sleeve gastrectomy (SG) indicate that weight gain and the occurrence of GERD may be long-term complications. In this regard, a single-center retrospective observational study of 104 patients undergoing SG showed a mean TBWL % of 29% after 13.4 years, but 43% experienced new-onset GERD symptoms [20]. Another similar study including 207 SG patients with a follow-up of more than 5 years observed new-onset GERD in 27.5% of cases [21].

In relation to the above, we can conclude that medium-term data suggest that Nissen sleeve gastrectomy (or sleeve gastrectomy with Nissen fundoplication) is a safe and effective intervention for obesity with GERD, demonstrating comparable rates of weight loss and GERD remission to other fundoplication techniques.

In addition, Nissen sleeve gastrectomy has shown promise in curing Barrett's esophagus.

While long-term data are still needed with studies specifically addressing Nissen sleeve gastrectomy, existing long-term studies of conventional sleeve gastrectomy indicate potential concerns regarding weight regain and new-onset GERD.

References

1. Brown WA, Liem R, Al-Sabah S, IFSO Global Registry Collaboration, et al. Metabolic bariatric surgery across the IFSO chapters: key insights on the baseline patient demographics, procedure types, and mortality from the eighth IFSO global registry report. Obes Surg. 2024;34:1764–77.
2. Dowgiałło-Gornowicz N, Lech P. The real occurrence of gastroesophageal reflux disease after sleeve gastrectomy—a prospective pH-monitoring study. Wideochir Inne Tech Maloinwazyjne. 2024 Jun;19(2):205–10. https://doi.org/10.5114/wiitm.2024.138521.
3. Felinska E, Billeter A, Nickel F, Contin P, Berlth F, Chand B, Grimminger P, Mikami D, Schoppmann SF, Müller-Stich B. Do we understand the pathophysiology of GERD after sleeve gastrectomy? Ann N Y Acad Sci. 2020 Dec;1482(1):26–35. https://doi.org/10.1111/nyas.14467.
4. Petersen WV, Meile T, Küper MA, Zdichavsky M, Königsrainer A, Schneider JH. Functional importance of laparoscopic sleeve gastrectomy for the lower esophageal sphincter in patients with morbid obesity. Obes Surg. 2012 Mar;22(3):360–6. https://doi.org/10.1007/s11695-011-0536-5.
5. Nocca D, Nedelcu M, Loureiro M, et al. The Nissen sleeve gastrectomy: technical considerations. J Laparoendosc Adv Surg Tech A. 2020;30(11):1231–6. https://doi.org/10.1089/lap.2020.0651.
6. Nocca D, Currie AC, Joumaa S, Brinas P, Nedelcu M, Gautier T. A video-based review of important technical concepts in the Nissen-sleeve gastrectomy. Obes Surg. 2023;33(4):1304–6. https://doi.org/10.1007/s11695-022-06429-7.
7. Lech P, Mysiorska D, Młyńska J, Szymborska E, Dowgiałło-Gornowicz N. Outcomes of Nissen sleeve gastrectomy in a short-term follow-up: a new future? Wideochir Inne Tech Maloinwazyjne. 2025;20(2):204–8. https://doi.org/10.20452/wiitm.2025.17945.
8. Amor IB, Casanova V, Vanbiervliet G, et al. The Nissen-sleeve (N-sleeve): results of a cohort study. Obes Surg. 2020;30(9):3267–72. https://doi.org/10.1007/s11695-020-04469-5.
9. Smith CR, Gardner JT, Vaughn LH, Kelly RJ, Whipple OC. Nissen fundoplication-preserving laparoscopic sleeve gastrectomy. Am Surg. 2019;85(2):173–6.
10. Carandina S, Andreica A, Danan M, Zulian V, Nedelcu M. The Nissen-sleeve: early postoperative complications. J Laparoendosc Adv Surg Tech A. 2021;31(2):141–5. https://doi.org/10.1089/lap.2020.0892.
11. Palermo M, Serra E, Duza G. N-sleeve gastrectomy: an option for obesity and gerd. Arq Bras Cir Dig. 2019;32(4):e1482. Published 2019 Dec 20. https://doi.org/10.1590/0102-672020190001e1482.
12. Fezzi M, Kolotkin RL, Nedelcu M, et al. Improvement in quality of life after laparoscopic sleeve gastrectomy. Obes Surg. 2011;21(8):1161–7.

13. Nocca D, Galtier F, Taleb S, et al. Peri-operative morbidity of Nissen sleeve gastrectomy: prospective evaluation of a cohort of 365 patients, beyond the learning curve. Obes Surg. 2022;32(7):1–7. https://doi.org/10.1007/s11695-022-06066-0.
14. Skalli EM, Parmar CD. Necrosis of the Nissen-Sleeve Gastrectomy (N-SG) wrap. Obes Surg. 2020;30(10):4174–5. https://doi.org/10.1007/s11695-020-04808-6.
15. Tusuntuoheti Y, Maimaitiming M, Maimaitiyusufu P, et al. The mid-term efficacy of sleeve-Nissen versus sleeve-Toupet fundoplication for the management of gastroesophageal reflux disease in patients with obesity. Obes Surg. Published online August 9. 2025. https://doi.org/10.1007/s11695-025-08141-8.
16. Li G, Jiang N, Chendaer N, Hao Y, Zhang W, Peng C. Laparoscopic Nissen versus Toupet fundoplication for short- and long-term treatment of gastroesophageal reflux disease: a meta-analysis and systematic review. Surg Innov. 2023;30(6):745–57. https://doi.org/10.1177/15533506231165829.
17. Salman MA, Salman A, Shaaban HE, et al. Nissen versus Toupet fundoplication for gastro-oesophageal reflux disease, short and long-term outcomes. A systematic review and meta-analysis. Surg Laparosc Endosc Percutan Tech. 2023;33(2):171–83. Published 2023 Apr 1. https://doi.org/10.1097/SLE.0000000000001139.
18. Lee Y, Tahir U, Tessier L, et al. Long-term outcomes following Dor, Toupet, and Nissen fundoplication: a network meta-analysis of randomized controlled trials. Surg Endosc. 2023;37(7):5052–64. https://doi.org/10.1007/s00464-023-10151-5.
19. Brinas P, Joumaa S, Currie A, et al. Efficacy of Nissen sleeve gastrectomy on mid-term Barrett's esophagus regression. Obes Surg. 2024;34(2):382–8. https://doi.org/10.1007/s11695-023-07034-y.
20. Kehagias I, Bellou A, Kehagias D, et al. Long-term (11 + years) efficacy of sleeve gastrectomy as a stand-alone bariatric procedure: a single-center retrospective observational study. Langenbeck's Arch Surg. 2022;408(1):4. Published 2022 Dec 29. https://doi.org/10.1007/s00423-022-02734-y.
21. Thiel AM, Plamper A, Kroll J, Alizai PH, Schmitz SM, Rheinwalt KP. Long-term outcomes of sleeve gastrectomy in a patient group with mainly high BMI: a single-center study. Updates Surg. Published online January 20. 2025; https://doi.org/10.1007/s13304-025-02076-6.

GPSR Compliance

The European Union's (EU) General Product Safety Regulation (GPSR) is a set of rules that requires consumer products to be safe and our obligations to ensure this.

If you have any concerns about our products, you can contact us on ProductSafety@springernature.com

In case Publisher is established outside the EU, the EU authorized representative is:

Springer Nature Customer Service Center GmbH
Europaplatz 3
69115 Heidelberg, Germany

Batch number: 10726060

Printed by Printforce, the Netherlands